MR Perfusion

Editors

ANANTH J. MADHURANTHAKAM
MAX WINTERMARK

MAGNETIC RESONANCE IMAGING CLINICS OF NORTH AMERICA

www.mri.theclinics.com

Consulting Editors
SURESH K. MUKHERJI
JENNY T. BENCARDINO

February 2024 • Volume 32 • Number 1

ELSEVIER

1600 John F. Kennedy Boulevard • Suite 1800 • Philadelphia, Pennsylvania, 19103-2899

http://www.mri.theclinics.com

MAGNETIC RESONANCE IMAGING CLINICS OF NORTH AMERICA Volume 32, Number 1
February 2024 ISSN 1064-9689, ISBN 13: 978-0-443-18394-2

Editor: John Vassallo (j.vassallo@elsevier.com)
Developmental Editor: Shivank Joshi

Magnetic Resonance Imaging Clinics of North America (ISSN 1064-9689) is published quarterly by Elsevier Inc., 360 Park Avenue South, New York, NY 10010-1710. Months of issue are February, May, August, and November. Business and Editorial Offices: 1600 John F. Kennedy Blvd., Ste. 1800, Philadelphia, PA 19103-2899. Customer Service Office: 3251 Riverport Lane, Maryland Heights, MO 63043. Periodicals postage paid at New York, NY and additional mailing offices. Subscription prices are $420.00 per year (domestic individuals), $100.00 per year (domestic students/residents), $455.00 per year (Canadian individuals), $579.00 per year (international individuals), $100.00 per year (Canadian students/residents), and $275.00 per year (international students/residents). For institutional access pricing please contact Customer Service via the contact information below. International air speed delivery is included in all *Clinics* subscription prices. All prices are subject to change without notice. **POSTMASTER:** Send address changes to *Magnetic Resonance Imaging Clinics*, Elsevier Health Sciences Division, Subscription Customer Service, 3251 Riverport Lane, Maryland Heights, MO 63043. Customer Service (orders, claims, online, change of address): Elsevier Health Sciences Division, Subscription **Customer Service, 3251 Riverport Lane, Maryland Heights, MO 63043. Tel:1-800-654-2452 (U.S. and Canada); 314-447-8871 (outside U.S. and Canada). Fax: 314-447-8029. E-mail: journalscustomerservice-usa@elsevier.com (for print support); journalsonlinesupport-usa@elsevier.com (for online support)**.

Reprints. For copies of 100 or more of articles in this publication, please contact the Commercial Reprints Department, Elsevier Inc., 360 Park Avenue South, New York, NY 10010-1710. Tel.: 212-633-3874; Fax: 212-633-3820; E-mail: reprints@elsevier.com.

Magnetic Resonance Imaging Clinics of North America is covered in the *RSNA Index of Imaging Literature, MEDLINE/PubMed (Index Medicus),* and *EMBASE/Excerpta Medica.*

Contributors

CONSULTING EDITORS

SURESH K. MUKHERJI, MD, MBA, FACR
Professor of Radiology and Radiation Oncology, University of Louisville, Peoria, Illinois, USA; Robert Wood Johnson Medical School, Rutgers University, New Brunswick, New Jersey, USA; Faculty, Otolaryngology–Head and Neck Surgery, Michigan State University, Farmington Hills, Michigan, USA; National Director of Head and Neck Radiology, ProScan Imaging, Carmel, Indiana, USA

JENNY T. BENCARDINO, MD
Vice Chair of Academic Affairs, Department of Radiology, Montefiore Medical Center, Bronx, New York, USA

EDITORS

ANANTH J. MADHURANTHAKAM, PhD
Associate Professor, Director of MR Research, Department of Radiology, Advanced Imaging Research Center, The University of Texas Southwestern Medical Center, Dallas, Texas, USA

MAX WINTERMARK, MD
Professor and Chair, Department of Neuroradiology, The University of Texas MD Anderson Cancer Center, Houston, Texas, USA

AUTHORS

DAVID C. ALSOP, PhD
Division of MRI Research, Department of Radiology, Beth Israel Deaconess Medical Center, Harvard Medical School, Boston, Massachusetts, USA

SHALINI A. AMUKOTUWA, PhD, MBBS
Department of Radiology and Radiological Sciences, Monash University, Associate Professor, Section Chief of Neuroradiology, Director of MRI, Monash Imaging, Monash Health, Clayton, Victoria, Australia

JENNY T. BENCARDINO, MD
Vice Chair of Academic Affairs, Department of Radiology, Montefiore Medical Center, Bronx, New York, USA

ROLAND BAMMER, PhD, MBA, MEE, FISMRM
Chair, Department of Radiology and Radiological Sciences, Monash University,

Monash Imaging, Monash Health, Clayton, Victoria, Australia

MELISSA M. CHEN, MD
Associate Professor, Department of Neuroradiology, The University of Texas MD Anderson Cancer Center, Houston, Texas, USA

DANIEL N. COSTA, MD
Associate Professor, Department of Radiology, Department of Urology, The University of Texas Southwestern Medical Center, Texas, USA

BAŞAK E. DOĞAN, MD
Associate Professor, Department of Radiology, Advanced Imaging Research Center, The University of Texas Southwestern Medical Center, Dallas, Texas, USA

CHRISTIAN FEDERAU, MD, MSc
AI Medical AG, Zollikon, Switzerland; University of Zürich, Zürich, Switzerland

JAMES F. GRIFFITH, MD, MRCP (UK), FRCR, FHKCR, FHKAM (Radiology)
Professor, Department of Imaging and Interventional Radiology, Prince of Wales Hospital, The Chinese University of Hong Kong

VIKAS GULANI, MD, PhD
Fred Jenner Hodges Professor and Chair, Department of Radiology, University of Michigan, Ann Arbor, Michigan, USA

JAMES H. HOLMES, PhD
Assistant Professor, Radiology, Biomedical Engineering, Holden Cancer Center, University of Iowa, Iowa City, Iowa, USA

WEI HUANG, PhD
Professor, Advanced Imaging Research Center, Oregon Health & Science University, Portland, Oregon, USA

HERO HUSSAIN, MD
Professor, Department of Radiology, University of Michigan, Ann Arbor, Michigan, USA

FERNANDO U. KAY, MD, PhD
Assistant Professor, Department of Radiology, The University of Texas Southwestern Medical Center, Dallas, Texas, USA

CHRISTOPHER M. KRAMER, MD
Ruth C. Heede Professor of Cardiology, Professor of Radiology, Departments of Medicine, and Radiology and Medical Imaging, Cardiovascular Division, University of Virginia Health, Charlottesville, Virginia, USA

VINODH A. KUMAR, MD
Professor, Department of Neuroradiology, The University of Texas MD Anderson Cancer Center, Houston, Texas, USA

JINA LEE, MS
Research Assistant, Department of Neuroradiology, The University of Texas MD Anderson Cancer Center, Houston, Texas, USA

HO-LING LIU, PhD
Professor, Department of Imaging Physics, The University of Texas MD Anderson Cancer Center, Houston, Texas, USA

ANANTH J. MADHURANTHAKAM, PhD
Associate Professor, Director of MR Research, Department of Radiology, Advanced Imaging Research Center, The University of Texas Southwestern Medical Center, Dallas, Texas, USA

DAVID J. MIKULIS, MD, FRCP(C)
Professor in the Joint Department of Medical Imaging, Senior Scientist, The Krembil Brain Institute, Full Member, Institute of Medical Science, Director of the Structural and Functional Neurovascular Lab, Department of Medical Imaging, The University of Toronto, The University Health Network, The Toronto Western Hospital, Toronto, Ontario, Canada

AMIT R. PATEL, MD
Departments of Medicine, and Radiology and Medical Imaging, Cardiovascular Division, University of Virginia Health, Charlottesville, Virginia, USA

ANUPAMA RAMACHANDRAN, MD, PhD
Fellow, Department of Radiology, University of Michigan, Ann Arbor, Michigan, USA

DEBORA Z. RECCHIMUZZI, MD
Assistant Professor, Department of Radiology, The University of Texas Southwestern Medical Center, Dallas, Texas, USA

NICOLE SEIBERLICH, PhD
Professor, Department of Radiology, University of Michigan, Ann Arbor, Michigan, USA

MANUEL TASO, PhD
Division of MRI Research, Department of Radiology, Beth Israel Deaconess Medical Center, Harvard Medical School, Boston, Massachusetts, USA

F. EYMEN UCISIK, MD
Assistant Professor, Department of Neuroradiology, The University of Texas MD Anderson Cancer Center, Houston, Texas, USA

DURGA UDAYAKUMAR, PhD
Assistant Professor, Department of Radiology, Advanced Imaging Research Center, UT Southwestern Medical Center, Dallas, Texas, USA

RAUL F. VALENZUELA, MD
Assistant Professor, Department of Musculoskeletal Imaging, The University of

Texas MD Anderson Cancer Center, Houston, Texas, USA

RIANNE A. VAN DER HEIJDEN, MD, PhD
Visiting Assistant Professor, Department of Radiology and Nuclear Medicine, Erasmus University Medical Center, Rotterdam, the Netherlands; Department of Radiology, University of Wisconsin-Madison, Madison, Wisconsin, USA

JOHN VASSALLO, BS, MS
Senior Clinics Editor, Clinics and Advances, Global Content Partners, Elsevier, Philadelphia, Pennsylvania, USA

MAX WINTERMARK, MD
Professor and Chair, Department of Neuroradiology, The University of Texas MD Anderson Cancer Center, Houston, Texas, USA

XIN LI, PhD
Associate Professor, Advanced Imaging Research Center, Oregon Health & Science University, Portland, Oregon, USA

DAVID K.W. YEUNG, PhD
Physicist, Department of Imaging and Interventional Radiology, Prince of Wales Hospital, The Chinese University of Hong Kong

MINGYAN WU, MD, PhD
Central Research Institute, UIH Group, School of Biomedical Engineering, ShanghaiTech University, Shanghai, China

STEFANIE W.Y. YIP, MBBS, FRCR, FHKCR, FHKAM (Radiology)
Associate Consultant, Department of Imaging and Interventional Radiology, Prince of Wales Hospital, The Chinese University of Hong Kong, Hong Kong

QING YUAN, PhD
Department of Radiology, The University of Texas Southwestern Medical Center, Dallas, Texas, USA

JEFF L. ZHANG, PhD
School of Biomedical Engineering, ShanghaiTech University, Shanghai, China

Contents

The measurement of blood flow has been a longstanding focus within the fields of medicine and physiology. The method of indicator dilution has gained widespread prominence due to the impracticality associated with using microspheres. Presently, nearly all perfusion-processing software packages employ a deconvolution-based approach. For medical practitioners, it is vital to meticulously assess deconvolution control parameters and possess a comprehensive understanding of how these parameters, as well as acquisition parameters, impact the generation of hemodynamic parameter maps.

In the companion article to this manuscript, a comprehensive theoretical explanation of perfusion analysis and fundamental concepts of DSC MR acquisition has been provided. We encourage you to explore that resource for a more in-depth understanding. Here, we demonstrate the practical implementation of DSC Perfusion Imaging in clinical settings. We place particular emphasis on scenarios where contrast material might traverse the vascular boundaries, affecting the DSC MRI signal's overall dynamics. We also address potential artifacts resulting from contrast leakage, strategies for their mitigation, and the valuable insights that can be gleaned from pharmacokinetic models that account for contrast material extravasation.

The non-invasive dynamic contrast-enhanced MRI (DCE-MRI) method provides valuable insights into tissue perfusion and vascularity. Primarily used in oncology, DCE-MRI is typically utilized to assess morphology and contrast agent (CA) kinetics in the tissue of interest. Interpretation of the temporal signatures of DCE-MRI data includes qualitative, semi-quantitative, and quantitative approaches. Recent advances in MRI technology allow simultaneous high spatial and temporal resolutions in DCE-MRI data acquisition on most vendor platforms, enabling the more desirable approach of quantitative data analysis using pharmacokinetic (PK) modeling. Many technical factors, including signal-to-noise ratio, temporal resolution, quantifications of arterial input function and native tissue T1, and PK model selection, need to be carefully considered when performing quantitative DCE-MRI. Standardization in data acquisition and analysis is especially important in multi-center studies.

Arterial Spin Labeling Perfusion Imaging

Manuel Taso and David C. Alsop

Noninvasive imaging of tissue perfusion is a valuable tool for both research and clinical applications. Arterial spin labeling (ASL) is a contrast-free perfusion imaging method that enables measuring and quantifying tissue blood flow using MR imaging. ASL uses radiofrequency and magnetic field gradient pulses to label arterial blood water, which then serves as an endogenous tracer. This review highlights the basic mechanism of ASL perfusion imaging, labeling strategies, and quantification. ASL has been widely used during the past 30 years for the study of normal brain function as well as in multiple neurovascular, neuro-oncological and degenerative pathologic conditions.

MR Perfusion Imaging for Gliomas

Jina Lee, Melissa M. Chen, Ho-Ling Liu, F. Eymen Ucisik, Max Wintermark, and Vinodh A. Kumar

Accurate diagnosis and treatment evaluation of patients with gliomas is imperative to make clinical decisions. Multiparametric MR perfusion imaging reveals physiologic features of gliomas that can help classify them according to their histologic and molecular features as well as distinguish them from other neoplastic and nonneoplastic entities. It is also helpful in distinguishing tumor recurrence or progression from radiation necrosis, pseudoprogression, and pseudoresponse, which is difficult with conventional MR imaging. This review provides an update on MR perfusion imaging for the diagnosis and treatment monitoring of patients with gliomas following standard-of-care chemoradiation therapy and other treatment regimens such as immunotherapy.

Clinical Interpretation of Intravoxel Incoherent Motion Perfusion Imaging in the Brain

Christian Federau

Intravoxel incoherent motion (IVIM) perfusion imaging extracts information on blood motion in biological tissue from diffusion-weighted MR images. The method is attractive from a clinical stand point, because it measures in essence local quantitative perfusion, without intravenous contrast injection. Currently, the clinical interpretation of IVIM perfusion maps focuses on the IVIM perfusion fraction maps, but improvements in image quality of the IVIM pseudo-diffusion maps, using advanced postprocessing tools involving artificial intelligence, could lead to an increased interest in this parameters, as it could provide additional local perfusion information in the clinical setting, not otherwise available with other perfusion techniques.

Cerebrovascular Reserve Imaging: Problems and Solutions

David J. Mikulis

The current standard of practice for assessing patients with cerebrovascular steno-occlusive disease is based on measuring resting blood flow metrics using MR imaging and CT perfusion imaging. However, the reliability of these methods decreases as the degree and number of stenoses increase. The reason for this is that measures of adequate baseline blood flow in highly collateralized circulations do not account for possible shortfalls in recruitable blood flow or increased metabolic demand. The following offers a clinically tested solution for this purpose using cerebrovascular reactivity methodology that applies a quantifiable vasodilatory stimulus improving reproducibility and repeatability essential for optimizing patient management.

Fernando U. Kay and Ananth J. Madhuranthakam

Lung perfusion assessment is critical for diagnosing and monitoring a variety of respiratory conditions. MRI perfusion provides a radiation-free technique, making it an ideal choice for longitudinal imaging in younger populations. This review focuses on the techniques and applications of MRI perfusion, including contrast-enhanced (CE) MRI and non-CE methods such as arterial spin labeling (ASL), fourier decomposition (FD), and hyperpolarized 129-Xenon (129-Xe) MRI. ASL leverages endogenous water protons as tracers for a non-invasive measure of lung perfusion, while FD offers simultaneous measurements of lung perfusion and ventilation, enabling the generation of ventilation/perfusion mapsHyperpolarized 129-Xe MRI emerges as a novel tool for assessing regional gas exchange in the lungs. Despite the promise of MRI perfusion techniques, challenges persist, including competition with other imaging techniques and the need for additional validation and standardization. In conditions such as cystic fibrosis and lung cancer, MRI has displayed encouraging results, whereas in diseases like chronic obstructive pulmonary disease, further validation remains necessary. In conclusion, while MRI perfusion techniques hold immense potential for a comprehensive, non-invasive assessment of lung function and perfusion, their broader clinical adoption hinges on technological advancements, collaborative research, and rigorous validation.

Amit R. Patel and Christopher M. Kramer

The use of myocardial perfusion imaging during a stress cardiac magnetic resonance (CMR) examination for the evaluation of coronary artery disease is now recommended by both US and European guidelines. Several studies have demonstrated high diagnostic accuracy for the detection of hemodynamically significant coronary artery disease. Stress perfusion CMR has been shown to be a non-invasive and cost-effective alternative to guide coronary revascularization.

Durga Udayakumar, Ananth J. Madhuranthakam, and Basak E. Doğan

Breast cancer is the most frequently diagnosed cancer among women worldwide, carrying a significant socioeconomic burden. Breast cancer is a heterogeneous disease with 4 major subtypes identified. Each subtype has unique prognostic factors, risks, treatment responses, and survival rates. Advances in targeted therapies have considerably improved the 5-year survival rates for primary breast cancer patients largely due to widespread screening programs that enable early detection and timely treatment. Imaging techniques are indispensable in diagnosing and managing breast cancer. While mammography is the primary screening tool, MRI plays a significant role when mammography results are inconclusive or in patients with dense breast tissue. MRI has become standard in breast cancer imaging, providing detailed anatomic and functional data, including tumor perfusion and cellularity. A key characteristic of breast tumors is angiogenesis, a biological process that promotes tumor development and growth. Increased angiogenesis in tumors generally indicates poor prognosis and increased risk of metastasis. Dynamic contrast-enhanced (DCE) MRI measures tumor perfusion and serves as an in vivo metric for angiogenesis. DCE-MRI has become the cornerstone of breast MRI, boasting a high negative-predictive value of 89% to 99%, although its specificity can vary. This review presents a thorough overview of magnetic resonance (MR) perfusion imaging in breast cancer, focusing on the role of DCE-MRI in clinical applications and exploring emerging MR perfusion imaging techniques.

MAGNETIC RESONANCE IMAGING CLINICS OF NORTH AMERICA

SERIES OF RELATED INTEREST

Advances in Clinical Radiology
www.advancesinclinicalradiology.com
Neuroimaging Clinics
www.neuroimaging.theclinics.com
PET Clinics
www.pet.theclinics.com
Radiologic Clinics
www.radiologic.theclinics.com

VISIT THE CLINICS ONLINE!
Access your subscription at:
www.theclinics.com

PROGRAM OBJECTIVE
The goal of *Magnetic Resonance Imaging Clinics of North America* is to keep practicing physicians up to date with current clinical practice by providing timely articles reviewing the state of the art in patient care.

TARGET AUDIENCE
All practicing physicians and healthcare professionals who provide patient care utilizing findings from Magnetic Resonance Imaging.

LEARNING OBJECTIVES
Upon completion of this activity, participants will be able to:
1. Review perfusion MRI's principles, techniques, and clinical applications.
2. Discuss the valuable insight dynamic contrast-enhanced magnetic resonance imaging (DCE-MRI) provides into tissue perfusion and vascularity.
3. Recognize the capability and clinical potential of imaging methods with the possibility of accelerating their adoption to clinical practice.

ACCREDITATION
The Elsevier Office of Continuing Medical Education (EOCME) is accredited by the Accreditation Council for Continuing Medical Education (ACCME) to provide continuing medical education for physicians.

The EOCME designates this journal-based CME activity enduring material for a maximum of 14 *AMA PRA Category 1 Credit*(s)™. Physicians should claim only the credit commensurate with the extent of their participation in the activity.

All other healthcare professionals requesting continuing education credit for this enduring material will be issued a certificate of participation.

DISCLOSURE OF CONFLICTS OF INTEREST
The EOCME assesses conflict of interest with its instructors, faculty, planners, and other individuals who are in a position to control the content of CME activities. All relevant conflicts of interest that are identified are thoroughly vetted by EOCME for fair balance, scientific objectivity, and patient care recommendations. EOCME is committed to providing its learners with CME activities that promote improvements or quality in healthcare and not a specific proprietary business or a commercial interest.

The planning committee, staff, authors, and editors listed below have identified no financial relationships or relationships to products or devices they or their spouse/life partner have with commercial interest related to the content of this CME activity:
Shalini A. Amukotuwa, PhD, MBBS; Melissa M. Chen, MD; Daniel N. Costa, MD; Başak E. Dogan, MD; James F. Griffith, MD, MRCP, FRCR, FHKCR, FHKAM; James H. Holmes, PhD; Wei Huang, PhD; Fernando U. Kay, MD, PhD; Kothainayaki Kulanthaivelu, BCA, MBA; Vinodh A. Kumar, MD; Jina Lee, MS; Xin Li, PhD; Michelle Littlejohn; Ho-Ling Liu, PhD; Ananth J. Madhuranthakam, PhD; Debora Z. Recchimuzzi, MD; F. Eymen Ucisik, MD; Durga Udayakumar, PhD; Raul F. Valenzuela, MD; Rianne A. van der Heijden, MD, PhD; Max Wintermark, MD; Mingyan Wu, MD, PhD; David K.W. Yeung, PhD; Stefanie W.Y. Yip, MBBS, FRCR, FHKCR, FHKAM; Qing Yuan, PhD; Jeff L. Zhang, PhD

The planning committee, staff, authors, and editors listed below have identified financial relationships or relationships to products or devices they or their spouse/life partner have with commercial interest related to the content of this CME activity:
David C. Alsop, PhD: Royalties/Patent Beneficiary: GE Healthcare, Siemens Healthineers, Philips, Hitachi, United Imaging

Roland Bammer, PhD, MBA, MEE, FISMRM: Ownership Interest: iSchemaView

Christian Federau, MD, MSc: Founder/CEO: AI Medical AG

Vikas Gulani, MD, PhD: Researcher: Siemens Healthineers: Consultant: Cook Medical

Hero K. Hussain, MD: Researcher: Siemens Healthineers

Christopher M. Kramer, MD: Researcher: Lilly; Consultant: Lilly, Xencor

David J. Mikulis, MD, FRCPC: Ownership Interest: Thornhill Medical

Amit R. Patel, MD: Researcher: GE Healthcare, Siemens Healthineers, Circle Cardiovascular Imaging, NeoSoft

Anupama Ramachandran, MD: Researcher: Siemens Healthineers

Nicole Seiberlich, PhD: Researcher: Siemens Healthineers

Manuel Taso: Employee: Siemens Healthineers

UNAPPROVED/OFF-LABEL USE DISCLOSURE
The EOCME requires CME faculty to disclose to the participants:

1. When products or procedures being discussed are off-label, unlabelled, experimental, and/or investigational (not US Food and Drug Administration [FDA] approved); and
2. Any limitations on the information presented, such as data that are preliminary or that represent ongoing research, interim analyses, and/or unsupported opinions. Faculty may discuss information about pharmaceutical agents that is outside of FDA-approved labelling. This information is intended solely for CME and is not intended to promote off-label use of these medications. If you have any questions, contact the medical affairs department of the manufacturer for the most recent prescribing information.

TO ENROLL

To enroll in the *Magnetic Resonance Imaging Clinics of North America* Continuing Medical Education program, call customer service at 1-800-654-2452 or sign up online at http://www.theclinics.com/home/cme. The CME program is available to subscribers for an additional annual fee of USD 270 for US individuals, and USD 281 for International individuals.

METHOD OF PARTICIPATION

In order to claim credit, participants must complete the following:
1. Complete enrolment as indicated above.
2. Read the activity.
3. Complete the CME Test and Evaluation. Participants must achieve a score of 70% on the test. All CME Tests and Evaluations must be completed online.

CME INQUIRIES/SPECIAL NEEDS

For all CME inquiries or special needs, please contact elsevierCME@elsevier.com.

Foreword

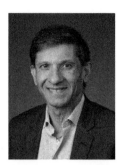 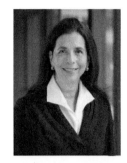

Suresh K. Mukherji, MD, MBA, FACR Jenny T. Bencardino, MD
Consulting Editors

Blood perfusion is an essential metabolic process responsible for the delivery of nutrients and removal of metabolic waste products. MR perfusion imaging is an important physiologic imaging that has been around since our residency years in the "last century!", perfusion imaging has been limited to academic centers and research trials. However, numerous technical innovations in MR hardware and software over the past 10 years have improved the quality of the MR perfusion data, resulting in new clinical applications that can be used in daily practice.

The goal of this issue of *Magnetic Resonance Imaging Clinics of North America* is to provide a state-of-the-art review of the current clinical applications of MR perfusion from "head to toe." We are grateful for Drs Ananth J. Madhuranthakam, PhD and Max Wintermark, MD for agreeing to edit this edition. As guest editors, they have created a comprehensive and practical issue covering different techniques and, more importantly, providing specific clinical applications of MR perfusion pertaining to imaging the brain, lungs, heart, breast, liver, kidneys, prostate, and musculoskeletal system…"head to toe!"

We want to thank Drs Madhuranthakam and Wintermark for accepting our invitation to guest edit this issue. Many thanks to the wonderful contributions of the article authors. The articles are complete and concise and provide pragmatic information that will allow greater use of MR perfusion in clinical practice. We are quite confident this issue will achieve the goals stated in Drs Madhuranthakam and Wintermark's Preface of creating a "quick reference but also as a comprehensive guide, advancing knowledge in MR perfusion imaging and providing answers to common questions in the field."

On a personal note, I (S.K.M.) have known Max Wintermark for many years and continue to be amazed by his talents, accomplishments, and humanity. Max is currently Chair of Neuroradiology at MD Anderson Cancer Center and serves as Editor-in-Chief of the *American Journal of Neuroradiology* and as President of the American Society of Neuroradiology. Max is a world-class radiologist and thought-leader, and despite his unrivaled notoriety, continues to be the same humble and approachable person I met over 20 years ago!

Suresh K. Mukherji, MD, MBA, FACR
University of Louisville &
University of Illinois
ProScan Imaging
Carmel, IN 46032, USA

Jenny T. Bencardino, MD
Vice Chair of Academic Affairs
Department of Radiology
Montefiore Medical Center
111 East 210th Street
Bronx, New York 10467-2401, USA

E-mail addresses:
sureshmukherji@hotmail.com (S.K. Mukherji)
jbencardin@montefiore.org (J.T. Bencardino)

Magn Reson Imaging Clin N Am 32 (2024) xv
https://doi.org/10.1016/j.mric.2023.09.013
1064-9689/24/© 2023 Published by Elsevier Inc.

Preface
MR Perfusion Imaging: Technical Advances and Clinical Applications

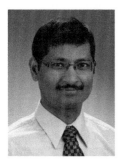
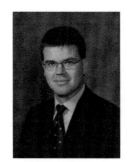

Ananth J. Madhuranthakam, PhD   Max Wintermark, MD

Editors

It has been both a pleasure and an honor to serve as the Guest Editors for this special issue of *Magnetic Resonance Imaging Clinics of North America*, which is focused on MR perfusion imaging. We extend our sincere gratitude to the Editors for entrusting us with this role and for providing us the latitude to curate this impressive collection of articles. We also wish to thank all contributing authors for their expertise, exceptional contributions, and timely submissions, which have made this issue possible. Each review article was meticulously crafted by international experts in the field of MR imaging, and we thoroughly enjoyed reading all articles.

Perfusion is a vital physiologic process responsible for the delivery of oxygen and nutrients to tissues while also facilitating the removal of waste products, such as carbon dioxide. Under normal physiologic conditions, perfusion is well regulated, and any disruption can lead to pathologic states. For instance, decreased perfusion can be a hallmark of conditions like stroke and myocardial infarction, while elevated perfusion can signify tumor growth and neo-angiogenesis. Noninvasive measurement of perfusion, therefore, holds significance for diagnosis, prognosis, and therapeutic

response assessment across various clinical applications. MR imaging offers a versatile modality for noninvasive, in vivo perfusion measurements. Since the early days of MR imaging, different imaging methods, both with and without the use of exogenous gadolinium-based contrast agent, have been developed for MR perfusion imaging. While the fundamental principles of MR perfusion imaging remain consistent, unique challenges arise when applying these methods to different anatomical regions. Technical advancements over the years have enabled MR perfusion imaging to become a routine part of clinical practice, covering a broad spectrum of applications. Recent emphasis has also been placed on quantitative imaging, and the majority of MR perfusion imaging techniques can now generate quantitative parameters. As a result, MR perfusion imaging is at the forefront of quantitative imaging and is a major part of the Quantitative Imaging Biomarker Alliance.

In this special issue, the earlier articles provide comprehensive reviews on various MR perfusion imaging methods, including dynamic susceptibility contrast MR imaging, dynamic contrast-enhanced MR imaging, and arterial spin-labeled MR imaging. These technical articles are followed by articles

Magn Reson Imaging Clin N Am 32 (2024) xvii–xviii
https://doi.org/10.1016/j.mric.2023.09.008
1064-9689/24/© 2023 Published by Elsevier Inc.

that delve into the clinical applications of MR perfusion imaging, covering topics such as perfusion imaging for gliomas, intravoxel incoherent motion applications in the brain, and problems and solutions in cerebrovascular reserve imaging. The issue also explores MR perfusion imaging in extracranial applications, including the lungs, heart, breast, liver, kidneys, prostate, and musculoskeletal system. Overall, this special issue serves as an excellent amalgamation of technical advances and clinical applications in the field of MR perfusion imaging.

We hope that this issue will serve not only as a quick reference but also as a comprehensive guide, advancing knowledge in MR perfusion imaging and providing answers to common questions in the field. In addition, we aspire for these expert reviews to inspire further research, enhancing the reliability of MR perfusion imaging and paving the way for innovative applications. We trust you will find these articles as insightful and engaging as we have.

Ananth J. Madhuranthakam, PhD
Department of Radiology and
Advanced Imaging Research Center
UT Southwestern Medical Center
5323 Harry Hines Boulevard
Dallas, TX 75390-9061, USA

Max Wintermark, MD
Department of Neuroradiology
MD Anderson Cancer Center
Houston, TX 77030, USA

E-mail addresses:
Ananth.Madhuranthakam@UTSouthwestern.edu
(A.J. Madhuranthakam)
max.wintermark@gmail.com (M. Wintermark)

Introduction

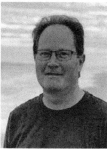
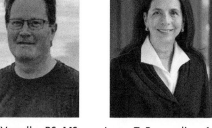

John Vassallo, BS, MS   Jenny T. Bencardino, MD

We are delighted to introduce our new co-Consulting Editor of *Magnetic Resonance Imaging Clinics of North America*, Dr Jenny Bencardino. She will join Dr Suresh Mukherji in guiding the editorial focus of the series.

Dr Bencardino is Vice-Chair of Academic Affairs at Montefiore Einstein in Bronx, New York. Her clinical interests focus on the imaging diagnosis, follow-up, and treatment of sports-related injuries of the musculoskeletal system and peripheral nerves.

After earning her Doctor of Medicine degree at Pontificia Universidad Javeriana in Bogota, Colombia, and completing her radiology residency at the Hospital of San Ignacio, Pontificia Universidad, Dr Bencardino came to the United States as a research musculoskeletal radiology fellow at NYU Hospital for Joint Diseases. She then completed residency training at the Long Island Jewish Medical Center, earning her American Board of Radiology certification in 2000.

Dr Bencardino's research efforts include the development and validation of MR imaging metrics for the diagnosis and follow-up of diseases affecting the microstructure and function of articular cartilage, bone, muscle, and nerves. Dr Bencardino is also a peer reviewer for several scientific journals, including *Skeletal Radiology*, *Radiology*, the *American Journal of Roentgenology*, and the *Journal of Magnetic Resonance Imaging*.

Dr Bencardino is board certified by the American Board of Radiology. She is a member of the International Skeletal Society (ISS), the Society of Skeletal Radiology (SSR), the Radiological Society of North America (RSNA), the American Roentgen Ray Society (ARRS), the European College of Radiology, and the American College of Radiology. She has received multiple accolades throughout her career, including the President's Medal from the International Skeletal Society in 2013, the Honored Educator Award from the Radiological Society of North America in 2014, and the Medal of the ISS in 2023.

Dr Bencardino will succeed Dr Lynne Steinbach of the University of California at San Francisco. Dr Steinbach was co-Consulting Editor of *Magnetic Resonance Imaging Clinics of North America* for a decade, and her expertise in musculoskeletal imaging was critical in maintaining the reputation and high-quality content for the series. We sincerely thank her for her dedication, diligence, and enthusiasm for *Magnetic Resonance Imaging Clinics of North America*.

John Vassallo, BS, MS
Senior Clinics Editor, *Clinics* and *Advances*
Global Content Partners | ELSEVIER
1600 JFK Boulevard, Suite 1800
Philadelphia, PA 19103, USA

Jenny T. Bencardino, MD
Vice Chair of Academic Affairs
Department of Radiology
Montefiore Medical Center
111 East 210th Street
Bronx, NY 10467-2401, USA

E-mail address:
j.vassallo@elsevier.com

Magn Reson Imaging Clin N Am 32 (2024) xix
https://doi.org/10.1016/j.mric.2023.09.009
1064-9689/24/© 2023 Published by Elsevier Inc.

mri.theclinics.com

Dynamic Susceptibility Contrast Perfusion, Part 1: The Fundamentals

Roland Bammer, PhD, MBA, MEE, FISMRM[a,b,]*,
Shalini A. Amukotuwa, PhD, MBBS[a,b]

KEYWORDS

- Diffusible tracers • Nondiffusible tracers • Gadolinium-based contrast agents • Cerebral blood flow
- Hemodynamic Parameter • Arterial spin label perfusion

KEY POINTS

- Long-standing interest: Measuring blood flow has been a subject of long-standing interest in the fields of medicine and physiology, with a focus on understanding circulation dynamics.
- Local nutrient delivery: Assessing capillary blood flow is a means to gauge the delivery of nutrients to specific tissue regions and the removal of metabolic by-products from these regions.
- Evolution of methods: The administration of gadolinium-based contrast agents in combination with rapid MR imaging of an anatomic location every 1 to 2 seconds allows the radiologist to measure signal intensity changes that can be relate to transient gadolinium concentration changes in large vessels as well as brain tissue, which in turn can be used to measure cerebral perfusion and blood volume.
- Computational approaches: The observed tracer concentration values in tissue are related to the arterial input of tracer material and a tissue-specific drainage function, known as residue function, by a mathematical relationship that is known as convolution. The residue function relates to blood flow and tracer transit times and is therefore of great interest.
- Deconvolution: To disentangle the inherent tissue response from the shape of the arterial bolus, a numerical method is used that is known as deconvolution. Because it is very sensitive to noise, it must be combined with another mathematical trick, which is known as regularization.

PART 1: THE FUNDAMENTALS
Background

Measuring blood flow has been of long-standing interest in medicine and physiology. Initially conceived to measure blood flow to the whole organ, attention turned quickly to measure capillary blood flow as a measure of local delivery of nutrients to a small region of tissue. Originally proposed with gases[1] and microspheres,[2] early on, the method of indicator dilution[3,4] has become the most prevalent approach because of the impracticality of using microspheres. After all, a technique that uses excised tissue to measure how many tracer microspheres per unit mass of tissue get trapped in the tissue's capillary bed would not have led to widespread and wildly enthusiastic adoption in humans.

Measuring blood flow, based on the indicator dilution theory, obviously requires an indicator, whose given concentration we know and can measure over time as it passes through the capillary bed. Here, the indicator is a substance that stands out from the normal signal, that is, some sort of contrasting agent. Various indicators have been used in the past, such as dyes, gas, temperature, iodine, magnetic susceptibility altering agents, T_1-shortening agents, or magnetically labeled spins

[a] Department of Radiology and Radiological Sciences, Monash University, Clayton, VIC, Australia; [b] Monash Imaging, Monash Health, Clayton, VIC, Australia
* Corresponding author.
E-mail address: roland.bammer@monash.edu

Magn Reson Imaging Clin N Am 32 (2024) 1–23
https://doi.org/10.1016/j.mric.2023.09.010

(aka arterial spin label [ASL] or spin tags) where magnetic spins are either saturated or inverted.[5]

Diffusible Versus Nondiffusible Tracers

At this point, the reader should become cognizant of the two main types of tracers.

1. Intravascular tracers, which are compounds that remain within the vasculature and are slowly excreted trough the kidneys. For example, gadofosveset trisodium, an albumin-bound intravascular agent, was used for contrast-enhanced MR angiography until it was withdrawn from the marked. It has an elimination half-life of 19 hours, which can increase to 49 hours in patients with severe renal impairment with glomerular filtration rates (GFRs) less than 30 mL/min/1.73 m.[2]
2. Diffusible tracers, which are not bound to the vascular system. This type of tracer leaves the capillary bed and distributes more or less freely in tissue. Examples for diffusible tracers are gases or water. A well-known example of gases that have been used to measure perfusion is unstable (and thus radioactive) Xenon $(Xe)^{133}$, which we can measure with gamma cameras. It turns out that stable (nonradioactive) Xe has an atomic number (54) that is close to that of iodine (53), thus yielding similar radio-opacity to iodine, and was therefore used in Xe-enhanced CT studies perfusion measurements.[6] Typical examples for diffusible water tracer methods are arterial spin labeling of water protons in MR imaging—as mentioned above—as well as ^{15}O-water PET. Given that at body temperature, water has a diffusion coefficient of 3200×10^{-6} mm^2/s, a water molecule travels a root-mean-square distance of around 3.5 mm in 10 minute according to Einstein's equation. This is roughly the upper limit that any aqueous or small particulate tracer molecule, including gadolinium-based contrast agents (GBCAs), would travel within a typical imaging time.

In case of blood-brain barrier (BBB) disruption, the assumption of a nondiffusible purely intravascular tracer may no longer hold, because the presumed intravascular tracer can seep into tissue. How easily a tracer can leave the capillary bed then depends on the "leakiness" of the vessel wall (referred to as permeability), and the molecular size, as well as other properties, of the tracer. Although tracers that are attached to a large ligand, such as gadofosveset trisodium or ferumoxytol, have a large enough molecular size that extravasation might be difficult, the molecular sizes of many of the standard commercially available MR contrast agents are not large enough to prevent the tracer molecules from escaping the capillary bed when the BBB is disrupted or impaired. In fact, this feature is why GBCAs are primarily used in MR. As we will discover later, these "escapee" tracer molecules mess a bit with our central volume principle. The presence of extravasation (ie, when contrast leaves the capillary bed) therefore warrants clever methods to address this problem in our MR (but also to some extent CT) perfusion measurements. Of note, both the rate at which the tracer "oozes" out into the tissue capillaries and how big its distribution volume might be can become diagnostic parameters by themselves and can be very useful to the neuroradiologist.

Gadolinium-based Contrast Agents

Although there are several materials that are used in MR imaging because of their ability to alter spin relaxation and/or magnetic susceptibility, such as dysprosium, manganese, or iron oxides, the tracer material used most prevalently in clinical practice is gadolinium (Gd). Among other alternatives, gadolinium stands out because of its high magnetic moment, its coordinated water lability, the availability of strong chelating agents, and having only a one available oxidation state.[7] With its seven unpaired electrons in the seven 4f orbitals, Gd^{3+} yields the largest paramagnetic moment. However, gadolinium in its free form is highly toxic and must therefore be combined with a (linear/ nonlinear | ionic/nonionic) chelating agent.[7] The molecular structure and molecular size of the chelating agent determines not only its chemical stability (eg, dissociation, pH-sensitivity, transmetalation), it also influences how strongly the gadolinium in the center of the chelate can affect relaxation processes and how easily it can extravasate from the capillary bed into the interstitial space.[7] For example, the molecular weight (as a surrogate for molecular size) for different compounds is as follows: gadofosveset trisodium (975.88 mg/mmol); gadoxetate disodium (725.72 mg/mmol); gadopentetate dimeglumine (938.00 mg/mmol); gadoteridol (558.70 mg/ mmol); gadobenate dimeglumine (1058.20 mg/ mmol); gadodiamide (573.66 mg/mL); gadoversetamide (661.77 mg/mmol); gadoterate meglumine (753.86 mg/mmol); and gadobutrol (604.72 mg/ mmol). These GBCAs are widely used in MR imaging and are therefore logical tracers to be used for measuring perfusion. Despite perfusion's ubiquitous use in clinical practice, do note however that dynamic susceptibility contrast (DSC) perfusion remains an off-label application for GBCAs.

MEASURING CONTRAST AGENT CONCENTRATION

When a tracer is injected into the blood stream, we can measure its concentration dynamically (ie, over time, every second) and observe how long it will take the tracer to pass through a region or voxel of interest. In MR imaging, we use a GBCA as such a tracer, and repeatedly acquire MR images of the same anatomic structures at multiple time points—generally at equidistant time intervals—with an MR acquisition technique that is fast enough to measure the transient MR signal changes that occur in response to the changes in underlying spin relaxation induced by the transient change in GBCA concentration levels as the tracer passes through the capillary bed (**Fig. 1**).

Of note here should be that the GBCA affects both T_1 and T_2^* relaxation times. However, as long as the contrast agent remains intravascular, the T_2^*-shortening effects are usually much more prominent than those from T_1-shortening; thus, changes in T_1 relaxation can usually be ignored with DSC MR imaging in the absence of contrast leakage. To understand this, one has to keep in mind that for T_1-shortening to occur in the presence of a GBCA, water protons need to get into close proximity of the gadolinium atom. This is obviously limited when the GBCA is confined to a tight intravascular compartment that occupies only a few percent of the voxel and—as we have seen from the calculation before—when diffusing water protons (which could pass through the BBB) do not cover a large distance, thus hindering proton exchange. The converse is true for T_2^*-shortening. The compartmentalization is actually helpful to exacerbate the susceptibility perturbation. As the susceptibility perturbations are far-reaching and do not require the protons to come into close proximity with the Gd atom, it explains why, with an intact BBB, the T_2^* effects dominate.

Setting Up Dynamic Susceptibility Contrast Perfusion

To measure dynamically transient magnetic susceptibility changes induced by GBCA, one needs an MR acquisition method that is T_2^*-weighted but also fast enough to produce images of the same anatomy every 1 to 2 seconds. An MR imaging method that is able to allow tracking GBCA in such way is DSC MR imaging. Here, the GBCA is usually administered as a short bolus through the (right) antecubital vein. The right side is normally preferred for a more direct access into the central venous system. Typical flow rates are between 4 to 6 mL/second through a large caliber venflon (20G). The GBCA should be injected at body temperature to avoid uncomfortable or painful experience to the patient and to lower viscosity. High viscosity, in conjunction with a limited venflon caliber, can lead to a significantly lower effective contrast injection flow rate than the desired one. Given the small volume that is usually injected, especially when using a 1-molar agent, it is critical to use a large enough saline chaser immediately after the contrast injection to ensure that all GBCA is pushed out of the injector tubing kit and well into the central circulation. A dual-piston power injector is required because of inconsistency of hand injection and because some of us might not even have the strength to push the syringe's plunger hard enough to achieve the desired flow rate.

Relating Changes in Relaxation Times to Contrast Concentration

We have learned that DSC MR imaging is the basis of GBCA-based perfusion measurements in MR imaging. The higher the concentration of the GBCA in the sample c, the more the MR imaging signal gets attenuated (**Fig. 2**); up to the point where there is no more signal left to be attenuated. In this context, the reader is advised to avoid to driving the T_2^*-weighted signal down so deeply that it starts bouncing off the noise floor (typically at signal-to-noise ratios ≤ 3) (nb, MR magnitude images hardly get to zero[8]). MR signal "blow out" can happen when the DSC sequence parameters are chosen to make it too sensitive to the expected range of Gd concentration, typically by selection of too long TE, and should be avoided by a clever choice of scan parameters. Driving the MR signal into saturation leads to a nonlinear association between the T_2^*-weighted MR imaging signal and underestimation of the underlying contrast concentration (see **Fig. 2**).

Regardless of T_1 or $T_2(^*)$ relaxation, in the presence of GBCA, the following general concepts apply, and we can drop the index "1," "2," or "2^*" for now:

If R_0 is the relaxation rate (s^{-1}) of the tissue in the absence of any GBCA, then in its most simplistic form, the relaxation rate constant in the presence of contrast material of concentration c in mmol/L or mM (and ignoring any issues of nonlinearity or exchange) is:

$$R(c(t)) = R_0 + r.c(t), \qquad (1)$$

where r (mM^{-1}s^{-1} or l mmol^{-1}s^{-1}) is the relaxivity of the contrast agent. The latter determines how strongly a specific contrast agent influences the relaxation rate relative to its concentration. The time variable t indicates that for a bolus injection

A

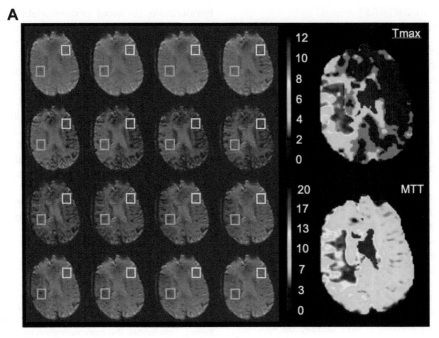

B

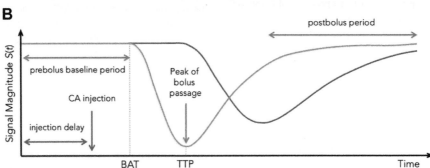

Fig. 1. (A) Left panel shows T_2^*-weighted images obtained every 2 second (time increases from left to right and top down) during passage of a bolus of GBCA. Owing to T_2^*-shortening of the GBCA, the images appear darker during bolus passage. From the time signal in each voxel, important parameters such as Tmax and MTT can be computed that highlight areas of hemodynamic abnormality. ROIs taken in normal (*gold*) and abnormal (*blue*) brain regions show T_2^*-weighted region of interest (ROI) signals over time in (B). Key parameters are labeled on these curves. (*Courtesy* of R Bammer, Melbourne, VIC, Australia.)

of contrast material, the contrast concentration changes over time and, as such, *R*.

Notice that most relaxivity values that are printed on package labels are obtained in homogeneous aqueous solutions at 37°C or 40°C. Particularly, the values for r_2 and r_2^*, if they are printed, need to be treated with some skepticism, as those values are dependent on tissue as well as vessel size and vessel orientation. For r_2, they are also dependent on MR pulse sequence parameters, such as spin echo time (**Fig. 3**) (as well as the underlying diffusion coefficient).

Equation 1 assumes a linear dependency although often, in reality, r_2 and r_2^* are not always linear (eg, see arterial concentration). Moreover, r_2

and r_2^* can be affected by extravasation (ie, when intravascular and extravascular Gd concentrations equilibrate, and GBCA-induced susceptibility gradients become less prominent). In such situations r_2 and r_2^* might become themselves a function of time. Therefore, measurement of absolute gadolinium concentrations remains a challenge and, as such, can influence the measurement of hemodynamic parameters in absolute values.

A Glance at Arterial Spin Label Perfusion MR Imaging

The alternative to DSC perfusion imaging is ASL perfusion MR imaging.[5] ASL uses magnetically

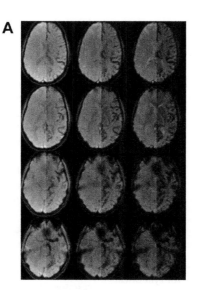

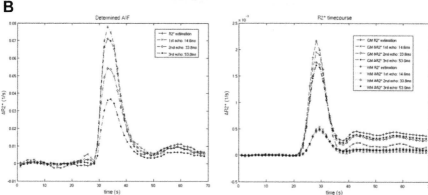

Fig. 2. (*A*) T_2*-weighted slice at four different anatomic levels (superior to inferior) at pre-bolus baseline (left half of images) and during peak of contrast bolus passage (right half of image) demonstrate the sensitivity of the GBCA at various echo times of TE_1 = 15 millisecond (left column), TE_2 = 34 millisecond (middle column) and TE_3 = 50msec (right column). (*B*) T_2*-weighted signal converted into ΔR_2*(t) courses, which reflect GBCA concentration at the three echo times (TE_1, TE_2, and TE_3), as well as the result when R_2* was determined directly from the three echoes, whereas (*B*) shows similar time courses for gray and white matter. There is a pronounced underestimation of ΔR_2*(t), and thus GBCA values, with higher echo times, especially in the large artery. This is due to the saturation of the T_2*-weighted signal, that is, when any further increase in GBCA no longer leads to measurable R_2* changes, as there is no more signal left to attenuate.

labeled blood as tracer; the label is introduced either by specific inversion or saturation radio frequency pulses. Similar to the aforementioned microsphere experiment, the label is washed into the tissue of the imaging volume (ie, diffusible tracer) and will alter T_1 relaxation of tissue, where the alteration is proportional to the underlying blood flow. With the exception that ASL uses a diffusible tracer, a lot of the advanced mathematics around calculating ASL perfusion shows strong similarities to the solutions shown for DSC perfusion.[9] In contradistinction to DSC, ASL has the advantage that it does not need an intravenous GBCA contrast injection and is not subject to the aforementioned tissue/vessel-dependent variations of *r*. This makes

ASL in theory more reproducible. However, the ASL can be affected by variations of the transmit field $B_1{}^+$ especially around dental or other surgical hardware (**Fig. 4**) and variations in label efficiency. The ASL also undergoes T_1 recovery, which limits the time the label is available for imaging, can be problematic for patients with long bolus arrival times (BATs) (eg, due to poor cardiac output and/or steno-occlusive disease). Although there are mathematical models to address some of those issues,[9] the parameter maps derived from ASL are not always as robust as those from DSC perfusion MR imaging and are usually of lower spatial resolution. Particularly, in the presence of very long bolus arrival delays, the T_1 decay of the label can lead

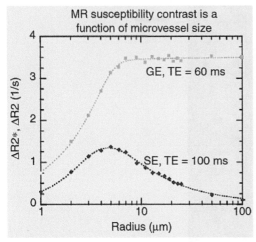

Fig. 3. Vessel size dependence of spin-echo (SE) (ΔR_2) and gradient-echo (GE) (ΔR_2^*) relaxivity for cylindrical magnetic field perturbers with 2% (blood) volume fraction and $\Delta\chi = 1 \times 10^{-7}$ at 1.5 T and with proton diffusion coefficient $D = 1 \times 10^{-5}$ cm^2/s. For the smallest perturbers, SE and GE relaxivities are nearly identical. For SE, ΔR_2 reaches a peak at approximately 5-mm radius. Unlike ΔR_2, however, ΔR_2^* does not fall off at a larger perturber size but plateaus for both experiment and simulation.

to significant overcall of blood flow reductions (see **Fig. 4**) or alternatively to arterial transit artifacts, that is, where the label remains in large vessel and arterioles and does not exchange with tissue.

When we talk about DSC perfusion, there are usually several other parameters that can be measured in addition to tissue perfusion and which, over the years, have become equally, if not more, important than frank tissue perfusion. We will discuss those parameters in more detail later in this article. To this point, the authors would like to point out that the literature is at times confusing when it comes to the correct use of units. Old publications, where tissue was excised from animals to determine the amount of tracer, use concentration per unit mass of excised tissue. However, the MR imaging signal is sensitive to the amount of tracer per unit volume. To add to the confusion, [plasma] blood flow, capillary permeability, and capillary surface area still relate to unit mass of tissue.

Contrast Concentration Measurements in Real Life

Before, we learned that relative to the susceptibility effect, the T_1-shortening effect of GBCA is usually much smaller, especially during the first pass of the tracer bolus. With an intact BBB, all tracer material is confined to the capillary bed. The volume that the capillary bed occupies in a voxel is called

the *blood volume*. In the brain, the cerebral blood volume (CBV) amounts to only a few percent of the entire voxel volume. In healthy gray matter, it is approximately twice that in health white matter.

Things get more complicated when the BBB is no longer intact and becomes (semi) permeable, which can occur due to formation of neovasculature with poorly formed endothelium (eg, tumors, metastases, membranes of chronic subdural hematomas) or the breakdown of tight junctions (eg, strokes). In that case, the contrast agent extravasates, that is, the tracer gradually diffuses—driven by intravascular/extravascular concentration gradients—into a much larger space, known as the extracellular–extravascular space (EES) (**Fig. 5**). Given that the EES is much larger as the intravascular space, the interactions of the GBCA with surrounding protons can increase and a greater T_1 effect can be observed. We also assume that the intracellular-extravascular space is off-limits for GBCA.

Unless the vessel wall is very permeable, in a first approximation, the tracer remains intravascular during the first passage of the bolus. In that case, the T_2^* effect is much stronger than the T_1 effect. Thus, most of the first-pass bolus perfusion methods are built around fast DSC MR imaging. Conversely, the extravasation often happens over several minutes and, because of the larger distribution volume T_1-effects, will eventually dominate T_2^* effects. For that reason, T_1-weighted sequences, such as 2D or 3D spoiled gradient-echo sequences (eg, spoiled gradient echo (SPGR), T1-weighted fast field echo (T1-FFE)), have been primarily used to measure the GBCA uptake in tissue and perform pharmacokinetic modeling.[10,11] This technique is widely known as dynamic contrast-enhanced (DCE) MR imaging.

It is worth pointing out that while with DSC, the MR imaging signal that is observed decreases with increased concentration due to transient T_2^*-shortening, with increased GBCA extravasation, T_1-shortening occurs. This is now more impactful for the measured signal because of its effect *not only in the blood plasma compartment but also in the much larger extravascular tissue space where all the protons now have easier access to the gadolinium atom.* This T_1-change is the underlying effect that DCE leverages with its T_1-weighted sequences. However, even with DSC, the T_1-shortening effect can be observed. In the presence of contrast leakage into tissue, all else being equal, the faster T_1-signal recovery toward equilibrium may dominate, or at least partially offset the T_2^*-signal decay. If not addressed, T_1 effects in the presence of BBB breakdown can therefore be a confounder. This

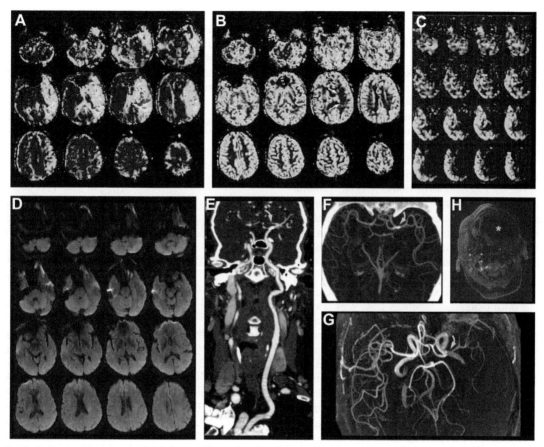

Fig. 4. Patient with a pronounced area of Tmax elevation (*A*), derived from DSC perfusion, and a widespread area of CBF reduction on ASL perfusion (*C*), despite only minor CBF reduction (*arrows*) on DSC CBF maps (*B*). diffusion-weighted imaging (DWI) acquired concurrently with CBF appears normal (*D*). CT angiography (*E, F*) shows patency of the neck vessels but reveals a chronic terminal internal carotid artery (ICA) occlusion (*curved arrow*), but with flow reconstitution after occlusion. The resultant delayed flow is not only seen on Tmax (*A*) but also seen as signal reduction on 3D time-of-flight magnetic resonance angiography (TOF MRA) (*G*). The severe CBF reduction on ASL (*C*) is likely due to a combination of both delayed bolus arrival and associated T_1 decay of arterial spin label, and a dental implant (*H*) (*asterisk*) that reduces labeling efficiency. (*Courtesy* of R Bammer, Melbourne, VIC, Australia.)

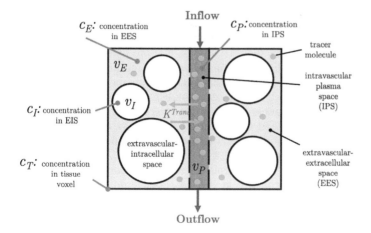

Fig. 5. Multicompartment model showing GBCA passage through tissue in the presence of GBCA extravasation. Dots represent GBCA within intravascular plasma space (IPS) and extravascular–extracellular space (EES) with volume fractions v_p and v_e, and GBCA concentrations c_P and c_E, respectively. The extravascular–intracellular space with volume fraction v_i is assumed to be impermeable to GBCA molecules; thus, the extravascular–intracellular CA concentration c_i is assumed to be equal to 0. K^{Trans} is the volume transfer constant.

effect is more pronounced in DSC sequences with shorter TR and larger flip angles, as both parameters yield more signal when signal recovery is driven by shorter T_1 times.

In acute ischemic stroke, we usually do not observe BBB breakdown in the early phase and would therefore not expect contrast leakage. However, in certain tumors, for example, where GBCA leakage occurs, a faster T_1 recovery during and after the first pass of the GBCA bolus can be expected. This can lead to errors in estimating the gadolinium concentration and, in turn, to an erroneous calculation of hemodynamic parameters, such as CBV. The calculation of cerebral blood flow (CBF) is usually not affected by leakage, as CBF is determined more by the early part of the tissue concentration curve where T_1 contamination is usually small.

Historically, DCE has been used mainly for characterizing the "leakiness" of tumors or multiple sclerosis (MS) plaques,[11] whereas DSC was primarily used for stroke and assessment of tumor grade. It can be shown, however, that DCE and DSC rely on many of the same fundamentals, and one can integrate extravasation and T_1 enhancement into DSC,[12] and vice versa. The two main differentiators are that T_1-based measurements are usually not good for the first pass when most of the contrast remains intravascular, whereas with increasing extravasation, the susceptibility differences between intravascular and extravascular compartments disappear. Sadly, for years, DSC and DCE have been treated by many clinicians and basic scientists in isolation. A major impediment to bringing the two methods together is the use of different nomenclature for similar or identical parameters and different units of measurement. Even within the DCE community, various investigators have used different terminology, which has led to some confusion.[13] There are, however, approaches now available that can leverage the benefits of DSC and DCE in one sequence.

Unlike CT density, the relationship between the MR imaging signal and GBCA concentration is rather complex. For a standard DSC sequence with echo time TE, repetition time TR, a GBCA concentration c, and a flip angle α, the steady-state signal equation is:

$$M(c) = m_0 \frac{sin(\alpha)[1 - exp(\text{-}TR\, R_1(c))]}{1 - cos(\alpha)\, exp(\text{-}TR\, R_1(c))} exp(\text{-}TE\, R_2^*(c)) =$$

$$= m_0 E_1(c)\, exp(\text{-}TE\, R_2^*(c)) =$$

$$= S_0(c)\, exp(\text{-}TE\, R_2^*(c)) \qquad (2)$$

The change in the MR signal that we observe and which is caused by the presence of the GBCA at concentration c, $M(c)$, relative to the signal in the absence of any GBCA, $M(0)$, can be computed from the ratio of both measurements and followed by taking the natural logarithm, that is,

$$ln\left[\frac{M(c)}{M(0)}\right] = ln\left[\frac{S_0(c)}{S_0(0)} exp\left(- TE\{R_2^*(c) - R_2^*(0)\}\right)\right]$$

$$= ln\left[\frac{S_0(c)}{S_0(0)}\right] - TE\left[\underbrace{R_2^*(c) - R_2^*(0)}_{\Delta R_2^*(c)}\right],$$

$$(3)$$

which yields the change in R_2^* dependent on c:

$$\Delta R_2^*(c) = -\frac{1}{TE} ln\left[\frac{M(c)}{M(0)}\right] + \frac{1}{TE} ln\left[\frac{S_0(c)}{S_0(0)}\right]. \qquad (4)$$

Notice that because the tracer concentration c in DSC MR imaging is a function of time, the change in R_2^* also implicitly becomes a function of time. In regular DSC imaging, when there is no extravasation, the T_1 effect reflected in the second term of Eq 4 is usually neglected.

Because the pre-bolus DSC signal $M(0)$ serves as a normalization reference, a correct estimate of $M(0)$ is important for an accurate calculation of ΔR_2^*. As all MR sample points of the DSC scan are contaminated by noise, instead of using just a single-point estimate of $M(0)$, a more accurate estimate of $M(0)$ is to take the average over several pre-bolus (baseline) time points. The larger the number of pre-bolus time points we average over (absent of any motion), the closer the estimation value of $M(0)$ gets to the true value of $M(0)$ that is free of any noise.[14] Historically, 20 to 40 baseline time points have been used to estimate $M(0)$. Unlike CT perfusion, where radiation dose is an issue, the only tradeoff for a longer pre-bolus acquisition period is total scan time. That said, even for CT perfusion (CTP), a few baseline points are usually not a bad idea as the same issues hold true. Note that it is not uncommon to see CTP studies that are timed so tightly that the bolus has already arrived at the first sample point. This ultimately defeats the purpose of radiation protection (ALARA—"as low as reasonable achievable"), when the remaining sample points lead to futile irradiation of the patient, because the study is rendered nondiagnostic because of a missing baseline.

In general, a linear dependence between the change in GBCA concentration and R_2^* is assumed,[15,16] so that

$$R_2^*(c) = R_{2,0}^* + r_2^* c \qquad (5)$$

and hence due to normalization to the pre-bolus reference point

$$\Delta R_2^*(c) = R_2^*(c) - R_{2,0} = r_2^* c. \qquad (6)$$

Although this linear relationship is widely used clinically and holds true for tissues, it starts to break down for arterial signal where a nonlinear relationship should be assumed, for example,

$$\Delta R_2^*(c) = ac + bc^2, \qquad (7)$$

with a and b being constants. Alternatively, the phase signal in a large artery can be measured. It has been demonstrated that there is a linear behavior in MR signal phase over the concentration range.[17] Phase-based measurements of arterial concentration changes are unfortunately difficult to perform in clinical practice, because in most DSC MR imaging examinations mainly magnitude data are stored. In addition, commercial DSC postprocessing tools only support magnitude data, which restricts this approach mainly to research applications.

Note also that in the presence of extravasation, Eq 6 is confounded by the second term shown in Eq 4, and the measured ΔR_2^* is an apparent $\Delta R_{2,app}^*$.

Concentration Measurements with Dynamic Echo-planar Imaging Sequences

For a dynamic multi-echo single-shot gradient-echo and spin-echo EPI sequence,[18] such as, in **Fig. 6**, the signal S that is acquired at given echo times TE (where TE_{SE} is the time the spin echo is

formed), and where R_2 and R_2^* are time-dependent due to the temporal chances of underlying GBCA changes, is defined by

$$S(t,TE) = \begin{cases} S_0(t)e^{-TE\,R_2^*(t)} & if\ TE < TE_{SE}/2 \\ \dfrac{S_0(t)}{\delta}e^{-TE_{SE}\,R_2^*(t)}e^{-TE\left(2R_2(t)-R_2^*(t)\right)} & if\ \dfrac{TE_{SE}}{2} < TE < TE_{SE} \end{cases} \qquad (8)$$

Here, δ is a correction factor for slice profile imperfections between excitation and refocusing pulse. Note if the DSC sequence is simply a gradient-echo EPI sequence or a multi-echo gradient-echo EPI sequence,[19] only the top portion of Eq 8 needs to be considered. With multiple echoes, one can do a parameter fit of Eq 8 to estimate $R_2^*(t)$, $R_2(t)$, and $S_0(t)$ for each time point of the bolus passage, thus eliminating the T_1-shortening effects. The latter are all contained in the $S_0(t)$ term. Even with two gradient echoes that are acquired at TE_1 and TE_2, and where $TE_2 > TE_1$, the T_1 effects can be eliminated (without a parameter fit) using the following expression:

$$\Delta R_2^*(c) = -\frac{1}{TE_2 - TE_1}\left[ln\left(\frac{M_{TE_2}(0)}{M_{TE_1}(0)}\right) - ln\left(\frac{M_{TE_2}(c)}{M_{TE_1}(c)}\right)\right]. \qquad (9)$$

INDICATOR DILUTION THEORY AND CENTRAL VOLUME PRINCIPLE

The basic concept of the indicator dilution theory[3,4] is that a small amount of the indicator is

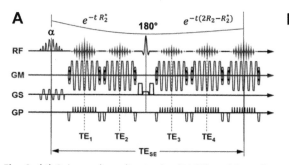
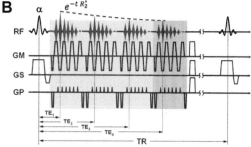

Fig. 6. (A) Spin- and gradient-echo (SAGE) multi-gradient echo and spin-echo EPI sequence. After an excitation radio-frequency (RF) pulse (flip angle is typically 90°), gradient echoes are formed at TE_1 and TE_2 which are readout by single-shot EPI trains. Thereafter, a 180° refocusing pulse rewinds the T_2^* decay to form a spin echo at TE_{SE}, which shows only T_2-weighting and is also readout by a single-shot EPI train. Between the refocusing pulse and the spin echo formation, two additional gradient echoes are formed at TE_3 and TE_4. (B) Multi-gradient-echo EPI sequence for DSC perfusion MR imaging. After an RF excitation pulse that is typically between 30° and 90°, multiple gradient echoes are formed at TE_1, ... TE_4, each will be readout by a single-shot EPI scan to form an image with increasing T_2^*-weighting. The standard T_2^*-weighted gradient-echo EPI sequence for DSC perfusion MR imaging uses a later echo time (*shaded in red*), leaving a period after the RF excitation pulse unused (*shaded in green*). The perfusion with multiple echoes and temporal enhancement (PERMEATE) multi-gradient-echo sequence uses this underused period to collect more echoes to achieve a more optimal weighting depending on the underlying T_2^* and the expected T_2^* changes during the GBCA bolus passage. (*Courtesy of* R Bammer, Melbourne, VIC, Australia.)

injected into the blood stream where we then can quantify the indicator's concentration over time.

Let us assume a very simplistic tissue model with a single arterial inlet and a single venous outlet. Between these is a voxel that contains a capillary network that connects the arterial with the venous side (**Fig. 7**). The capillary vessels occupy only a small fraction of this voxel. Individual capillary vessels within this voxel are of variable length, so that—under the assumption of equal flow through each capillary vessel—tracer molecules will have different path length and take more or less time to pass from the arterial to the venous side, dependent on which capillary pathway they took.

If the bolus $c_A(t)$ on the arterial side is super short (aka infinitesimal), we measure at the venous outlet a dispersed bolus shape $c_V(t)$, that is very different from the initial shape at the input. Depending on the length of individual capillary segments, parts of the bolus will appear at the venous side with more or less lag (**Fig. 8**). The concentration curve that we measure at the venous outlet $c_V(t)$ —if there were an infinitesimally short bolus at the arterial input (ie, $c_A(0) = 1$)—is in essence the probability density function (PDF) $h(t)$ of all the durations t, the tracer molecules need to pass through the individual capillary pathways. From a systems theory perspective, $h(t)$ is the *impulse response function* of the underlying vascular network of this voxel. This system also underlies the principle of conservation of mass, that is, everything that flows into the voxel from the arterial side, must eventually come out of the venous side. The area under the curve of $h(t)$ needs to be equal to the arterial input. For convenience, the area under the curve of $h(t)$ is usually normalized to "1."

If we stay with the PDF and basic statistics for a moment, we can compute the *first moment* of $h(t)$, which is by definition the mean time that tracer molecules will take to pass through the capillary bed from the arterial to the venous side of the voxel (ie, mean transit time [MTT]). Later, we will discuss that the first moment needs to be treated carefully if the arterial input is not infinitesimally short (as is always the case in the

real-world clinical practice) and $c_V(t)$ is no longer just $h(t)$.

For any arterial input function (AIF) $c_A(t)$ into our voxel, the quantity of contrast material that has reached the arterial inlet by the time t is the sum of arterial concentration at each point in time weighted by the CBF:

$$q_A(t) = CBF \int_0^t c_A(\tau)\, d\tau, \qquad \textbf{(10)}$$

whereas the amount of contrast material that has reached the venous outlet by the time t is:

$$q_V(t) = CBF \int_0^t c_V(\tau)\, d\tau. \qquad \textbf{(11)}$$

If $t \to \infty$, then the entire amount of tracer material that went in must have also come out of the voxel. In more general terms, the amount of contrast remaining in the voxel at time t is determined by Fick's principle,[1] that is, the CBF-weighted time integral of the arterio-venous difference in contrast concentration:

$$q(t) = q_A(t) - q_V(t) = CBF \int_0^t (c_A(\tau) - c_V(\tau))d\tau. \quad \textbf{(12)}$$

The Maximum Slope Method

If we look at Eq 12 at very short times t (ie, when t is less than the time it takes the tracer to pass to the venous side) then Eq 12 can be simplified, which is broadly known in the literature as the *no outflow* assumption[20]:

$$q(t) = q_A(t) - 0 = CBF \int_0^t c_A(\tau)\, d\tau \qquad \textbf{(13)}$$

Note that the *no outflow* condition was assumed to be achieved with high injection flow rates (eg, 20 mL/s) and became the basis for the *maximum slope method*[20] that has been used in the past to

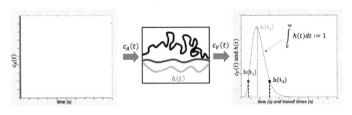

Fig. 7. Simple capillary model with three capillary pathways in one voxel. A very short bolus of unit height "1" at the arterial inlet c_A will cause a dispersed response at the venous outlet c_V due to the different capillary paths that fractions of the unit bolus will take. For an infinitesimally short bolus of unit hight, $c_V(t)$ becomes the impulse response of the voxel, which is also the probability density function of transit times that the contrast molecules take to travel through the capillaries within the voxel. (*Courtesy* of R Bammer, Melbourne, VIC, Australia.)

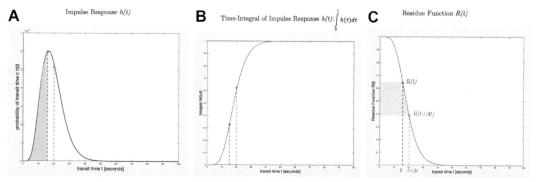

Fig. 8. Impulse response function $h(t)$ (*A*), its corresponding time integral (*B*) and the corresponding residue function $R(t)$ (*C*) for various times t. (*Courtesy* of R Bammer, Melbourne, VIC, Australia.)

determine perfusion and works as follows: First, one takes the time derivative of Eq 13 to determine the rate of contrast accumulation:

$$\left[\frac{d(q(t))}{dt}\right]_{t=\tau} = CBF\ c_A(\tau). \tag{14}$$

Next, one takes the second derivative of Eq 13, that is,

$$\frac{d^2(q(t))}{dt^2} = CBF\ \frac{d(c_A(t))}{dt}. \tag{15}$$

Then, we know from calculus that at the time δ when the second derivative of a curve becomes zero, the slope of the curve has its maximum. In other words, Eq 15 becomes zero when $d(c_A(\delta))/dt$ is zero. Hence, CBF can be computed from the ratio of the maximum rate of contrast accumulation in tissue, that is, the maximum slope of $q(t)$ and the maximum arterial concentration:

$$CBF = max\left[\frac{d(q(t))}{dt}\right] / max[c_A(t)]. \tag{16}$$

Comparing Eqs 12 and 13 shows that if the venous outflow starts before the arterial concentration peaked, CBF is underestimated when determined with the maximum slope method. Owing to the short capillary transit times, this is particularly problematic for brain tissue. In addition, compared with other computation methods that we will discuss later, the maximum slope method relies on differentiating the tissue concentration curve and is therefore noisier. It also does not provide additional hemodynamic parameters, such as Tmax.

The Residue Function

One problem we have not mentioned thus far is the fact that we usually do not have access to the venous outlet to measure $c_V(t)$, let alone $h(t)$.

Even the true arterial input $c_A(t)$ into a tissue voxel is difficult to observe and measure, although seminal work has been silent about this fact. There have been some incidental applications of local AIF applications[21] but this approach has never found broad adoption. What is accessible to us with both CT and MR imaging, though, is the tracer concentration in the voxel over time. As such, following an instantaneous bolus injection, we can determine the amount of tracer that remains within the voxel at a particular point in time, which is commonly known as the tissue *residue function* $r(t)$ (see **Fig. 8**C).

Please remember that we normalized the complete area under the $h(t)$ curve to "1," and that at $t = 0$, no tracer molecule has made it yet to the venous outlet and $r(t = 0) = 1$. We can therefore compute the residue function for any time point as follows:

$$r(t) = 1 - \int_0^t h(\tau)d\tau. \tag{17}$$

Because of this, $r(t)$ must be a positive, decreasing function of time. If the bolus at the arterial input differs from an instantaneous bolus, we will show in a moment how the residue function relates to the observable tissue signal $c_T(t)$. But let us first address the blood volume as it is easy to understand.

Cerebral Blood Volume

CBV is probably the simplest hemodynamic parameter to calculate. In many cases, it is reported as the proportion (or in percent) of blood within a voxel when compared with a reference voxel that contains exclusively blood (ie, no tissue), such as a large artery. Sometimes CBV is multiplied with the density of brain tissue (ie, 1.04 g/ mL) to put CBV on a quantitative basis, that is, report it in units of mL per 100 mg brain tissue (recall our earlier discussion about old parameters being reported in units of tissue mass):

$$CBV = \frac{1mL}{1.04g} \frac{\int_0^t c_T(\tau)d\tau}{\int_0^t c_A(\tau)d\tau} . \tag{18}$$

Here, the time variable t is chosen such that it usually denotes the end of the first pass to avoid recirculation or, more conveniently, the whole length of the dynamic acquisition window when the duration of the dynamic acquisition is chosen to be so long that the recirculation effects and their respective tissue responses have abated. A common source for CBV underestimation is to choose t too short. This is often the case when the DSC scan is terminated prematurely, for example, due to patient motion or—in case of CT perfusion—to minimize radiation dose.

Particularly in regions with delayed bolus arrival, this can lead to significant CBV underestimation and consequently also in paradox MTT reductions (**Fig. 9**).

Rather than absolute CBV quantitation, based on our practical experience, CBV is used most often in the context of regional changes, either by assessing hemispheric differences, differences in vascular territories, or just changes within parts of a lesion (eg, enhancing part of a tumor) (**Fig. 10**) relative to a reference point or tissue.

Of note, here also is that historically, when CT scanners had limited coverage and covered mostly the basal ganglia, arteries in this scanning area were too small in caliber, and measurements of the AIF, that is, $c_A(t)$, thus suffered from partial volume artifacts. Consequently, arterial concentration measurements got underestimated. A remedy for such situations was to normalize the AIF area under the curve to a large vein, such as the sagittal or transverse sinuses. After all, the only thing that is needed to determine the proportion of the voxel that contains blood is knowledge of

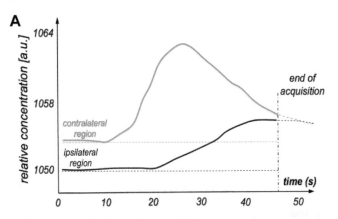

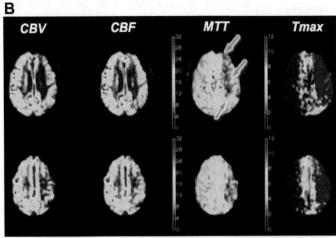

Fig. 9. (*A*) Relative tracer concentration curves from a perfusion study taken in a brain region with prolonged bolus arrival and tracer transit through tissue in comparison with the patient's normal hemisphere (contralateral region). The perfusion study was stopped prematurely, whereas the contrast agent was still going through the healthy tissue, but to an even greater extent the hemodynamically challenged region. (*B*) Consequently the CBV was significantly underestimated in the hemodynamically challenged area and led to a paradoxically low MTT value. (*Courtesy* of R Bammer, Melbourne, VIC, Australia.)

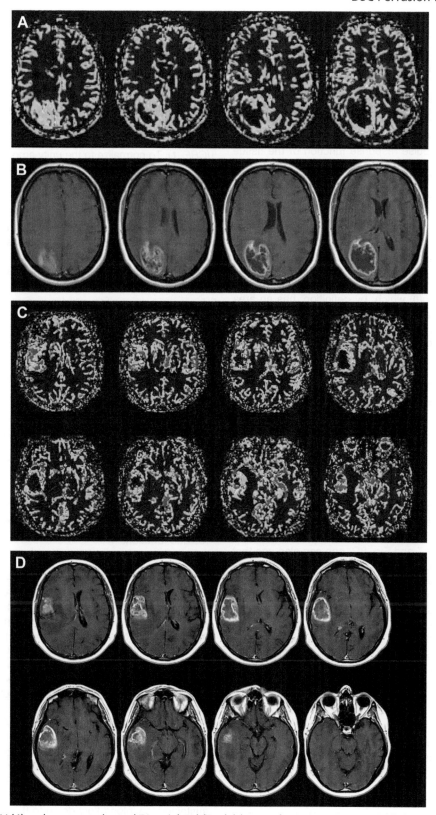

Fig. 10. CBV (*A*) and contrast-enhanced T1-weighted (T1w) (*B*) scan of a patient with a right occipital mass consistent with a high-grade glioma. The homogenous rim of T1-enhancement appears heterogenously on CBV maps. CBV (*C*) and contrast-enhanced T1w (*D*) scan of a patient with a glioblastoma. Again, the homogenous rim of T1 enhancement is rather heterogenous on the CBV maps, suggesting areas which inhomogeneous neovessel proliferation. (*Courtesy* of R Bammer, Melbourne, VIC, Australia.)

the concentration-over-time curve in a voxel that contains just blood, hence the choice of the large vein for scaling purposes.

Mean Transit Time

The mean (tracer) transit time is another key hemodynamic parameter and can be directly derived from the impulse response function of the tissue voxel $h(t)$. As mentioned before, $h(t)$ can be seen as the PDF of tracer transport times across the voxel of interest. Hence, the first moment of $h(t)$ is the center of the distribution of transit times, or the mean, hence the name *mean transit time*:

$$MTT = \int_0^\infty \tau \cdot h(\tau) d\tau. \tag{19}$$

Although $h(t)$, which, by definition, has an area under the curve that equals 1, is not directly observable, if we could achieve an instantaneous bolus, one could compute MTT as:

$$MTT = \frac{\int_0^\infty \tau \cdot c_T(\tau) d\tau}{\int_0^\infty c_T(\tau) d\tau}, \tag{20}$$

where the denominator in Eq 20 is simply for normalization (remember that the area under $h(t)$ is 1 but $c_T(t)$ is not). However, one should be cautioned that this equation does not hold true for non-instantaneous arterial injections, which is the case in clinical practice.[22] More on that in a minute.

From Eq 17 and **Fig. 8C**, one can also see that the difference between $r(t + dt)$ and $r(t)$ is the fraction of tracer that has the transit time t, that is, $h(t)$. From **Fig. 8C**, we also see that the area under the $r(t)$ curve is the area under "the product of the transit time, t, and the fraction of tracer material taking the time t to transit," that is, equivalent to Eq 19. Thus, MTT can be calculated alternatively by the area under the residue curve, that is,

$$MTT = \int_0^\infty r(\tau) d\tau, \tag{21}$$

which is more practical, because $r(t)$ is accessible to measurements and is corrected for situations when the arterial input is not instantaneous.

Central Volume Principle

If we go back to our initial single-voxel model in **Fig. 7** and look at the individual capillary pathways, we can also derive one of the most

fundamental relationships in perfusion imaging: the central volume principle.[23] Although everyone uses this relationship, the origin of it is rarely explained, which is why we will review it here.

Under the assumption of constant equal blood flow, that is, CBF through each capillary thread (see **Fig. 7**), the volume that the ith capillary thread covers if the tracer seems at the outlet at t_i is $(CBF \cdot t_i)$. To normalize to the unity amount of tracer material, this covered thread volume is weighted by the fraction of total tracer material that was initially injected instantaneously at $t = 0$ and arrived at the venous outlet at t_i, so that $\Delta V_i = (CBFt_i)h(t_i)$

If we sum over all the subvolumes of capillary threads across the voxel, this equals the CBV, that is, the proportion of the voxel containing blood, and we can express it in integral form as:

$$CBV = CBF \int_0^\infty \tau \cdot h(\tau) d\tau. \tag{22}$$

If we substitute the integral in Eq 22 with the definition of MTT from Eq 19, voila! we immediately get the familiar expression for the *central volume principle*:

$$CBV = CBF \cdot MTT. \tag{23}$$

Using the central volume principle as defined by Eq 23 and substituting MTT with Eq 21, we can use

$$CBV = CBF \int_0^\infty r(\tau) d\tau \tag{24}$$

as an alternative to Eq 18 to calculate CBV via the residue function.

Cerebral Blood Flow

A lot has been written about the correct way to calculate CBF. We have already discussed one way to determine CBF: the maximum slope method[20] and its strengths and weaknesses. We will devote a whole section (below) to CBF calculation, but in short, CBF is the rate at which blood flows through the capillary bed and therefore the determining factor for both delivering nutrients and disposing metabolic waste.

Normal blood flow is in the range of 40 to 60 mL/min per 100g (brain tissue).[24] CBF values above that are considered as hyperperfusion. CBF is one of the key parameters in stroke, where a prolonged and significant CBF reduction is usually a surrogate for poor tissue outcome. For example, sustained low blood flow down to 8 to 12 mL/sec per 100 mg brain tissue[24] or a reduction of CBF down to less than 30% of its contralateral healthy value (ie, a 70% CBF reduction)[25] is deemed to be a surrogate for irreversibly damaged tissue, if blood flow cannot restored within a short period after the occlusion. A milder CBF reduction, within the range between 20 and 40 mL/min/100g, is called benign oligemia; this is a condition which patients can tolerate well, and the tissue is not at risk of infarction under normal conditions[24] unless the patient deteriorates and there is a reduction in CBF, for example, due to a reduction in cerebral perfusion pressure. All these values have been empirically determined, and CBF values differ between gray and white matter as well as with age and other factors. Thus, the exact thresholds should not be assumed and must be treated with caution.

It is important to point out that unlike diffusion-restriction, which in stroke reflects tissue injury due to the cumulative effects of sustained hypoperfusion, blood flow is a snapshot view. Any short transient reduction of CBF, even if severe, would normally not lead to lasting tissue damage. Conversely, when a previously occlusive arterial clot dissolves or is dislodged, the CBF may appear normal or even increased in already infarcted tissue. CBF has also demonstrated to be of important diagnostic utility in seizures, migraines, brain tumors, or chronic occlusive disease.

We would like to point out, again from experience and similar to CBV, that it is often the changes relative to a reference point or region, such as normal contralateral hemisphere, that is most often much more revealing and useful than focusing on absolute CBF numbers. Applications where absolute values are probably more important is the assessment of CBF values over time such as dementia,[26,27] cerebral vascular reserve testing, or intersubject comparisons. However, even here, relative numbers are important at the end. The only difference is that intersubject variations or test–retest variability within one subject may need to be considered, and absolute CBF values are harder to accomplish with DSC perfusion due to confounding factors, such as variability in injection rate and head (and thus large vessel) orientation relative to B_0, which can affect the estimation of (arterial) GBCA concentration and thus CBF than ASL-based measurements.

Dynamic Tissue Signal Changes in Response to Arbitrary Arterial Inputs

The previous sections laid the general foundation for CBV, CBF, and MTT and connected these parameters via the central volume principle. We also mentioned that $h(t)$ and $r(t)$ are difficult to obtain when the arterial input differs from an instantaneous bolus. In a clinical practice, even with very high flow rates, as required for the maximum slope method, an instantaneous bolus is impossible to achieve. The contrast material is usually injected intravenously, typically in the right antecubital vein, with flow rates between 4 and 8 mL/second and then followed by at least 20 mL of saline chaser to push the contrast agent through the injector tubing and the arm vein, all the way into the central circulation. There, the bolus undergoes further delay and dispersion in the lung circulation and then the left heart. The bolus which arrives at the brain therefore looks significantly different from the injected bolus profile and is far from an instantaneous bolus.

So how does the tissue signal look like if the bolus is more spread out (ie, dispersed)? — The answer to that was already provided by Meier and Zierler in their seminal paper[23] in 1954 but was forgotten or overlooked by others. From **Fig. 6**, we know that the response to an instantaneous bolus of nondiffusible tracer at the arterial inlet, $c_A(0) = \delta$, is usually a protracted response at the venous outlet that usually abates after a few seconds, when all portions of the tracer have cleared all capillary pathways. We have described this before by $h(t) = [h(t_0), h(t_1), h(t_2),...]$. Now, if we assume that another instantaneous bolus follows the first one, say at $t = \Delta$, then the response to this bolus, $c_A(\Delta)=\delta$ will be observed at the outlet, similar to the first one, but with a delay Δ. A third instantaneous bolus played out 2Δ from the first one, that is, $c_A(2\Delta) = \delta$, would cause a response that follows $h(t)$, just with a delay of 2Δ, and so on. For each point in time, the individually delayed responses to the boli, will add up and form the net response at the output. When we make Δ very small and replace δ at each point in time of c_A with the true arterial concentration $c_A(t)$ and then multiply $c_A(t)$ with the individually time-shifted $h(t)$ functions, we derive the net response to the arbitrary AIF at the venous output (**Fig. 11**).

To better understand that concept let us use a discrete representation shown with the simple equations in **Fig. 12**. For $t = 3$, in this figure, the venous signal at the output, $c_V(t = 3)$, is the sum of: the first time point of the AIF, $c_A(t = 0s)$, weighted by $h(t = 3s)$; plus the second time point of the AIF, $c_A(t = 1s)$, weighted by $h(t = [3s - 1s])$, as the arterial input came 1s later; plus the third time point of the AIF, $c_A(t = 2s)$, weighted by $h(t = [3s - 2s])$, as the arterial input came 2s later; and plus the fourth time point of the AIF, $c_A(t = 3s)$, weighted by $h(t = [3s - 3s])$. If then Δ becomes infinitesimal small, we can

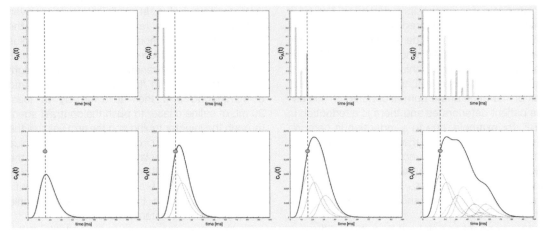

Fig. 11. Discretizing the arterial input $c_A(t)$ into short boli of height $c_A(t)$, showing the individual responses to these boli at the venous output, where they are add up to show their net effect. Top graphs show the individual instantaneous boli that resample the continuous waveform of concentration time course of the arterial input in a discretized fashion, whereas the bottom figure shows the responses to the individual time-shifted boli at the venous output and what the overall response looks like at a particular point in time. (*Courtesy* of R Bammer, Melbourne, VIC, Australia.)

write the signal at the venous outlet in integral form as:

$$c_V(t) = \int_0^t c_A(\tau)\,h(t-\tau)d\tau = c_A(t) \otimes h(t). \quad \textbf{(25)}$$

This integral type is also known as convolution, that is, the AIF, $c_A(t)$, is convolved with the impulse response function $h(t)$. The convolution operator "$\otimes$" has been introduced to avoid always writing the lengthy integral expression.

As mentioned previously, we usually cannot measure $c_V(t)$ for each voxel. What is accessible to us is the overall tissue concentration curve $c_T(t)$ associated with the residue function:

$$c_T(t) = CBF \int_0^t c_A(\tau)\,r(t-\tau)d\tau$$
$$= CBF\,[c_A(t) \otimes r(t)]. \quad \textbf{(26)}$$

The inverse operation of convolution is deconvolution, which is denoted by "$\otimes.^{-1}$" If we

deconvolve the tissue concentration curve from the AIF, we get the flow-weighted residue function:

$$c_T(t) \otimes^{-1} c_A(t) = CBF\,r(t). \quad \textbf{(27)}$$

Because the residue function r at $t = 0$ is by definition equal to 1, we can compute CBF from the first time point of Eq 27, which yields CBF·1.

Solving Eq 27 is not entirely trivial. It requires us to deconvolve two (noisy) time courses from each other, which is also known as an "inverse problem," because we infer the internal information $r(t)$ from the entities $c_T(t)$ and $c_A(t)$, that can be measured, by inverting the characteristic Eq 25. Owing to the measurement noise on the data, the solution is highly unstable and requires a mathematical trick, which also known as regularization, to address an otherwise erratically oscillating result and generate useful results.[28]

There are different ways of implementing deconvolution and performing regularization,[29] which can be categorized into *Fourier transformation-*based applications[30–32] in the frequency domain and singular value decomposition (SVD)-based

$t=0:\ C_V(0) = C_A(0) \cdot h(0)$

$t=1:\ C_V(1) = C_A(0) \cdot h(1) + C_A(1) \cdot h(0)$

$t=2:\ C_V(2) = C_A(0) \cdot h(2) + C_A(1) \cdot h(1) + C_A(2) \cdot h(0)$

$t=3:\ C_V(3) = C_A(0) \cdot h(3) + C_A(1) \cdot h(2) + C_A(2) \cdot h(1) + C_A(3) \cdot h(0)$

$\vdots$

$t=n:\ C_V(n) = C_A(0) \cdot h(n) + C_A(1) \cdot h(n-1) + \cdots + C_A(n) \cdot h(0)$

Fig. 12. Mathematical representation of the principles shown in **Fig. 11.** The concentration at the venous output at the 4th time point $c_V(3)$ is the summation of the individual contributions from four boli at the input that made their way to the output. How much each bolus will show at the output depends on $h(t)$. (*Courtesy* of R Bammer.)

applications[28,33] in the time domain. SVD is also just a transformation, similar to the more commonly known Fourier transform, just based on a different set of so-called basis functions.[29] Inherent to both approaches is the fact that the high-frequency components that are contained in both the arterial input and tissue concentration signal and yield a division of two mainly noisy signals, which in turn gives raise to erratic signal behavior of the estimated residue function and which is filtered out by regularization. The effect of this regularization "filter" on the residue function is that the true shape of $r(t)$ gets more or less smoothed out, depending on how aggressive of a regularization filter has been applied. This is especially noticeable around $t = 0$, when the residue function transitioned from 0 at $t < 0$ to its maximum value at $t = 0$. With increasing degree

of regularization, this transition gets flattened out and the time when the maximum of the residue function occurs gets shifts away from $t = 0$.

As we determine CBF from the maximum of $r(t)$ (see Eq 27), the regularization causes an underestimation of CBF. Moreover, the time of the maximum of $r(t)$, which is commonly referred to as Tmax and is another important hemodynamic parameter, will be increased by this regularization step.

Fig. 13A shows the relative weights of the individual singular values and a typical filter threshold for regularization values. It can be seen that the weights taper off relatively quickly and have little contributions to the overall signal; most of the information is stored in a small subset of (low frequency) basis functions. Therefore, with regularization, singular values below this threshold are simply ignored (ie,

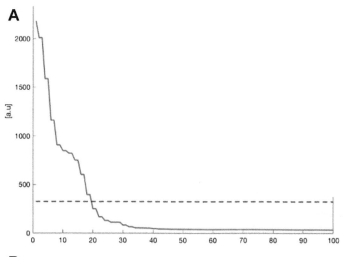

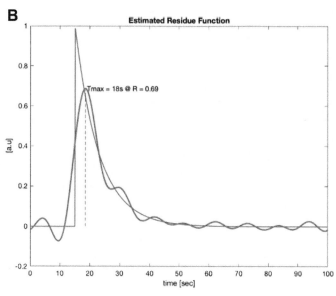

Fig. 13. (A) Singular values derived from an AIF function with 100 time points. Each singular value is associated with a unique singular vector. The higher corresponding singular value, the more its singular vector is contributing to the AIF. At a certain level, the singular vectors contribute very little. Therefore, to stabilize the solution of the inverse problem, a threshold is set (usually a percentage of the maximum singular value) (dashed red line) below which singular values are set to zero after inversion. (B) Original residue function (assume model $R = \exp(-t/MTT)$) (blue) that was included in the forward model $c_T(t) = AIF(t) *R(t) +$ noise and calculated residue function $R'(T) = (AIF(t)+noise) \otimes^{-1} c_T(t)$ after truncated SVD regularization (red). Without regularization, the residue function would oscillate wildly and would be rendered useless. The truncated SVD regularization stabilizes the solution at the expense of an underestimation of the peak of the residue function. The peak of the residue function is also delayed relative to the true peak and there are remaining oscillations. (Courtesy of R Bammer, Melbourne, VIC, Australia.)

nulled out) when solving the inverse problem.[28] **Fig. 13B** shows a model residue function and the corresponding regularized residue function using the aforementioned threshold, which in this case was 15% of the maximum singular value. **Fig. 13B** shows the effect of regularization on both the residue function and Tmax.

Tmax

Tmax has become one of the most powerful parameters that is used in perfusion imaging, mainly because it is a robust indicator of at-risk tissue in stroke.[25] Thus, Tmax has been used as an important tissue marker in almost all stroke landmark trials.[25,34–37] Under physiologic conditions, Tmax maps are relatively flat, that is, the maps demonstrate very little contrast between gray and white matter. Following an arterial occlusion or stenosis, blood arrives in the vascular territory distal to the clot with significant delay relative to the AIF reference point and thus stands out as a high-contrasting lesion relative to the surrounding tissue (**Figs. 14 and 15**).

Because of this strong image contrast in the presence of steno-occlusive disease, areas of abnormal hemodynamics are much more conspicuous on Tmax maps than CBF and CBV maps, where subtle lesions can be masked by normal gray/white matter differences or "blooming" caused by partial volume effects of large vessels adjacent to the tissue of interest (**Figs. 16 and 17**). The degree of Tmax elevation is often used to draw conclusions about which regions are at risk of infarction or still receive favorable collateral blood supply and may therefore be salvageable. Moreover, Tmax has proven extremely helpful in directing the neuroradiologist to the specific site of occlusion, which is particularly useful in a busy emergency setting with a large volume of scans to read for the neuroradiologist. Particularly for distal-to-medium vessel occlusions (**Figs. 15–17**) of both the anterior and posterior circulation, Tmax can help to identify occlusions within seconds as compared with several minutes.[38,39]

At this point, it is important to differentiate between MTT and Tmax. Both are time parameters that are derived from DSC perfusion scans. However, as we have seen in previous paragraphs, although MTT describes the mean time that a unit amount of tracer takes to *pass through the voxel* from the arterial to the venous side, Tmax measures—relative to an arterial reference point—how long it takes the tracer to *arrive at the voxel*. Understanding the differences between those two parameters can be an important "survival skill" for the practicing neuroradiologist.

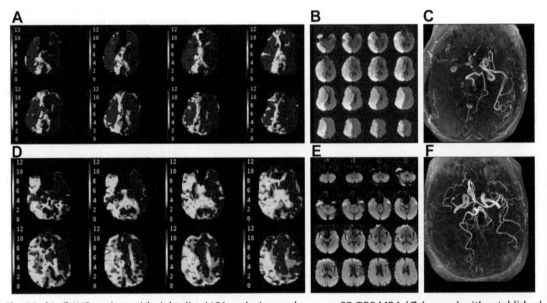

Fig. 14. (*A–C*) LVO patient with right distal ICA occlusion as shown on 3D TOF MRA (*C*) (*arrows*) with established infarct seen on DWI (*B*) and fully matched penumbra as evidenced by the area of Tmax elevation (*A*). The right anterior cerebral artery (ACA) territory was spared thanks to cross-flow via the Acom. (*D–F*) Another LVO patient with a right distal M1 occlusion, shown on 3D TOF MRA (*F*) (*arrow*), sparing the anterior perforators as seen on Tmax (*D*) with several minor areas of infarction seen on DWI (*E*). The DWI-Tmax mismatch suggests a considerable area of salvageable tissue. Moreover, the heterogenous pattern of Tmax elevation with large areas of only mild Tmax prolongation is also suggestive of good collateral supply. (*Courtesy* of R Bammer, Melbourne, VIC, Australia.)

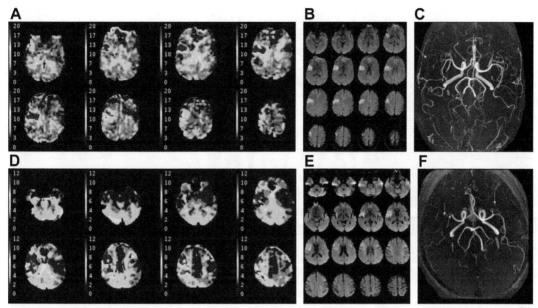

Fig. 15. (*A–C*) Patient with right distal–medium vessel occlusion (M3 segment of the MCA) as shown on 3D TOF MRA (*C*) (*arrow*), with an established infarct seen on DWI (*B*) and fully matched penumbra, as evidenced by the area of Tmax elevation (*A*). The occlusion was initially difficult to identify on the TOF MRA, but both Tmax and DWI helped to narrow down the occluded vessel. (*D–F*) Another LVO patient with a right proximal M2 occlusion shown on 3D TOF MRA (*F*) (*arrow*) and better evidenced on Tmax (*D*), with matching areas of infarction seen on DWI (*E*). This patient had also a distal vessel occlusion (M4 MCA branch) in the left hemisphere. (*Courtesy* of R Bammer, Melbourne, VIC, Australia.)

Tmax, for example, can be elevated despite MTT being normal, for example, in patients with robust collaterals. Here, an elevated Tmax simply means that the blood arrives later, that is, longer arterial transit times (see **Fig. 4**). In stroke patients with Tmax elevation, it has been shown that if there is a significant proportion of high Tmax relative to the entire Tmax region—also known as hypoperfusion intensity ratio (HIR)—evidence suggests that these patients usually have poor collaterals, and the elevated HIR thus predicts infarct progression and poor functional outcome.[40] On the other hand, MTT can be elevated, whereas Tmax is normal. This means that the blood gets to the voxel, but for example, its venous outflow might be obstructed.

The question often arises how Tmax differs from other arrival time parameter, such as time to peak (TTP) or BAT of the tissue contrast concentration

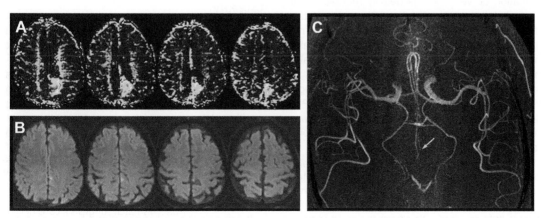

Fig. 16. (*A*) Patient with a distal vessel occlusion on Tmax (distal left A5 segment) with a punctuate DWI lesion (*B*) that one could have easily overlooked. (*C*) 3D TOF MRA also demonstrates occlusion (*arrow*). (*Courtesy* of R Bammer, Melbourne, VIC, Australia.)

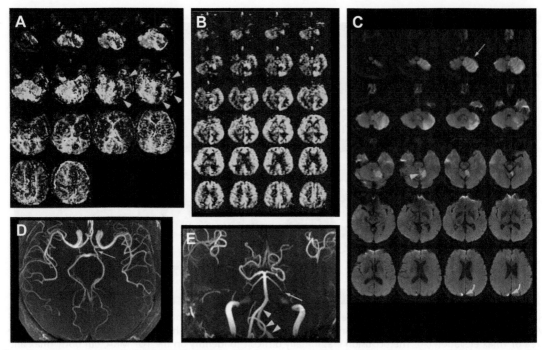

Fig. 17. Patient with a left fetal PCA demonstrating Tmax times (*A*) in the left PCA territory that are comparable to those of the anterior circulation (*arrowheads*). The fetal PCA is seen on 3D TOF MRA (*D*) (*arrow*). The patient also suffered from a left-sided superior cerebellar artery occlusion (*E*) (*arrow*) and occlusion of the left V2/3 segments, with delayed flow further distally as seen reduced TOF effect (*arrowheads*), which led to infarcts seen on DWI (*C*) in the left superior cerebellar artery (SCA) and posterior inferior cerebellar artery (PICA) territories (*arrowhead and arrow*). Tmax maps (*A*) showed also a small area of delayed flow in the right distal PCA territory (*curved arrow*) that corresponds to a small focus of DWI hyperintensity (*C*). (*Courtesy* of R Bammer, Melbourne, VIC, Australia.)

curve $c_T(t)$. The key difference and strength of Tmax is its independence from the shape of the AIF and MTT, as Tmax is derived from the inherent system response of the underlying voxel.

In contrast, TTP—defined as $\max[c_T(t)] = c_T(TTP)$ —is directly derived from the tissue contrast concentration curve, which is heavily modulated by the underlying residue function. Closer inspection of Eq 21 shows that $c_T(t)$ and its peak are not only dependent on the shape of the AIF but also the MTT. This is because MTT determines also the residue function with which the AIF is convolved. Thus, TTP elevation can be fraught with ambiguity. One cannot tell whether TTP is elevated due to a delayed tracer arrival, the way the GBCA was injected, an increased MTT, or a combination of these factors.

BAT—defined as $c_T(t = BAT) > C_{T,\ arrival\ threshold}$ for $0 < t < TTP$—on the other hand, tries to determine the inflection point of the tissue uptake curve. At the inflection point of $c_T(t)$, one can assume that there is little contamination from the residue function. However, one has to bear in mind the facts that a potentially slow/low attacking AIF ramp, as

well as an overall poor contrast-to-noise signal of the tissue concentration curve (even at peak concentration) makes it very difficult to find the inflection point of the tissue signal uptake curve, thus yielding very noisy BAT maps.

Causality

The equations above have assumed that the arterial cause of a bolus is followed by a measurable effect in the tissue tracer concentration change. Regularization adds another offset to the maximum of r. This offset depends on the degree of SVD regularization and is a relatively constant offset (**Fig. 18**A). Small, positive delays cause, however, a nonlinear increase in Tmax with SVD-based deconvolution (see **Fig. 18**A, blue curve). Because we cannot determine the true AIF to each voxel, the more practical solution, that is widely used, is a global AIF, which is selected from a large feeding artery, such as the ICA or MCA.

It can sometimes happen that a "surrogate" AIF is chosen such that the blood arrives in the tissue before the start of the AIF. Although this AIF violates

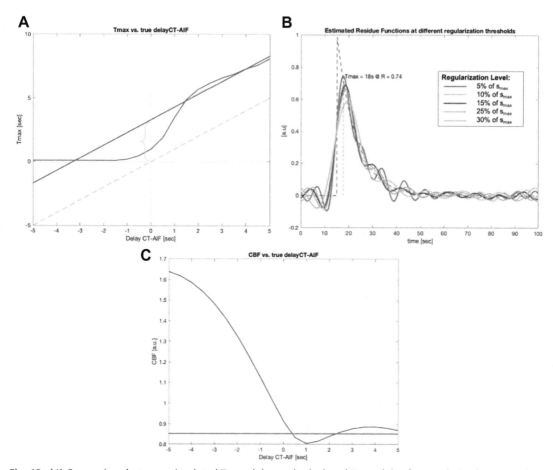

Fig. 18. (*A*) Comparison between simulated Tmax delay and calculated Tmax delay for regularized truncated SVD (delay variant) (*blue*) and circular SVD (delay invariant) (*red*) deconvolution for a set regularization threshold (eg, 10% maximum singular value). For positive delays, the two regularization schemes perform Tmax prediction comparably. For negative delays between AIF and C_T (causality violation), delay sensitive deconvolution falls apart, whereas circular deconvolution is able to identify negative delays. There is, however, an offset between the true delay between AIF and C_T (*golden dashed line*) and the computed Tmax. This offset (*curly gray brace*) depends on the degree of regularization. With increasing regularization, the estimated residue function gets increasingly smoothened. (*B*) Estimated residue function depending on the degree of regularization relative to the original residue function that was used in the forward simulation (*dashed blue line*). With increasing regularization, the residue function peak gets smaller and also shifted to the right, increasing the estimated Tmax. (*C*) Error in CBF calculation as a function of delay between AIF and CT with delay-invariant (*red*) and delay-variant regularization (*blue*). Although delay-invariant regularization keeps for a specific regularization threshold the calculated CBF at 0.87 of its original value, regardless of the delay, the delay-variant regularization leads to CBF estimates that vary over a wide range, especially with negative delays. (*Courtesy* of R Bammer, Melbourne, VIC, Australia).

any causality rules and is obviously not the true AIF into that voxel, it is still a good enough approximation with regard to shape and arterial concentration (especially when corrected for partial volume effects), just not in terms of arrival timing.

A typical example for such scenario would be if the basilar artery is chosen as AIF for the anterior circulation. Under normal conditions, the posterior circulation lags the anterior one a few second or so. Thus, when selecting an AIF from the anterior circulation, the slight delay in the posterior circulation is not a problem. We see this normally as a slight increase Tmax unless the patient has a fetal posterior cerebral artery (PCA) (see **Fig. 17**, where the vascular territory supplied by the fetal PCA has Tmax values similar as the anterior circulation under normal conditions). However, the standard SVD-based deconvolution would fall apart when the causality principle is violated, and for example, the AIF trails the tissue uptake such as seen when we pick a basilar artery AIF (see **Fig. 18A**, blue curve for negative AIF delays). For that reason, circular SVD-based deconvolution[33] or Fourier-based deconvolution[30–32] methods are recommended. These techniques are also referred to as delay-invariant deconvolution, which is in contradistinction to the delay-variant standard SVD method, which is—to the authors' surprise—still used in hospitals and commercial products. The profound impact that delay-variant deconvolution can have on CBF calculation (relative to delay-invariant versions) can be seen in **Fig. 18C**. **Fig. 18B** shows how increased levels of regularization reduce the degree of oscillations on the estimated residue function while simultaneously $r(t = \text{Tmax})$ decreases and Tmax increases. The degree of regularization also influences the global Tmax offset in **Fig. 18A**. Although not shown specifically in this figure, the higher the degree of regularization, the greater the Tmax offset.

REFERENCES

1. Fick A. Ueber die Messung des Blutquantums in den Herzventrikeln. Verhandlungen der Physikalisch-medizinischen Gesellschaft zu Wuerzburg. Sitzungsberichte fuer das Gesellschaftsjahr 1870. XIV, Sitzung am 8. Juli 1870. Wuerzburg, Germany: 2: XVI–XVII. hdl:2027/mdp.39015076673493; 1870.
2. Prinzen FW, Bassingthwaighte JB. Blood flow distributions by microsphere deposition methods. Cardiovasc Res 2000;45:13–21.
3. Hering A. Versuche, die Schnelligkeit des Blutlaufs und der Absonderung zu Bestimmen. Ztschr. Physiol. 1829;3:85–126.
4. Stewart GN. Researches on the Circulation Time and on the Influences which affect it. J Physiol 1897;22:159–83.
5. Detre JA, Leigh JS, Williams DS, et al. Perfusion imaging. Magn Reson Med 1992;23:37–45.
6. Yonas H, Gur D, Wolfson SK Jr, et al. Xenon-enhanced computerised tomographic cerebral blood flow mapping. Lancet 1984;1:1357.
7. Thomsen HS, Dawson P, Tweedle MF. MR and CT Contrast Agents for Perfusion Imaging and Regulatory Issues. In: Bammer R, editor. MR and CT perfusion and pharmacokinetic imaging: clinical applications and theory. Philadelphia, PA, U.S.A: Wolters Kluwer; 2016. p. 85–102.
8. Gudbjartsson H, Patz S. The Rician distribution of noisy MRI data. Magn Reson Med 1995;34:910–4.
9. Parkes LM. Quantification of cerebral perfusion using arterial spin labeling: two-compartment models. J Magn Reson Imag 2005;22:732–6.
10. Tofts PS, Kermode AG. Measurement of the blood-brain barrier permeability and leakage space using dynamic MR imaging. 1. Fundamental concepts. Magn Reson Med 1991;17:357–67.
11. Larsson HB, Stubgaard M, Frederiksen JL, et al. Quantitation of blood-brain barrier defect by magnetic resonance imaging and gadolinium-DTPA in patients with multiple sclerosis and brain tumors. Magn Reson Med 1990;16:117–31.
12. Schmiedeskamp H, Andre JB, Straka M, et al. Simultaneous perfusion and permeability measurements using combined spin- and gradient-echo MRI. J Cerebr Blood Flow Metabol 2013;33:732–43.
13. Tofts PS. Modeling tracer kinetics in dynamic Gd-DTPA MR imaging. J Magn Reson Imag 1997;7:91–101.
14. Boxerman JL, Rosen BR, Weisskoff RM. Signal-to-noise analysis of cerebral blood volume maps from dynamic NMR imaging studies. J Magn Reson Imag 1997;7:528–37.
15. Kjolby BF, Ostergaard L, Kiselev VG. Theoretical model of intravascular paramagnetic tracers effect on tissue relaxation. Magn Reson Med 2006;56:187–97.
16. Fisel CR, Ackerman JL, Buxton RB, et al. MR contrast due to microscopically heterogeneous magnetic susceptibility: numerical simulations and applications to cerebral physiology. Magn Reson Med 1991;17:336–47.
17. van Osch MJ, Vonken EJ, Viergever MA, et al. Measuring the arterial input function with gradient echo sequences. Magn Reson Med 2003;49:1067–76.
18. Schmiedeskamp H, Straka M, Newbould RD, et al. Combined spin- and gradient-echo perfusion-weighted imaging. Magn Reson Med 2012;68:30–40.
19. Newbould RD, Skare ST, Jochimsen TH, et al. Perfusion mapping with multiecho multishot parallel imaging EPI. Magn Reson Med 2007;58:70–81.
20. Klotz E, Konig M. Perfusion measurements of the brain: using dynamic CT for the quantitative assessment of cerebral ischemia in acute stroke. Eur J Radiol 1999;30:170–84.
21. Calamante F, Morup M, Hansen LK. Defining a local arterial input function for perfusion MRI using independent component analysis. Magn Reson Med 2004;52:789–97.
22. Weisskoff RM, Chesler D, Boxerman JL, et al. Pitfalls in MR measurement of tissue blood flow with intravascular tracers: which mean transit time? Magn Reson Med 1993;29:553–8.
23. Meier P, Zierler KL. On the theory of the indicator-dilution method for measurement of blood flow and volume. J Appl Physiol 1954;6:731–44.
24. Baron JC. Perfusion thresholds in human cerebral ischemia: historical perspective and therapeutic implications. Cerebrovasc Dis 2001;11(Suppl 1):2–8.
25. Albers GW, Goyal M, Jahan R, et al. Ischemic core and hypoperfusion volumes predict infarct size in SWIFT PRIME. Ann Neurol 2016;79:76–89.

26. Capizzano AA, Schuff N, Amend DL, et al. Subcortical ischemic vascular dementia: assessment with quantitative MR imaging and 1H MR spectroscopy. AJNR Am J Neuroradiol 2000;21:621–30.

27. Johnson NA, Jahng GH, Weiner MW, et al. Pattern of cerebral hypoperfusion in Alzheimer disease and mild cognitive impairment measured with arterial spin-labeling MR imaging: initial experience. Radiology 2005;234:851–9.

28. Ostergaard L, Weisskoff RM, Chesler DA, et al. High resolution measurement of cerebral blood flow using intravascular tracer bolus passages. Part I: Mathematical approach and statistical analysis. Magn Reson Med 1996;36:715–25.

29. Hansen PC, O'Leary DP. The use of the L-curve in the regularization of discrete ill-posed problems. SIAM J Sci Comput 1993;14:1487–503.

30. Straka M, Albers GW, Bammer R. Real-time diffusion-perfusion mismatch analysis in acute stroke. J Magn Reson Imag 2010;32:1024–37.

31. Rempp KA, Brix G, Wenz F, et al. Quantification of regional cerebral blood flow and volume with dynamic susceptibility contrast-enhanced MR imaging. Radiology 1994;193:637–41.

32. Gobbel GT, Fike JR. A deconvolution method for evaluating indicator-dilution curves. Phys Med Biol 1994;39:1833–54.

33. Wu O, Ostergaard L, Weisskoff RM, et al. Tracer arrival timing-insensitive technique for estimating flow in MR perfusion-weighted imaging using singular value decomposition with a block-circulant deconvolution matrix. Magn Reson Med 2003;50:164–74.

34. Albers GW, Marks MP, Kemp S, et al. Thrombectomy for Stroke at 6 to 16 Hours with Selection by Perfusion Imaging. N Engl J Med 2018;378:708–18.

35. Nogueira RG, Jadhav AP, Haussen DC, et al. Thrombectomy 6 to 24 Hours after Stroke with a Mismatch between Deficit and Infarct. N Engl J Med 2018;378:11–21.

36. Lansberg MG, Straka M, Kemp S, et al. MRI profile and response to endovascular reperfusion after stroke (DEFUSE 2): a prospective cohort study. Lancet Neurol 2012;11:860–7.

37. Saver JL, Goyal M, Bonafe A, et al. Stent-retriever thrombectomy after intravenous t-PA vs. t-PA alone in stroke. N Engl J Med 2015;372:2285–95.

38. Amukotuwa SA, Wu A, Zhou K, et al. Distal Medium Vessel Occlusions Can Be Accurately and Rapidly Detected Using Tmax Maps. Stroke 2021;52:3308–17.

39. Amukotuwa SA, Wu A, Zhou K, et al. Time-to-Maximum of the Tissue Residue Function Improves Diagnostic Performance for Detecting Distal Vessel Occlusions on CT Angiography. AJNR Am J Neuroradiol 2021;42:65–72.

40. Olivot JM, Mlynash M, Inoue M, et al. Hypoperfusion intensity ratio predicts infarct progression and functional outcome in the DEFUSE 2 Cohort. Stroke 2014;45:1018–23.

Dynamic Susceptibility Contrast Perfusion, Part 2: Deployment With and Without Contrast Leakage Present

Roland Bammer, PhD, MBA, MEE, FISMRM[a,b,*],
Shalini A. Amukotuwa, PhD, MBBS[a,b]

KEYWORDS

- DSC MR imaging • large vessel occlusion • MeVO • Contrast leakage • Extravascular • Brain tumor
- Metastasis/es • Pharmacokinetic Model

KEY POINTS

- Choosing the right MR imaging sequence: DSC MR imaging relies on MR imaging pulse sequences that are sensitive to magnetic susceptibility changes to capture contrast concentration alterations during the passage of GBCA through both capillary beds and large vessels (ie, MR imaging pulse sequences that are T_2*- or T2-weighted and able to capture image every 1–2 second).
- Signal saturation: Choose optimal echo time (TE) to avoid signal saturation when GBCA concentration is high or alternatively use a multi-echo sequence with long TE for tissue and short TE for arteries and veins.
- Contrast leakage alters cerebral blood volume (CBV) but not CBF measurements: CBF measurements are determined by the initial part of the bolus where little leakage occurs, whereas CBV measurements depend on large portions of DSC scan where contrast leakage into tissue can cause T1-base signal enhancement that counters the T_2*-base signal attenuation, thus leading to CBV underestimation. Therefore, pre-dosing a few minutes before DSC scanning is recommended.
- With leakage, area under the tissue concentration time course is NOT CBV: tissue concentration is a weighted (plasma volume and extravascular–extracellular volume) contribution plasma and extravascular–extracellular concentration. The concentration in the plasma can be determined via convolution of the AIF with the residue function, whereas the extravasucalar–extracellular concentration is determined by volume transfer rates from the vascular system into the extracellular space (and back).
- Simplifications: Some DCE models assume that the plasma volume space is negligible (Larsson Model). Some DSC leakage correction models assume not backdiffusion occurring (Boxerman–Weisskoff).

PART 2: DEPLOYMENT WITH AND WITHOUT CONTRAST LEAKAGE

How to Perform DSC

A very thorough description of perfusion analysis and basic DSC MR acquisition concepts has been described in the companion article to this article, which the interested reader may also find useful.

DSC MR imaging requires an MR imaging pulse sequence that is sensitive to magnetic susceptibility changes to register the contrast concentration changes when GBCA passes through the capillary bed (**Figs. 1** and **2**). Any pulse sequence that has T_2*-weighting can be used to pick up these changes, provided that the sequence is fast enough to acquire an image of that slice of tissue

---

[a] Department of Radiology and Radiological Sciences, Monash University, Clayton, VIC, Australia; [b] Monash Imaging, Monash Health, Clayton, VIC, Australia
* Corresponding author.
E-mail address: roland.bammer@monash.edu

Magn Reson Imaging Clin N Am 32 (2024) 25–45
https://doi.org/10.1016/j.mric.2023.09.011

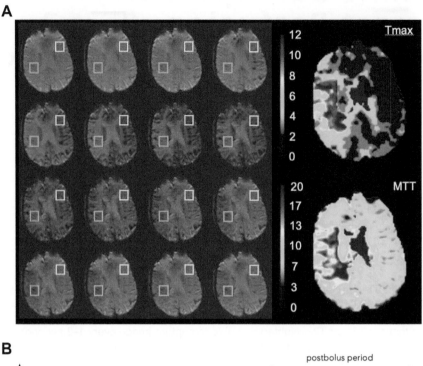

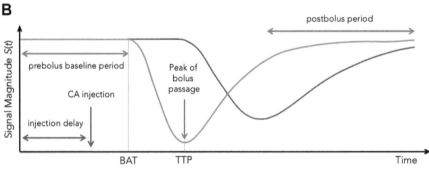

Fig. 1. (A) Left panel shows T_2*-weighted images obtained every 2 second (time increases from left to right and top down) during passage of a bolus of GBCA. Owing to T_2*-shortening of the GBCA, the images appear darker during bolus passage. From the time signal in each voxel, important parameters such as Tmax and MTT can be computed that highlight areas of hemodynamic abnormality. ROIs taken in normal (gold) and abnormal (blue) brain regions show T_2*-weighted ROI signals over time in (B). Key parameters are labeled on these curves. (*Courtesy* of R Bammer, Melbourne, VIC, Australia).

at least every 1 to 2 seconds.[1,2] In general, it is not recommended to have sampling intervals more than 4 to 5 seconds[3,4] as it is leads to problems with short MTT tissues and greater motion sensitivity. It also puts higher SNR requirements on the remaining fewer sample points as their point estimates for tracer concentration must make up for the loss of sample points. Cerebral blood volume (CBV) calculations suffer from the loss of data fidelity if the curves are sampled more sparsely as well as from the lack of commensurate SNR increase of individual sample points in case the sampling interval was increased. Rapid readout sequences are therefore needed to capture the bolus passage at high fidelity, especially

the narrow AIF, which may be only few seconds long. Conversely, sampling too frequently with MR imaging, that is, at short repetition times (TRs), renders the DSC more sensitive to transient T_1 relaxation changes and may offset the effect of the desired T_2* signal apodization, especially when there is leakage (see Eq 6).

Aside from a high temporal sampling rate, another key parameter is how long the read out of each image should takes. For a time series, such as acquired with DSC MR imaging, this is called the dwell time. The shorter the dwell time, the better the point estimate that is taken represents the underlying concentration value. The longer the dwell time, the more of an average of the underlying

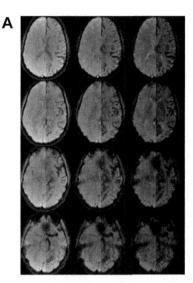

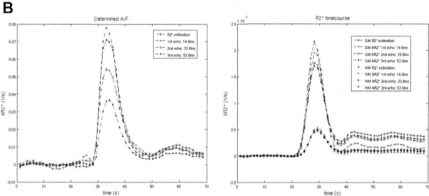

Fig. 2. (A) T_2*-weighted slice at four different anatomic levels (superior to inferior) at pre-bolus baseline (left half of images) and during peak of contrast bolus passage (right half of image) demonstrates the sensitivity of the GBCA at various echo times of TE_1 = 15 millisecond (left column), TE_2 = 34 millisecond (middle column), and TE_3 = 50 millisecond (right column). (B) T_2*-weighted signal converted into ΔR_2*(T) courses, which reflect GBCA concentration at the three echo times (TE_1, TE_2, and TE_3), as well as the result when R_2* was determined directly from three echoes, whereas (B) shows similar time courses for gray and white matter. There is a pronounced underestimation of ΔR_2*(T) and thus GBCA values, with higher echo times, especially in the large artery. This is due the saturation of the T_2*-weighted signal, that is, when any further increase in GBCA no longer leads to measurable R_2* changes, as there is no more signal left to attenuate.

concentration is measured. This is particularly important for rapid contrast concentration changes, such as seen with the arterial input function.

There are only a few MR imaging pulse sequences that have these capabilities and allow one to capture a fast bolus passage. Although fast variants of gradient-echo sequences, such as PRESTO,[5] are offered by some vendors, the most widely adopted sequence for DSC is single-shot T_2*-weighted gradient-echo EPI (**Fig. 3**). Depending on the performance of the imaging gradient set (ie, slew rate and peak gradient strength) of the MR imaging scanner, the acquisition matrix, and whether some acceleration methods are used (eg, parallel imaging and partial Fourier imaging), a single slice can be acquired in

typically much less than 100 millisecond on a modern clinical scanner. These EPI scans are usually performed in 2D interleaved slice acquisition mode. Interleaved slice acquisition means that multiple slices are excited and readout successively within 1 TR. Here, the desired TR, echo time (TE), and EPI readout times determine how many slices (each ~100 millisecond) can be fit within 1 TR, and thus how much brain can be covered (number of slices in 1 TR) × (slice thickness + slice gap). For example, with a 100-millisecond dwell time (ie, combination of TE and EPI readout time) and a 2-second TR, one can interleave a maximum of 20 slices. Prescribing more slices than what one can fit in 1 TR is not recommended, because the leftover

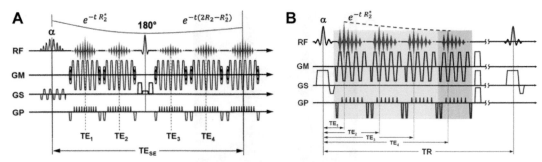

Fig. 3. (*A*) SAGE multi-gradient-echo and spin-echo EPI sequence. After an excitation RF pulse (flip angle is typically 90°), gradient echoes are formed at TE_1 and TE_2 which are read out by single-shot EPI trains. Thereafter, a 180° refocusing pulse rewinds the T_2^* decay to form a spin-echo at TE_{SE}, which shows only T_2-weighting and is also read out by a single-shot EPI train. Between the refocusing pulse and the spin echo formation, two additional gradient echoes are formed at TE_3 and TE_4. (*B*) Multi-gradient-echo EPI sequence for DSC perfusion MR imaging. After an RF excitation pulse that is typically between 30° and 90°, multiple gradient echoes are formed at TE_1, ... TE_4, each will be read out by a single-shot EPI scan to form an image with increasing T_2^*-weighting. The standard T_2^*-weighted gradient-echo EPI sequence for DSC perfusion MR imaging uses a later echo time (shaded in red), leaving a period after the RF excitation pulse unused (shaded in green). The PERMEATE multi-gradient-echo sequence uses this underused period to collect more echoes to achieve a more optimal weighting depending on the underlying T_2^* and the expected T_2^* changes during the GBCA bolus passage. (*Courtesy* of R Bammer, Melbourne, VIC, Australia.)

slices would need to fit in the next TR and so forth, which would double, triple, and so forth the temporal footprint of the perfusion sequence. This is not desirable and it often confuses the vendor's perfusion analysis packages. If we stick with the previous example (TR 2 second, 100 millisecond dwell time), and prescribe thirty 5 mm slices (+no gap) to achieve whole brain coverage, which is often done by keen MR operators to match the coverage of an accompanying DWI or FLAIR scan, 10 slices would not fit into the 2-second TR interval. Modern MR imaging scanners would pack these 10 slices into the next TR, thus doubling the sampling interval from 2 to 4 seconds.

Aside from striving to fit as many slices as possible into 1 TR and thus allowing maximum brain coverage, choosing the right TR is obviously also critical. Although the longer we make TR, the more the spins return to their equilibrium state, which improves SNR and makes the DSC sequence less T_1-sensitive, we cannot make TR too long to fit a lot of slices either, as we also want to sample the bolus passage as often as possible. On the other hand, as we discussed in the previous paragraphs, too short of a TR not only limits slice coverage, it also renders the DSC scan more T_1-sensitive.

Choosing TR and other scan parameter, such as TE, acquisition matrix and flip angle, can also depend on the different use cases for DSC. For example, a lot of DSC studies that we do are for brain tumors and are optimized to measure CBV.[6,7] For CBV measurements, the recommendations are usually to use shorter TR, to sample the bolus passage

more frequently and get better CBV estimates.[7] To address T_1 sensitivity of DSC that arises from contrast leakage during the DSC and which causes the longitudinal MR imaging signal to come back stronger after the bolus than before, one can inject a small amount of GBCA several minutes before the DSC scan. With this approach, the GBCA will leak from the vascular bed into tissue where it shortens its T_1 relaxation time already before the DSC scan and, thus, avoids any significant transient T_1-shortening that could confound CBV measurement.[8] This is often referred to as "pre-dosing." Boxerman and colleagues[7] discuss a wide range of predose volumes and flip angle and TR combinations in their consensus paper. For relatively low flip angles around 35° and 1.5-second TR, one might even get away without pre-dosing for reliable CBV calculations, but at the price of significantly lower SNR. The overall consensus for the choice of flip angles sits around 60° and 1.5-second TR and TEs of 30 and 50 millisecond for 3 and 1.5 T, respectively. Why lowering the flip angles makes DSC less T_1-sensitive is evident from the standard steady-state signal equation for DSC MR imaging, which for an echo time *TE*, repetition time *TR*, a GBCA concentration *c*, proton-density m_0, and a flip angle α, yields:

$$M(c) = m_0 \frac{sin(\alpha)[1 - exp(-TR\,R_1(c))]}{1 - cos(\alpha)exp(-TR\,R_1(c))}.$$
$$\cdot exp(-TE\,R_2^*(c)) =$$
$$= m_0 E_1(c)exp(-TE\,R_2^*(c)) =$$
$$= S_0(c)exp(-TE\,R_2^*(c))$$

$$(1)$$

and is also visualized in **Fig. 4**. Here, $R_2^*I = R_{20}^* + r_2^* c$ is the change in $R_2^* = 1/T_2^*$ dependent on the GBCA concentration c. R^*20 is without contrast on board. r_2^* is the relaxivity of the contrast agent. A similar expression can be given for $R_1(c) = R_{10} + r_1 c$. In addition, **Fig. 5A** shows simulated data for normalized steady-state signals as a function of TR and underlying T_1 relaxation times for different excitation flip angles. As evident from both **Figs. 4** and **5A**, one must keep in mind that both shorting TRs and lowering flip angles lead to a considerable signal reduction and thus reduced SNR.

Interestingly, for flip angles of 60° and 1.5-second TR, Boxerman and colleagues[7] reported that the best results could be achieved when the pre-dosing GBCA amount was 50% to 100% of the amount of bolus volume that they used for the DSC scan. Although pre-dosing is a necessary step, it is no panacea. Later, we discuss further steps that are needed to address other issues that arise with GBCA leakage.

In acute stroke, where extravasation is rather rare, things are a bit easier. We normally use different DSC protocols that rely on higher flip angles that are close to the Ernst angle, because that yields optimal signal for brain tissue at a given field strength (**Fig. 5B**). Relative to tumor DSC imaging, one can also be more generous with TR times, having a sweet spot around 1.8 second (range: 1.6–2 second). Moreover, for stroke applications,

in particular large vessel occlusions, the expected areas of abnormalities are generally more widespread. We usually do not need to push the acquisition matrix/voxel resolution too hard. Typical acquisition matrices for stroke DSC range between 80^2 and 128^2, with a preference toward the lower end. Larger voxels, and thus better SNR that yields better CNR of parameter maps, is often desirable. One disadvantage of larger voxels with gradient-echo EPI is increased intra-voxel dephasing, manifesting as more pronounced and widespread T_2^*-induced signal loss adjacent to air tissue interfaces (eg, above auditory canals, nasal cavities, resection cavities, or surgical hardware).[9] These DSC scan parameter choices need to be contrasted to those we use in brain tumor imaging, where the question is often whether there are, for example, small amounts of residual tumor or tumor recurrence that need to be attended to. For that purpose, and to be less sensitive to T_2^*-induced signal loss adjacent to the area of interest, smaller voxels, that is, larger acquisition matrices, may be more appropriate, such as 96^2 to 128^2, with a tendency toward the higher end.

We therefore recommended the use of different DSC sequence parameters, which are tailored and optimized for the clinical indication.

Partial Fourier Imaging

Partial Fourier (PF)[10] imaging is used to shorten the EPI readout and possibly to shorten TE. Although the use of PF is common practice with DWI, it is usually not recommended for DSC. PF methods rely on the estimation of the image phase from a central k-space region. As the GBCA is a magnetic susceptibility agent, it alters the image phase profoundly and depends on the underlying GBCA concentration.[11] Unfortunately, the higher spatial frequency phase information is not well represented with PF methods and can be confounded during the GBCA passage. In addition, PF-accelerated scans take a relatively high SNR-hit relative to the unaccelerated scan, which can limit the dynamic range of GBCA concentrations that can be measured without saturation effects.

Parallel Imaging

Another way to shorten the EPI readout and thus to reduce both image distortions and dwell time, is parallel imaging.[12–14] With EPI, image distortions[15] (eg, stretched or squeezed brains or signal pile up), T_2^* image blurring, and off-resonance-induced arterial voxel shifts during bolus passage all depend on how quickly k-space can be traversed along the phase-encode direction.[16] With classical parallel imaging methods, such as

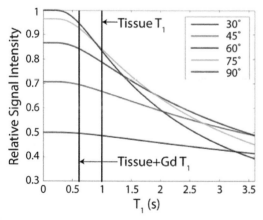

Fig. 4. Change in relative DSC signal intensity for tissue with and without GBCA on board dependent on excitation flip angle. The presence of GBCA, when leaking into tissue, shortens T_1 of tissue. With increasing excitation flip angle, the faster relaxation of longitudinal magnetization leads to a larger signal intensity effect (pre- vs post-GBCA). Thus, lower flip angles, such as 30°, demonstrate very little dependence on T_1 changes. However, overall baseline signal is also only a fraction of that when using a 90° flip angle. (*Courtesy of R Bammer, Melbourne, VIC, Australia.*)

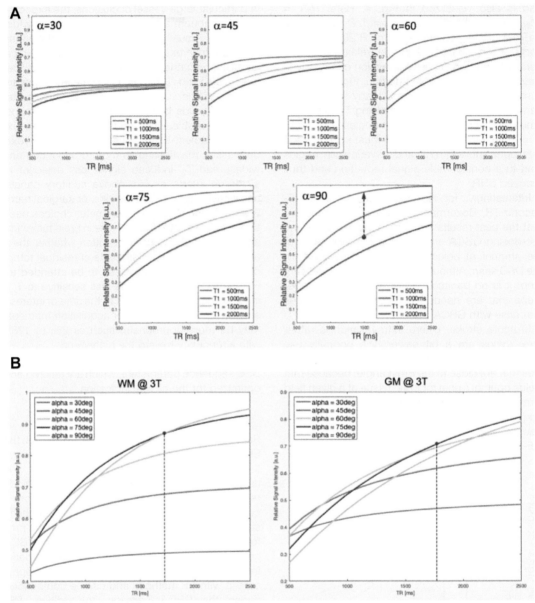

Fig. 5. (*A*) DSC steady-state signal dependency of tissues with different T_1 times for different excitation flip angles. Similar to Fig. 3, there is little sensitivity to T_1 for low flip angles. The overall signal also does not depend too much on TR because only a fraction of the longitudinal signal is tipped into the transverse plane, whereas the rest remains in equilibrium. Matters are different for larger flip angles where there is profound dependency on T_1 times and TR intervals. As more and more magnetization is tipped into the transverse plane. Signal recovery depends on either how quickly the spins can relax back to equilibrium (T_1), or how much time we give them to do so (TR). The red dashed arrow shows the transition of a pre-bolus signal level for a 90° excitation and TR of 1500 millisecond after GBCA tissue enhancement, which suggests that post-bolus signal values can become substantially higher than pre-bolus values if there is leakage. (*B*) Determination of the flip angle that yields optimal (maximal) signal (aka Ernst angle) for a DSC sequence with a given TR of 1800 millisecond and underlying T_1 relaxation time. This angle is slightly different for GM and WM and computes from arccos (exp(–TR/T_1)). (*Courtesy of R Bammer.*)

SENSE[12] or GRAPPA,[13] k-space traversal can be made two to four times faster. This can reduce the presence of these artifacts significantly. However, similar to the aforementioned PF imaging,

parallel imaging acceleration comes at a significant SNR cost. Relative to an unaccelerated scan, the SNR penalty is at least the square root of the parallel imaging acceleration factor. This

SNR penalty gets further exacerbated by the so-called g-factor, which depends on the choice RF coil array (eg, size and location of individual receiver coil elements) and other factors.[12] With the exception of multi-echo sequences (see next section), it has been our practice to minimize the use of parallel imaging for DSC, and if used, resort to relatively modest acceleration factors (eg, $2\times$ acceleration at 3T and avoid it at 1.5 T).

The reason why we try to avoid high SNR penalties from PF or parallel imaging, despite their obvious benefits, is that DSC relies on (1) T_2^*-based signal attenuation (where we need a reasonable dynamic range) and (2) is fraught by small effect sizes due to the relatively small CBV of normal tissue voxels of a few percent, especially in white matter. Regarding the first point, we therefore do not want high GBCA concentrations which drive the signal so low that it bounces off the noise floor of MR imaging magnitude images (nb, MR noise in magnitude images is nonzero mean[17]) in turn causing significant underestimation of high tracer concentration values. Regarding the second point, we also do not want the noise level to be too high, to ensure that the contrast change over time can be detected even in white matter, especially with poor bolus injections or patients with poor cardiac output. Getting a reasonable T_2^* response in white matter that stands out from the noise is also the reason we want a relatively compact bolus, which warrants injection at a high flow rate. Although the CNR, or signal-to-fluctuation noise ratio, measures noise in the time domain of the DSC concentration time course based on ergodicity, the spatial noise (absent g-factor noise) is comparable to noise in the temporal domain (absent physiologic noise).

In this context, it is worth mentioning that an interesting variant of parallel imaging, which can be used to increase the number of slices per TR, is *simultaneous multi-band imaging*, especially blipped-CAIPI[18] or a variant thereof. With this method, several slices are simultaneously excited and then recorded. The blips create interslice image shifts in the phase-encode direction to increase the distance between aliased pixels. The separation of the individual slices works due to fact that the different slices are "seeing" different coil sensitivities and can therefore be separated at little SNR expense.[18]

T2-Shortening and Spin-Echo Sequences

Although the inherent effect on spin–spin relaxation due to the GBCA is generally negligible,[19] a transient pronounced "apparent" T_2-shortening can be observed with a T_2-weighted DSC approach when a magnetic susceptibility altering agent, such as gadolinium, passes through the capillary network.[2,20] The local difference in magnetic susceptibility and the associated B_0 field perturbation that the GBCA causes in the vicinity of the capillaries can be seen as local field gradients, which are small in extent but relatively high in strength. (Think of it as analogous to GBCA switching "on" diffusion-encoding gradients due to its presence).

Static magnetic spins, which do not move around in tissue but are exposed to these local gradients, will experience regular dephasing and thus undergo the classic T_2^* decay. The dephasing can be unwound by a spin-echo 180° refocusing pulse. Driven by thermal energy, magnetic spins in tissue will also undergo diffusive motion. When spins are randomly moving in the strong local gradient field that is established around the capillaries by the GBCA, they will experience diffusion-weighting by these local magnetic field gradients, even when no external diffusion-encoding gradients are switched on. This diffusion-weighting on long-TE sequences in the presence of GBCA is so strong that it can be observed on T_2-weighted spin-echo sequences, such as single-shot T_2-weighted spin-echo EPI. Hence, the observed signal attenuation in the presence of GBCA is not really T_2-weighting, that is, in the classical sense due to spin–spin relaxation. It is an apparent T_2-shortening and merely caused by the diffusion of water protons in the presence of strong static field gradients that are switched "ON" for the entire time that GBCA is present in the capillaries. This is known as "dynamic dephasing," and is in contradistinction to "static dephasing" which is what we are used to seeing normally with standard gradient-echo imaging due to the magnetic field inhomogeneities asserted onto the static spins in the tissue.

The keen reader will ask now, "What will happen in stroke or tumors where ADC values are changed?"—With restricted diffusion, such as seen in these pathologies, spins move less freely around; thus, the effect of dynamic dephasing and hence r_2 relaxivity will be suppressed. In other words, for the same contrast agent concentration, one can expect less pseudo-T_2 attenuation, which in turn may mean that we will underestimate the contrast concentration in tissue with a reduced diffusion coefficient relative to normal tissue. The authors are not aware of any publications that have investigated the effect of change in r_2-relaxivity subject to pathologic ADC changes in stroke or highly cellular tumors, although the general sensitivity of T_2-weighted spin-echo sequences by diffusion-weighting, and as such its dependence on apparent diffusion coefficient, diffusion time (: = TE/2 for a constant gradient diffusion-weighted spin-echo sequence), and vessel size is well known (also in the context of functional MR imaging, where the magnetic susceptibility agent is deoxygenated vs oxygenated hemoglobin aka BOLD effect).

A keen reader may also ask: "What will happen when GBCA extravasates and the intravascular and extravascular magnetic susceptibilities start to equilibrate?" —Relative to no extravasation, the local field gradients would indeed become less, and hence relaxivity or the sensitivity to the presence of contrast agent will be less. This is a known effect.[21,22] In many cases, we assume however an adiabatic condition, that is, where we the rate of change in the intravascular space (IS) is much higher than in the extravascular–extracellular space (EES) (Fig. 6).[23] Nevertheless, the reader should keep in mind as GBCA extravasates, the intra- and extravascular susceptibility gradients will decrease, and as such, so will both $T_2{}^*$- and T_2-shortening effects. This gets exacerbated by concurrent T_1 enhancement. Together, these two effects lead to an underestimation of GBCA concentration and therefore blood volume.

Vessel Size Imaging

The different sensitivity to the capillary vessel sizes of spin-echo sequences vis-à-vis to gradient echo sequences also forms the basis of vessel size imaging (VSI).[24] It allows one to create maps that inform the neuroradiologist about abnormally engorged capillaries, such as seen in brain tumors[25] (Fig. 7) and may add additional information to work up these patients. A DSC pulse sequence with combined gradient-echo/spin-echo EPI, such as spin echo and gradient echo (SAGE) (see Fig. 3A), can be used for VSI.[26] A VSI parameter

image can be computed as the ratio between the CBV obtained from gradient-echo and spin-echo images of such a scan, that is, VSI = 100% CBV_{GRE}/CBV_{SE}

Do note that the relative sensitivity of spin echoes to the same amount of GBCA is only a fraction of that from gradient echoes.[20] Thus, the lower CNR leads to noisier parameter maps. However, gradient-echo-based maps are usually fraught with partial volume effects from large vessel blooming (eg, cortical vessels) that extends into adjacent tissue and can confound measurements.[9] Similarly, surgical material or blood can cause frank susceptibility changes around resection cavities impairing the quality of gradient-echo-based maps. Fig. 8 shows a comparison of gradient-echo and spin-echo-based parameter maps.

Multi-gradient Echo EPI (PERMEATE) and Multi-Echo Spin-echo and Gradient-Echo EPI

Gradient-echo sequences with more than one echo time after each RF excitation (ie, multi-gradient echo sequences) have been introduced to mitigate the problem of signal saturation in the presence of high GBCA concentrations.[27,28] To optimize the DSC signal, the TE of a gradient-echo EPI sequence should be roughly equivalent to the underlying $T_2{}^*$ time.[29] This is obviously a challenge with a single gradient echo, where one needs to trade high sensitivity to small traces of contrast agent in the capillaries within white matter against not saturating out the signal in the presence of large amounts of contrast in the feeding arteries.

Using multiple gradient echoes reduces this challenge and makes it is easier to achieve the optimal T2* sensitivity for both white matter and arteries. With multi-echo sequences, less heavily

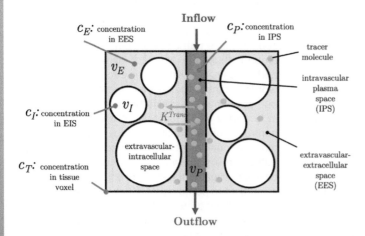

Fig. 6. Multicompartment model showing GBCA passage through tissue in the presence of GBCA extravasation. Dots represent GBCA within intravascular plasma space (IPS) and extravascular–extracellular space (EES) with volume fractions v_p and v_e and GBCA concentrations c_P and c_E, respectively. The extravascular–intracellular space with volume fraction v_i is assumed to be impermeable to GBCA molecules; thus, the extravascular–intracellular CA concentration c_i is assumed to be equal to 0. K^{Trans} is the volume transfer constant.

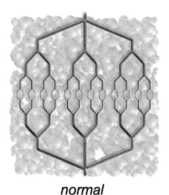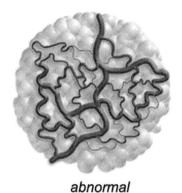

normal   *abnormal*

Fig. 7. Model representation of a normal tissue capillary bed (left) and one in cancer (*red*). The latter usually contains neovessels that are engorged and either lack a BBB (metastases) or have an impaired BBB (high-grade tumors).

$T2^*$-weighted echoes can be used for regions where a significant susceptibility contrast is expected (eg, distal ICA or M1 MCA), whereas stronger $T2^*$-weighted echoes can be used for tissue where we would expect less susceptibility contrast. Typically, multi-echo gradient-echo EPI sequences need to be 2 to 3 times accelerated to allow placement of multiple EPI readout trains at two to three different echo times.[28] Of note here is that standard gradient-echo EPI sequences usually have a relatively long TE time, for example, 50 millisecond on 1.5 T, where between the RF excitation pulse and the EPI readout nothing happens. It is therefore to no detriment regarding additional scan time to place extra gradient-echo EPI acquisitions before the standard gradient-echo readout (see **Fig. 3**B). Moreover, "listening" to the MR imaging signal longer, that is, with more than one echo, also confers SNR benefits. Further, the multi-echo approach allows us to directly determine $T2^*$ relaxation times and therefore eliminates T1-sensitivities entirely.[28]

A variant to the aforementioned PERMEATE multi-gradient-echo EPI sequence[28] is SAGE.[26] Here, a spin-echo EPI sequence is used, where between one to two additional gradient-echo EPI readouts straddle the 180° spin-echo refocusing pulse on each side (see **Fig. 3**B) yielding one spin-echo image and two to four gradient-echo images with different TEs and therefore different contrast weightings. SAGE therefore allows simultaneous gradient-echo and spin-echo-based DSC imaging to leverage the different sensitivities of spin and gradient echoes to vessel (sizes) as well as to reduce confounding T_1 effects. Here, the gradient-echo EPI images at TEs located after the excitation pulse, but before the refocusing pulse, follow a regular T_2^* decay, that is, the signal drops with increasing TE (**Fig. 9**). Similarly, the EPI image that is acquired at the TE when spin-echo forms, follows a standard T_2-weighted behavior. However, the EPI images after the refocusing pulse but before the spin-echo formation, follow a mixture of inverted T_2^* decay and regular T_2

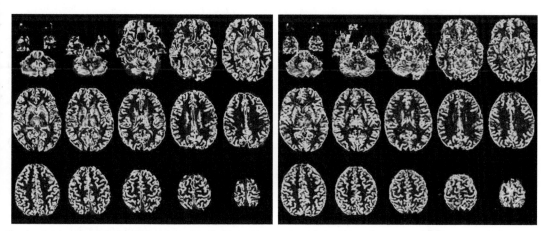

Fig. 8. CBV maps using gradient-echo EPI (left) and spin-echo EPI (right). The gradient-echo scans are characterized by less noise in the parameter maps; however, the blooming around the circle of Willis and large cortical vessels is very small on spin-echo EPI. (*Courtesy* of R Bammer, Melbourne, VIC, Australia.)

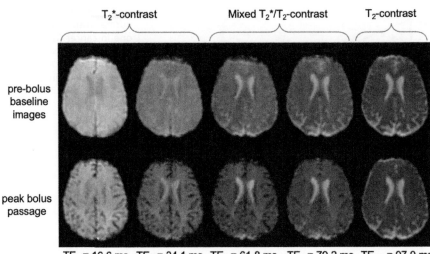

T_2^*-contrast   Mixed T_2^*/T_2-contrast T_2-contrast

pre-bolus
baseline
images

peak bolus
passage

$TE_1 = 16.6$ ms $TE_2 = 34.1$ ms $TE_3 = 61.8$ ms $TE_4 = 79.2$ ms $TE_{SE} = 97.0$ ms

Fig. 9. Individual echo images of SAGE. Top row shows the image contrast without any contrast on board, whereas bottom row shows the image contrast at peak bolus concentration. From left to right are the images as they are acquired after each excitation. First two images are regular gradient-echo images. The image on the right is the spin-echo image. Notice the lack of large vessel blooming at the peak bolus. The third and fourth rows are gradient-echo images occurring after the refocusing pulse. The third image has stronger T_2^*-weighting than the fourth image as its TE is closer to the time when the spin-echo form, that is, when all T_2^*-dephasing is unwound and only T_2 decay remains. (*Courtesy* of R Bammer, Melbourne, VIC, Australia.)

decay as described in Eq 2. Specifically, for a dynamic multi-echo single-shot gradient-echo and spin-echo EPI sequence,[18] such as, that in **Fig. 8**, the signal S that is acquired at given echo times TE (where TE_{SE} is the time the spin echo is formed), and where R_2 and R_2^* are time-dependent due to the temporal chances of underlying GBCA changes, is defined by

basic principles of perfusion analysis and DSC MR acquisition concepts that these authors have been described in the companion article to this article and which the interested reader may also find useful. The basis for the computation of the tissue concentration time curve $c_T(t)$ was that the GBCA remains in the capillary bed, that is, (blood) plasma and can be expressed as the convolution

$$S(t, TE) = \begin{cases} S_0(t)e^{-TE\,R_2^*(t)} & if\ TE < TE_{SE}/2 \\ \dfrac{S_0(t)}{\delta}e^{-TE_{SE}\,R_2^*(t)}e^{-TE\,\left(2R_2(t) - R_2^*(t)\right)} & if\ \dfrac{TE_{SE}}{2} < TE < TE_{SE} \end{cases}. \tag{2}$$

Here, δ is a correction factor for slice profile imperfections between excitation and refocusing pulse. Note if the DSC sequence is simply a gradient-echo EPI sequence or a multi-echo gradient-echo EPI sequence,[19] only the top portion of Eq 2 needs to be considered.

CONTRAST EXTRAVASATION, LEAKAGE CORRECTION, AND PHARMACOKINETIC MODELING

Until now our perfusion analysis formulas have assumed that the GBCA is nondiffusible and thus remains in the vascular compartment. This has been the focus of a very thorough review of the

between the arterial input function into the voxel of interest $c_A(t)$ and the tissue residue function $r(t)$, that is,

$$c_T(t) = CBF \int_0^t c_A(\tau)\,r(t-\tau)d\tau =$$
$$CBF\,[c_A(t) \otimes r(t)]. \tag{3}$$

In case of a breakdown of the blood brain barrier (BBB), however, GBCA diffuses into the extravascular space. Thus, the tissue concentration that we measure can no longer be described as shown in Eq 3. If the contrast leakage happens rapidly, we observe shorter tissue T_1 relaxation already during the first pass of the bolus.[8] Because of the faster T_1 recovery, the signal during the bolus passage may become paradoxically higher than the pre-bolus baseline signal and the calculated concentration curve will underestimate CBV (**Fig. 10**).

The change in the MR signal that we observe and which is caused by the presence of the GBCA at concentration c, $M(c)$, relative to the signal in the absence of any GBCA, $M(0)$, can be computed from the ratio of both measurements and followed by taking the natural logarithm, that is,

$$\ln\left[\frac{M(c)}{M(0)}\right] = \ln\left[\frac{S_0(c)}{S_0(0)}exp\left(-TE\{R_2^*(c)-R_2^*(0)\}\right)\right]$$

$$= \ln\left[\frac{S_0(c)}{S_0(0)}\right]-TE\underbrace{\left[R_2^*(c)-R_2^*(0)\right]}_{\Delta R_2^*(c)},$$

$$\text{(4)}$$

which yields the change in R_2^* dependent on c:

$$\Delta R_2^*(c) = -\frac{1}{TE}\ln\left[\frac{M(c)}{M(0)}\right]+\frac{1}{TE}\ln\left[\frac{S_0(c)}{S_0(0)}\right]. \quad \text{(5)}$$

Notice that since the tracer concentration c in DSC MR imaging is a function of time, the change in R_2^* also implicitly becomes a function of time. In regular DSC imaging, when there is no extravasation, the T_1 effect reflected in the second term of Eq 4 is usually neglected. However, in the presence of contrast extravasation, the second part Eq 5 becomes nonzero. Using Eq. 2, $R_{10} = 1/T_{10}$ and a flip angle (α) of 90°, one gets an expression for the apparent change in R_2^*, which reflects what we normally observe with DSC MR imaging:

$$\Delta\tilde{R}_2^*(t) = -\frac{1}{TE}\ln\left(\frac{S(t)}{S_0}\right) =$$

$$= \Delta R_2^*(t)-\frac{1}{TE}\ln\left[\frac{1-exp(-TR(R_{10}+r_1 c_T(t)))}{1-exp(-TR\,R_{10})}\right].$$

$$\text{(6)}$$

As a remedy to minimize the contribution from the second term in Eq 6 to $\Delta\tilde{R}_2^*(t)$, one can resort to lower flip angles and apply pre-dosing, as discussed previously, or resort to multi-echo sequences, which eliminates T_1 sensitivity entirely (eg, by determining ΔR_2^* through a parameter fit).[28] For small T_1 enhancements (<30%), Eq 6 can be simplified further. If $TR \cdot r_1 \cdot c_T$ is small, then $exp(-TR \cdot r_1 \cdot c_T)$ becomes approximately $1-TR \cdot r_1 \cdot c_T$. Using furthermore the approximation $\ln(1+\alpha/\beta) \approx \alpha/\beta$, where $\alpha = TR \cdot r_1 \cdot c_T \cdot exp(-TR \cdot R_{10})$ and $\beta = 1-exp(-TR \cdot R_{10})$, Eq 6 reduces to[30]:

$$\Delta\tilde{R}_2^*(t) \approx \Delta R_2^*(t)-\frac{TR}{TE}\cdot\frac{exp(-TR\,R_{10})}{1-exp(-TR\,R_{10})}\cdot r_1\cdot c_T(t), \quad \text{(7)}$$

an expression that we will revisit soon when discussing the Boxerman–Weisskoff approach.

Important for the reader is however to understand that correcting the T_1 effects will still not address the issue that the contrast agent is no longer just bound to in the intravascular (plasma) space (IS). With an impaired BBB, GBCA starts to accumulate in the EES (see **Fig. 10**). Most importantly, the area under the tissue concentration curve is no longer CBV, as it also contains the contribution from the EES. The tracer concentration in tissue c_T is the combination of contributions from tracer concentration in plasma c_P, the tracer concentration in the EES c_E, and the tracer concentration in the extravascular–intracellular

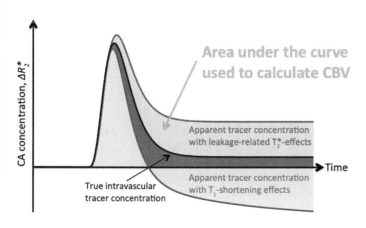

Fig. 10. Measured GBCA concentration in tissue. The gray curve shows the situation when the tracer remains truly intravascular, whereas the blue curve shows a situation when tracer leaks into the tissue and shortens T_1 relaxation times. For the latter, the faster T_1 recovery can lead to a higher signal after the bolus than before. When converted into concentration values, this leads to what is shown in the blue curve. Consequently, the area under the curve, which is used to compute CBV, is less than that without leakage. Therefore, CBV calculations from DSC MR imaging without leakage correction generally underestimate the true CBV. We can only measure an apparent CBV. After the T_1-shortening due to GBCA leakage has been addressed, we still observe an increased post-bolus tail (red curve). This is because tracer material is not only in the intravascular space but distributes also in extravascular–extracellular space. (*Courtesy* of R Bammer.)

space c_I, weighted by the individual volume fractions v_P, v_E, and v_I,[31] so that

$$c_T(t) = v_P c_P(t) + v_E c_E(t) + v_I c_I(t). \qquad (8)$$

We can assume that GBCA does not enter cells, so the plasma volume represents the blood volume corrected for hematocrit. Therefore, the last term $v_I c_I$ of Eq 8 becomes zero, and the unit proportions of the contrast agent distributes are therefore $v_P + v_E = 1$.

Cerebral Blood Volume -Mapping with Blood-Pool Agents

In tumors, the expression of VEGF and other promotors stimulates the formation and growth of neovessels. Compared with a regular capillary bed, these neovessels can be abundant and engorged, which in aggregate can lead to an increased intravascular fraction, that is, increased CBV, in a tumor containing voxel compared with a voxel containing healthy tissue. Before we move on to explain how we can computationally solve the problem of leakage, it is worthwhile to draw the reader's attention to alternatives, in case only CBV is of interest. One alternative to avoid confounding effects from GBCA leakage into the EES is to resort to blood-pool agents, such as ferumoxytol[32,33] (a superparamagnetic iron oxide nanoparticle with a polyglucose sorbitol carboxymethylether coating). Until 2017, gadofosveset was another blood-pool agent option available on the market. Gadofosveset binds to human serum albumin and can be used to determine CBV without extravasation.[34] CBV maps can be simply computed from two regular structural scans before and after the contrast administration. Since rapid, EPI-based DSC scanning is not needed, such CBV maps can be generated with much higher spatial resolution than DSC (**Fig. 11**).

Pharmacokinetic Modeling

Two key parameters when we want to describe flux across a semipermeable vessel membrane are *permeability* (P) and membrane *surface area per unit mass of tissue* (S). P and S are difficult to measure individually, so in practice physiologists measure the *permeability–surface area product* (PS) per unit mass of tissue [cm^3 min^{-1} g^{-1}]. The proportion of tracer that leaves the blood plasma and entered the tissue in one pass through the capillary bed is called the *extraction fraction* (E) and is related to PS and blood flow (F) or CBF as follows:

$$E = 1 - e^{-\frac{PS}{F}} = 1 - e^{-\frac{PS\,\rho}{CBF\,k_H}}, \qquad (9)$$

where k_H accounts for the hematocrit differences between capillaries and large vessels.

$$k_H = \frac{1 - Hct_{art}}{1 - Hct_{cap}}, \qquad (10)$$

ρ denoting the brain density (approximately 1.04 g/mL) and the relationship between F (given in mL min^{-1} g^{-1}) and CBF (in units of mL min^{-1} per 100 g brain tissue):

$$CBF = \frac{k_H}{\rho} F. \qquad (11)$$

The ratio $(1\text{-}Hct_{art})/(1\text{-}Hct_{cap})$ is around 0.733 but can vary under pathologic conditions, severe dehydration, and with age.

Equation 9 teaches us that if permeability if high ($PS \gg F$), then most of the tracer is extracted in one pass ($E \sim 1$), PS cannot be determined because the tracer flux across the capillary membrane is driven by the flow F and independent of PS. Conversely, if extraction is low then the flow is sufficient to replace tracer that passes through the capillary wall with fresh tracer molecules (ie, $F \gg PS$), and the blood plasma compartment has a well-defined concentration. In that case PS is equal to EF.

In the simplest bidirectional pharmacokinetic model that considers contrast influx and backflux (or backdiffusion), the rate of contrast enhancement in the EES is driven by the concentration gradient, $c_P(t) - c_E(t)$, between the intravascular (plasma) GBCA concentration and the GBCA concentration in the EES $c_E(t)$, across the vessel wall[35]:

$$v_E \left(\frac{d(c_E(t))}{dt} \right) = PS\,\rho\,(c_P(t) - c_E(t)), \qquad (12)$$

where v_E is the proportion of the voxel that is occupied by the EES (see **Fig. 6**).[36,37] In other words, v_E is the additional volume fraction—on top of the IS—where contrast material can be found if the blood-brain barrier is not intact. At this stage, we introduce the familiar *volume transfer constant* K^{Trans}, which is given in units of min^{-1}:

$$K^{Trans} = PS\,\rho = E\,F\,\rho. \qquad (13)$$

In other words, K^{Trans} is the permeability–surface area product per unit volume of tissue. Under the assumption that the plasma volume is negligible compared with v_E, we get $c_T = v_E c_E$, and Eq 12 can be expressed in the more familiar differential equation:

$$\frac{d(c_T(t))}{dt} = K^{Trans} \left(c_P(t) - \frac{c_T(t)}{v_E} \right). \qquad (14)$$

A key parameter in DSC MR imaging is the CBV which is derived from the area under the curve of

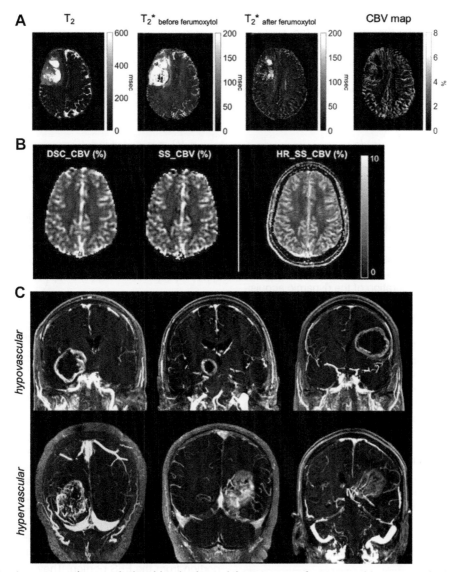

Fig. 11. Various approaches to calculate blood volume. (*A*) MR images of a 59-year-old women with glioblastoma (WHO 4): from left to right: quantitative T_2 map, quantitative T_2* maps before and after ferumoxytol infusion, and blood volume fraction map (modified from Maralani and colleagues). (*B*) Volunteer undergoing dual-gradient echo EPI and 3D multi-echo (16 echoes) gradient-echo imaging during and after injection of ferumoxytol. The image on the left is obtained from regular CBV calculation of the DSC MR imaging scan. The middle and right images are computed from a steady-state method, where T_2* maps are computed from the multi-echo acquisition before and after ferumoxytol administration. Changes in R_2* of tissue where then normalized to a vessel containing only blood (eg, sagittal sinus), so that steady-state CBV was calculated as $100\% * \Delta R_2^*_{,\ tissue}/(\Delta R_2^*_{,\ sag\ sinus})^{0.5}$ The square root is used to address the quadratic relationship between concentration and R_2* changes. For the middle CBV maps, 15 time points of the DSC scan were average before and after the bolus and R_2* computed from the two echoes. The right image was computed from R_2* maps using the 16 echoes (From Christen T, Ni W, Qiu D, et al. High-resolution cerebral blood volume imaging in humans using the blood pool contrast agent ferumoxytol. Magn Reson Med. 2012).(*C*) High-resolution 3D contrast-enhanced MRA 5 minute after administration of 0.03 mmol/kg body weight of gadofosveset in six patients with glioblastoma (top row: hypovascular; bottom row: hypervascular [more than three vessels]). (*From* Puig J, Blasco G, Daunis IEJ, et al. High-resolution blood-pool-contrast-enhanced MR angiography in glioblastoma: tumor-associated neovascularization as a biomarker for patient survival. A preliminary study. Neuroradiology. 2016;58:17-26).

the tracer concentration in tissue over time and then normalized by the area under the curve of the tracer concentration a large artery (or vein). This ratio is then is multiplied by the density of brain tissue (ie, 1.04 g/mL) to put CBV on a quantitative basis, that is, report it in units of mL/100 mg brain tissue, such that:

$$CBV = \frac{1ml}{1.04g} \cdot \frac{\int_0^T c_T(\tau)d\tau}{\int_0^T c_A(\tau)d\tau}. \qquad (15)$$

Here, the time variable T is chosen such that it usually denotes the end of the first pass of the bolus to avoid recirculation or, more conveniently, the whole length of the dynamic acquisition window when the duration of the dynamic acquisition is chosen to be so long that the recirculation effects and their respective tissue responses have abated.

Now, we would like to emphasize that calculating the area under the tissue contrast concentration time curve $c_T(t)$ to determine CBV, as defined by Eq 15, is no longer correct as $c_T(t)$ no longer represents the tracer concentration in the capillary or plasma space, as is evident from Eq 14. Instead, it yields an apparent CBV, that is, CBV_{app}, as the summation (or integration) over $c_T(t)$ would measure contributions from both IS (v_P) and EES (v_E). Referring to the area under $c_T(t)$ curve as CBV is therefore a misnomer and should be avoided.

Making Things Easier: No Backflux Assumption

During the first pass of the GBCA bolus, we can assume that there is a very high concentration gradient between the IS and the EES, that is, $c_P >> c_E$, where contrast diffuses only in one direction (from IS into EES) without backdiffusion (from EES to IS). These assumptions hold if the observation time t is longer than the first pass (eg, <1 minute) but much shorter than any renal clearance time.[35] In that case, the second term of Eq 12 can be assumed to be zero and the uptake in the EES can be found through integration of the thus simplified Eq 12:

$$v_E c_E(t) = K^{Trans} \int_0^t c_P(\tau)d\tau. \qquad (16)$$

As described above, what we observe through DSC imaging in $c_T(t)$ is therefore the combined (weighted) effect (see Eq 8) from the proportion

of contrast agent that resides in the intravascular plasma space $v_P \cdot c_P$ and the proportion of contrast agent that has leaked into the EES $v_E \cdot c_E$. The observable contrast concentration time course is therefore the famous Patlak equation,[38] which is (by substitution of Eqs 15 and 16) only dependent on the intravascular (plasma) tracer concentration:

$$c_T(t) = v_P c_P(t) + v_E c_E(t) =$$
$$= v_P c_P(t) + K^{Trans} \int_0^t c_P(\tau)d\tau. \qquad (17)$$

In case of back diffusion of tracer from EES to IS, Eq 17 would need to be replaced by the convolution approach by Tofts and Kermode[39]:

$$c_T(t) = v_P c_P(t) + K^{Trans} c_P(\tau) \otimes \exp\left(-\frac{K^{Trans}}{V_E}t\right). \qquad (18)$$

Here, we assumed isodirectional permeability. If isodirectionality is not given K^{Trans} in the exponential of Eq 18 would need to be replaced by the volume transfer constant for outflux from the EES into IS, and the first K^{Trans} term would become the volume transfer constant for the initial influx from IS into the EES.

Boxerman–Weisskoff leakage correction

It is important to notice that when we image a patient with BBB breakdown, in the region of leakage, we cannot extract either the first or second term of Eq 17, we measure the combined effect with $c_T(t)$. What we observe with DSC is the apparent change in R_2^*, $\Delta \tilde{R}_2^*(t)$, as described in Eq 6. Boxerman and colleagues[30] introduced a clever approximation to separate the intravascular portion from the EES portion. They assumed that the concentration time course of the intravascular component remains unchanged and can be approximated by $c_T(t)$ of the healthy contralateral side. This holds because, in the absence of leakage, $\Delta \tilde{R}_2^*(t)$ becomes $\Delta R_2^*(t)$ again. To improve the robustness of their method, they used the concentration time course of the average over a larger region, $\overline{\Delta R_2^*(t)}$, so that Eq 17 can be rewritten as an expression of $\Delta \tilde{R}_2^*(t)$ (ie, the DSC surrogate of $c_T(t)$):

$$\Delta \tilde{R}_2^*(t) \approx K_1 \overline{\Delta R_2^*(t)} - K_2 \int_0^t \overline{\Delta R_2^*(\tau)} \, d\tau. \qquad (19)$$

The negative sign between the two terms when comparing Eq 17 with Eq 19 comes from the fact that the T_1 effects in Eq 6 weakens the effective R_2^* effect.

The Boxerman–Weisskoff approach in Eq 19 approximates the observable R_2^* changes, $\Delta \tilde{R}_2^*(t)$, in a leaky voxel by the linear combination of two basis functions. The first is $\overline{\Delta R_2^*(t)}$ and the second is its time integral $\int_0^t \overline{\Delta R_2^*(\tau)}\, d\tau$, representing contrast accumulation. If each basis function is multiplied with a weight K_1 and K_2, respectively these weights are adjustable for each voxel, so that the weighted combination of the basis functions resembles the time course of $\Delta \tilde{R}_2^*(t)$ for that voxel. This is usually done by a least-squares fitting routine that tries to find in each voxel a K_1 and K_2 value, so that the difference between the measured $\Delta \tilde{R}_2^*(t)$ and the model $K_1 \overline{\Delta R_2^*(t)} - K_2 \int_0^t \overline{\Delta R_2^*(\tau)}\, d\tau$ becomes a minimum (in a least-squares sense). **Fig. 12** shows an example of a patient presenting with a disrupted BBB where we have applied this method. Using Eq 7 (for mild T_1 enhancement, ie, <30%), K_2 can be expressed as a function of MR parameters such as[32]:

$$K_2 = \frac{TR}{TE} \frac{e^{-TR\, R_{10}}}{1 - e^{-TR\, R_{10}}} r_1\, k\, PS, \qquad (20)$$

where R_{10} is the relaxation rate without GBCA on board, r_1 is the spin-lattice relaxivity of the GBCA, PS is the permeability–surface area product, and k is an undetermined constant that depends on CBV, vessel size, and other physiologic factors. K_2 is not exactly a physiologic quantity, such as K^{Trans}, because it also relies on the underlying native relaxation times T_{10} (ie, before GBCA arrival) and relaxivities r_1, which both can change

between tissues or in pathologic tissue, it is nevertheless useful information.

Using Eq 19, we can than get an expression of an approximate change in R_2^* that is corrected for leakage:

$$\Delta \tilde{R}_2^*(t)_{leakcorr} = \Delta \tilde{R}_2^*(t) + K_2 \int_0^t \overline{\Delta R_2^*(\tau)}\, d\tau. \qquad (21)$$

If we integrate Eq 21 over time, we get a corrected estimate of the blood volume. If $\int_0^t \Delta \tilde{R}_2^*(t)\, d\tau$ is the flawed CBV, i.e., CBV_{app}, that we cautioned you to avoid, then the CBV corrected for leakage $CBV_{leakcorr}$ that should approximately reflect the capillary blood volume is:

$$CBV_{leakcorr} = CBV_{app} + K_2 \int_0^T \left[\int_0^t \overline{\Delta R_2^*(\tau)}\, d\tau \right] dt. \qquad (22)$$

The original Boxerman–Weisskoff approach assumes no backflux. In case of backflux, Eq 22 can be expanded by the Tofts-Kermode approach, which includes an expression for the volume transfer from EES to IS[40]:

$$CBV_{leakcorr} = CBV_{app} + K_2 \int_0^T \left[\int_0^t \overline{\Delta R_2^*(\tau)} \cdot \exp\left(-\frac{K^{Trans}}{v_E}(t-\tau) \right) d\tau \right] dt. \qquad (23)$$

Leigh and colleagues[41] have pointed out that sometimes, $c_P(t)$ at the pathologic site might differ in shape (ie, due to dispersion and different MTT) and arrival time relative to the contralateral side, so that using the two basis functions in Eq 19 makes

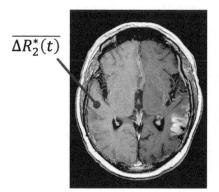
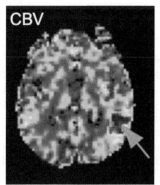
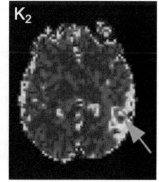

$\overline{\Delta R_2^*(t)}$ CBV K_2

Fig. 12. Patient with a subacute left middle cerebral artery infarct (parietal M4 branch) demonstrating contrast enhancement in the left hemisphere on post-contrast T_1-weighted imaging. The yellow overlay shows the area chosen to take a surrogate $\Delta R_2^*(T)$ basis function where no contrast enhancement is suspected. The middle image shows the CBV after leakage correction. The right image shows the corresponding K_2 parameter map. (*Courtesy* of R Bammer, Melbourne, VIC, Australia).

it difficult to approximate $\Delta \tilde{R}_2^*(t)$ and offered a variant to the Boxerman–Weisskoff method that addresses this problem. This applies in acute ischemic stroke, in the 24-hour treatment window.

Building the Bridge Between DCE and DSC

Using a dynamic multi-echo gradient-echo or spin- and gradient-echo DSC sequence, such as PERMEATE or SAGE, in combination with a quick T_1-mapping scan (eg, IR EPI ideally with same EPI readouts as SAGE to match distortions with inversion times of 50, 150, 250, 350, 450, 750, and 1050 millisecond as suggested in previous work[26]) to obtain pre-bolus tissue T_1 relaxation times T_{10}, allows us to merge DSC and DCE imaging.

The signal change of a DSC sequence due to T_1-shortening can be written as

$$S_0(t) = S_{0,baseline} \frac{1 - exp\left(-TR\left(R_{10} + r_1 c_T^{R_1}(t)\right)\right)}{1 - exp(-TR \cdot R_{10})}, \quad \textbf{(24)}$$

where the longitudinal relaxivity r_1 of the contrast agent can be usually found in the literature (eg, 6.3 L per mmol per second for gadobenate dimeglumine in human blood plasma at 37°C). As both PERMEATE and SAGE allow that computation of $S_0(t)$ and $S_{0,baseline}$ is the pre-bolus baseline, one can solve Eq 24 for $c_T^{R_1}(t)$, that is, the tissue concentration time course from T_1 effects using a nonlinear least-squares fit. Note that prior saturation of tissue with GBCA is not needed, it is, in fact, unwanted, to ensure a sufficient T_1 effect in tissue.

Now vascular permeability parameters can be computed using $c_T^{R_1}(t)$ and the previously mentioned adiabatic approximation (ie, $d_{c_E}(t)/dt \ll d_{c_P}(t)/dt$) of the tissue homogeneity model[23]:

$$c_T^{R_1}(t) = FR'(t) \otimes c_A(t) +$$
$$+ K^{Trans} exp\left(-\frac{K^{Trans}}{v_E}(t - T_C)\right) \otimes c_A(t), \quad \textbf{(25)}$$

where T_C is the transit time of the GBCA through the capillary network and $R'(t)$ is a model-based intravascular residue function, which can be approximated by $R'(t) = exp(-t/T_C)$. For this model, T_C is also the MTT. Equation 27 can be solved for T_C, K^{Trans}, v_E, and F. The latter is tissue flow in units of 1/second, which can be converted to CBF by a scaling factor that factors in small and large vessel hematocrit and the blood-brain partition coefficient. The T_1 enhancement curve of the patient from **Fig. 12** can be seen in **Fig. 13**.

Next, for perfusion data processing on GBCA-induced T_2^*-shortening, we need to first separate the effects of different compartments of brain tissue from the change of R_2^* depending on the GBCA concentration. (We restrict our formulas below to PERMEATE and T_2^* changes for simplicity, but they apply also for T_2 changes in SAGE as shown in the original publication by Schmiedeskamp and colleagues[26]). Thus, to model perfusion MR data in the presence of leakage, one can use the following expression[42]:

$$\Delta R_{2,m}^*(t) = r_{2,P}^* v_P c_P(t) + r_{2,E}^* v_E c_E(t) + \\ + k v_P v_E |c_P(t) - c_E(t)|, \quad \textbf{(26)}$$

where k is a scaling factor. The third term in Eq 26 can be assumed to be small, compared with the first two terms and is therefore neglected. Then, the adiabatic approximation of the tissue homogeneity model can be used to determine the leakage-corrected R_2^*-based perfusion parameters from the intravascular and extravascular–extracellular contributions and put into the simplified version of Eq 26[31]:

$$\Delta R_{2,m}^*(t) = r_{2,P}^* v_P c_P(t) + r_{2,E}^* v_E c_E(t) =$$
$$= r_{2,P}^* FR(t) \otimes c_A(t) +$$
$$+ r_{2,E}^* K^{Trans} exp\left(-\frac{K^{Trans}}{v_E}(t - T_C)\right) \otimes c_A(t) =$$
$$= \left[r_{2,P}^* FR(t) + \right.$$
$$\left. + r_{2,E}^* K^{Trans} exp\left(-\frac{K^{Trans}}{v_E}(t - T_C)\right)\right] \otimes c_A(t) =$$
$$= H(t) \otimes c_A(t) \quad \textbf{(27)}$$

Here, $H(t)$ is the vascular transfer function[45],

$$H(t) = r_{2,P}^* FR(t) + \\ + r_{2,E}^* K^{Trans} exp\left(-\frac{K^{Trans}}{v_E}(t - T_C)\right), \quad \textbf{(28)}$$

which can be estimated by deconvolving the changes in R_2^* from the AIF using $r_{2,P}$ (eg, 20.4 L/mmol/second) and $r_{2,P}^*$ (eg, 87.0 L/mmol/second) relaxivity values from the literature. The complete separation of the intravascular part (first term) and extravascular–extracellular part (second term) of Eq 28 would only work if $R(t)$ is a so-called "boxcar" function, that is, where $R(t) = 1$ if $t < T_C$ and zero thereafter. As we have seen in previous sections, however, the tracer material does not leave the capillary paths all at once and $R(t)$ is typically a monotonically decreasing function (**Fig. 14C**) so that the intravascular and the

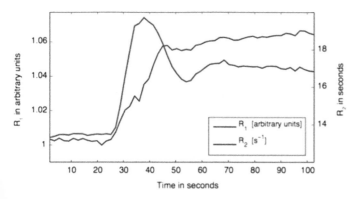

Fig. 13. Corresponding time course of T_1 enhancement (*blue* curve), reflective of contrast accumulation in tissue due to BBB breakdown, in the patient shown in Fig. 12. Also note that the apparent R_2 curve does not return to pre-bolus baseline reflecting the same contrast accumulation. (*Courtesy* of R Bammer, Melbourne, VIC, Australia.)

extravasation phase will overlap, and T_C becomes MTT. At times, when t becomes significantly larger than T_C, that is, when all the tracer has left the capillary bed, $H(t)$ becomes dominated by the extravasation phase, that is, the first term of Eq 28 vanishes. Moreover, if we assume that there is no backdiffusion of contrast material $H(t)$ reduces to

$$H(t) = r^*_{2,E} \, K^{Trans} \, for \ t \gg T_C. \tag{29}$$

From this insight into Eq 28, we also see that cerebral blood flow is little affected by extravasation, because for times much shorter than T_C (or MTT), $H(t)$ is not dependent on K^{Trans}. Since K^{Trans}, v_E, and T_C where already determined with Eq 25, Eq 29 allows us to estimate $r^*_{2,E}$.[26] With all other parameters known, we can then compute the intravascular residue function $R(t)$ and estimate blood flow F, which then can be converted into CBF using Eq 11.

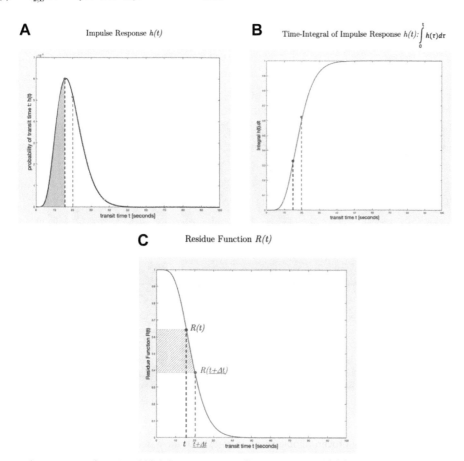

Fig. 14. Impulse response function $h(t)$ (*A*), its corresponding time integral (*B*), and the corresponding residue function $R(t)$ (*C*) for various times t. (*Courtesy* of R Bammer, Melbourne, VIC, Australia.)

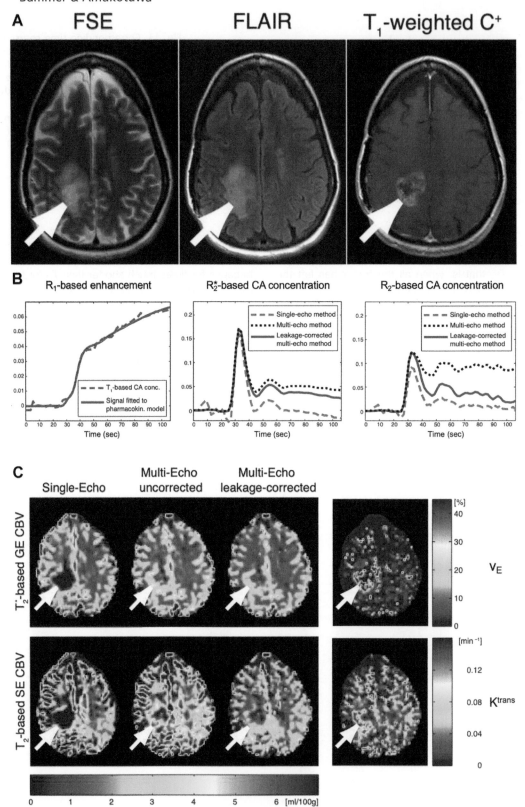

Fig. 15. (*A*) Patient with biopsy-proven glioblastoma (*arrow*) with increased signal on T_2w-FSE, T_2w-FLAIR and post-contrast T1w imaging suggesting tumor progression. (*B*) T_1-based contrast agent (CA) concentration time curve (*blue dashed*) and fit of the pharmacokinetic model to the data (*red solid*) are shown in (*left*), with a sub-stantial post-bolus GBCA concentration increase due to BBB leakage. Moreover, T^*_2-based (*middle*) and T_2-based (right) GBCA concentrations using uncorrected single-echo data (*green dashed*), uncorrected multi-echo data (black dotted), as well as leakage-corrected multi-echo data (*red solid*) are shown. (*C*) Uncorrected single-echo

Fig. 15 shows a patient with a biopsy-proven glioblastoma post-chemoradiation treatment and bevacizumab.[26] Multi-echo DSC was performed without pre-dosing. Single-echo data show a concentration time course in the enhancing lesion where the post-bolus concentration change returns to normal and then trends to negative concentration values due to the competing T_1 enhancement, which is shown in a separate plot. CBV calculation of single-echo DSC scans without pre-dosing or any leakage correction can therefore lead to significant CBV underestimation, as seen in this figure in the region of the GBM. Using multi-echo data to determine $R_2(t)$ values, the T_1 effects can be eliminated, and the post-bolus increase of tissue tracer concentration can be seen reflecting GBCA extravasation. The area under the tissue concentration curves is now elevated relative to normal tissue. Note that this apparent CBV is $\frac{k_H}{\rho}(v_P + v_E)$,[43] that is,

$$\frac{k_H}{\rho}v_T(t) \approx CBF \int\limits_0^{T_C} R(\tau)d\tau +$$

$$+\frac{k_H}{\rho}K^{Trans} \int\limits_{T_C} exp\left(-\frac{K^{Trans}}{v_E}(\tau - T_C)\right)d\tau.$$

(30)

Using the DSC/DCE framework described above, these values can be further refined and separate maps for v_E, leakage-corrected CBV and K^{Trans} can be provided. If we assume that for $t > 2T_C$, the intravascular component in Eq 30 can be neglected, and the second term is proportional to $\frac{k_H}{\rho}K^{Trans}$.[26,43] Thus, the leakage-corrected CBV can be computed by subtracting the second term of Eq 18, $\frac{k_H}{\rho}v_E$, from CBV$_{app}$.

Further work is, however, needed to tackle the challenges of nonlinear responses in the DSC signal relative to the underlying contrast concentrations as well as decreasing r_2^* relaxivity with decreasing intravascular and extravascular–extracellular tracer concentration differences. Using this framework, we wanted to give the reader the opportunity to connect the dots between DSC and DCE imaging and appreciate that both techniques can in theory be combined.

DISCLOSURE

The authors have no conflicts of interest to disclose.

REFERENCES

1. Weisskoff RM, Rosen BR. Noninvasive determination of regional cerebral blood flow in rats using dynamic imaging with Gd(DTPA). Magn Reson Med 1992;25: 211–2.
2. Rosen BR, Belliveau JW, Aronen HJ, et al. Susceptibility contrast imaging of cerebral blood volume: human experience. Magn Reson Med 1991;22:293–9 [discussion: 300-293].
3. Wintermark M, Smith WS, Ko NU, et al. Dynamic perfusion CT: optimizing the temporal resolution and contrast volume for calculation of perfusion CT parameters in stroke patients. AJNR Am J Neuroradiol 2004;25:720–9.
4. Ganguly A, Fieselmann A, Marks M, et al. Cerebral CT perfusion using an interventional C-arm imaging system: cerebral blood flow measurements. AJNR Am J Neuroradiol 2011;32:1525–31.
5. Liu G, Sobering G, Olson AW, et al. Fast echo-shifted gradient-recalled MRI: combining a short repetition time with variable T2* weighting. Magn Reson Med 1993;30:68–75.
6. Essig M, Nguyen TB, Shiroishi MS, et al. Perfusion MRI: the five most frequently asked clinical questions. AJR Am J Roentgenol 2013;201: W495–510.
7. Boxerman JL, Quarles CC, Hu LS, et al. Consensus recommendations for a dynamic susceptibility contrast MRI protocol for use in high-grade gliomas. Neuro Oncol 2020;22:1262–75.
8. Paulson ES, Schmainda KM. Comparison of dynamic susceptibility-weighted contrast-enhanced MR methods: recommendations for measuring relative cerebral blood volume in brain tumors. Radiology 2008;249:601–13.

data (left column) show decreased cerebral blood volume (CBV) due to severe T1-shortening caused by GBCA leakage. This might be interpreted as no evidence to suggest tumor recurrence. However, both multi-echo data with (3rd column) and without (2nd) leakage correction suggest considerable CBV elevation (*arrow*). Of note here is that the uncorrected multi-echo data measure the apparent CBV, not the corrected CBV. Thus, just computing the area under the curve of multi-echo data would suggest to the uninitiated that there is increased vascular volume from neovessels and/or engorged vessels. After application of the leakage correction described here, one can see by comparing the second with the third column that the corrected CBV is much less elevated than the uncorrected multi-echo data. Much of the enhancement is coming from the tracer distribution in the EES, as seen by the increased v_E in this area (4th column, top), and the significantly increased volume transfer constant K^{Trans} in this area, which explains the rapid T_1 enhancement (4th column, bottom) seen in (*B*).

9. Amukotuwa S, Straka M, Aksoy D, et al. Cerebral Blood Flow Predicts the Infarct Core: New Insights From Contemporaneous Diffusion and Perfusion Imaging. Stroke 2019;50:2783–9.

10. Noll DC, Nishimura DG, Macovski A. Homodyne detection in magnetic resonance imaging. IEEE Trans Med Imag 1991;10:154–63.

11. van Osch MJ, Vonken EJ, Viergever MA, et al. Measuring the arterial input function with gradient echo sequences. Magn Reson Med 2003;49:1067–76.

12. Pruessmann KP, Weiger M, Scheidegger MB, et al. SENSE: sensitivity encoding for fast MRI. Magn Reson Med 1999;42:952–62.

13. Griswold MA, Jakob PM, Heidemann RM, et al. Generalized autocalibrating partially parallel acquisitions (GRAPPA). Magn Reson Med 2002;47:1202–10.

14. Brau AC, Beatty PJ, Skare S, et al. Comparison of reconstruction accuracy and efficiency among autocalibrating data-driven parallel imaging methods. Magn Reson Med 2008;59:382–95.

15. Farzaneh F, Riederer SJ, Pelc NJ. Analysis of T2 limitations and off-resonance effects on spatial resolution and artifacts in echo-planar imaging. Magn Reson Med 1990;14:123–39.

16. Scheffler K. A pictorial description of steady-states in rapid magnetic resonance imaging. Concepts Magn Reson 1999;11:291–304.

17. Gudbjartsson H, Patz S. The Rician distribution of noisy MRI data. Magn Reson Med 1995;34:910–4.

18. Setsompop K, Gagoski BA, Polimeni JR, et al. Blipped-controlled aliasing in parallel imaging for simultaneous multislice echo planar imaging with reduced g-factor penalty. Magn Reson Med 2012;67:1210–24.

19. Thomsen HS, Dawson P, Tweedle MF. MR and CT contrast agents for perfusion imaging and regulatory issues. In: Bammer R, editor. MR and CT perfusion and pharmacokinetic imaging: clinical applications and theory. Philadelphia, PA, U.S.A: Wolters Kluwer; 2016. p. 85–102.

20. Boxerman JL, Hamberg LM, Rosen BR, et al. MR contrast due to intravascular magnetic susceptibility perturbations. Magn Reson Med 1995;34:555–66.

21. Donahue KM, Weisskoff RM, Burstein D. Water diffusion and exchange as they influence contrast enhancement. J Magn Reson Imag 1997;7:102–10.

22. Schmiedeskamp H, Andre JB, Straka M, et al. Simultaneous perfusion and permeability measurements using combined spin- and gradient-echo MRI. J Cerebr Blood Flow Metabol 2013;33:732–43.

23. St Lawrence KS, Lee TY. An adiabatic approximation to the tissue homogeneity model for water exchange in the brain: I. Theoretical derivation. J Cerebr Blood Flow Metabol 1998;18:1365–77.

24. Kiselev VG, Strecker R, Ziyeh S, et al. Vessel size imaging in humans. Magn Reson Med 2005;53:553–63.

25. Jain RK. Normalizing tumor vasculature with anti-angiogenic therapy: a new paradigm for combination therapy. Nat Med 2001;7:987–9.

26. Schmiedeskamp H, Straka M, Newbould RD, et al. Combined spin- and gradient-echo perfusion-weighted imaging. Magn Reson Med 2012;68:30–40.

27. Vonken EJ, van Osch MJ, Bakker CJ, et al. Measurement of cerebral perfusion with dual-echo multi-slice quantitative dynamic susceptibility contrast MRI. J Magn Reson Imag 1999;10:109–17.

28. Newbould RD, Skare ST, Jochimsen TH, et al. Perfusion mapping with multiecho multishot parallel imaging EPI. Magn Reson Med 2007;58:70–81.

29. Jochimsen TH, Newbould RD, Skare ST, et al. Identifying systematic errors in quantitative dynamic-susceptibility contrast perfusion imaging by high-resolution multi-echo parallel EPI. NMR Biomed 2007;20:429–38.

30. Boxerman JL, Schmainda KM, Weisskoff RM. Relative cerebral blood volume maps corrected for contrast agent extravasation significantly correlate with glioma tumor grade, whereas uncorrected maps do not. AJNR Am J Neuroradiol 2006;27:859–67.

31. Quarles CC, Gochberg DF, Gore JC, et al. A theoretical framework to model DSC-MRI data acquired in the presence of contrast agent extravasation. Phys Med Biol 2009;54:5749–66.

32. Christen T, Ni W, Qiu D, et al. High-resolution cerebral blood volume imaging in humans using the blood pool contrast agent ferumoxytol. Magn Reson Med 2012. https://doi.org/10.1002/mrm.24500.

33. Maralani PJ, Das S, Mainprize T, et al. Hypoxia detection in infiltrative astrocytoma: ferumoxytol-based Quantitative BOLD MRI with intraoperative and histologic validation. Radiology 2018;288:821–9.

34. Puig J, Blasco G, Daunis IEJ, et al. High-resolution blood-pool-contrast-enhanced MR angiography in glioblastoma: tumor-associated neovascularization as a biomarker for patient survival. A preliminary study. Neuroradiology 2016;58:17–26.

35. Larsson HB, Stubgaard M, Frederiksen JL, et al. Quantitation of blood-brain barrier defect by magnetic resonance imaging and gadolinium-DTPA in patients with multiple sclerosis and brain tumors. Magn Reson Med 1990;16:117–31.

36. Kety SS. The theory and applications of the exchange of inert gas at the lungs and tissues. Pharmacol Rev 1951;3:1–41.

37. Landau WM, Freygang WH Jr, Roland LP, et al. The local circulation of the living brain; values in the unanesthetized and anesthetized cat. Trans Am Neurol Assoc 1955;125–9.

38. Patlak CS, Blasberg RG, Fenstermacher JD. Graphical evaluation of blood-to-brain transfer constants from multiple-time uptake data. J Cerebr Blood Flow Metabol 1983;3:1–7.

39. Tofts PS, Kermode AG. Measurement of the blood-brain barrier permeability and leakage space using dynamic MR imaging. 1. Fundamental concepts. Magn Reson Med 1991;17:357–67.

40. Leu K, Boxerman JL, Cloughesy TF, et al. Improved leakage correction for single-echo dynamic suscep-tibility contrast perfusion MRI estimates of relative cerebral blood volume in high-grade gliomas by ac-counting for bidirectional contrast agent exchange. AJNR Am J Neuroradiol 2016;37:1440–6.

41. Leigh R, Jen SS, Varma DD, et al. Arrival time correction for dynamic susceptibility contrast MR permeability imaging in stroke patients. PLoS One 2012;7:e52656.

42. Quarles CC, Ward BD, Schmainda KM. Improving the reliability of obtaining tumor hemodynamic pa-rameters in the presence of contrast agent extrava-sation. Magn Reson Med 2005;53:1307–16.

43. Bjornerud A, Sorensen AG, Mouridsen K, et al. T1- and T2*-dominant extravasation correction in DSC-MRI: part I--theoretical considerations and implica-tions for assessment of tumor hemodynamic prop-erties. J Cerebr Blood Flow Metabol 2011;31:2041–53.

Dynamic Contrast-Enhanced (DCE) MRI

Xin Li, PhD[a], Wei Huang, PhD[a], James H. Holmes, PhD[b],*

KEYWORDS

- Dynamic contrast-enhanced magnetic resonance imaging • DCE-MRI • Permeability • Perfusion
- K^{trans} • Pharmacokinetic modeling • Contrast agent • T_1-weighted bolus tracking

KEY POINTS

- Dynamic contrast-enhanced MRI (DCE-MRI) uses T_1-weighted imaging method to track the passage of the exogenously administered contrast agent (CA) through the tissue of interest.
- The signal change is driven by the T_1-shortening effect from the CA on water protons, making DCE-MRI an indirect method in detecting CA concentration change.
- Interpretation of DCE-MRI time-course data for evaluation of CA kinetics includes qualitative, semi-quantitative, and quantitative approaches, with the quantitative method expected to play an important role in future precision medicine.
- Technical factors such as signal-to-noise ratio, temporal resolution, arterial input function, etc. need to be carefully considered for data acquisition and analysis when performing quantitative DCE-MRI.

BACKGROUND

Dynamic contrast-enhanced (DCE) MRI is an integral part of several standard of care MRI protocols for disease diagnosis, such as in the breast[1] and the prostate.[2] DCE-MRI data acquisition generally involves continuous and repeated acquisition of T_1-weighted images over a period of time, during which a bolus injection of contrast agent (CA) is administered intravenously. For the tissue of interest, such as a tumor, DCE-MRI usually provides important information on both morphology and CA kinetics for the purposes of disease screening and diagnosis, preoperative staging, therapeutic monitoring, residual disease evaluation, and recurrence assessment. For example, morphologic assessment is routinely performed in liver cancer diagnosis, where rim enhancement of the tumor is typically associated with hepatocellular carcinoma (**Fig. 1**); other morphologic information including size, shape, margin, and internal enhancement pattern plays an important role in breast cancer diagnosis.[1] To extract CA kinetics information from the DCE-MRI signal time-course data, which reflects the underlying microvascular properties of perfusion and permeability in the tissue of interest, there are 3 common approaches: qualitative,[3,4] semi-quantitative (or heuristic),[5,6] or quantitative.[7–11]

Despite recent advances in rapid imaging methods which are becoming commercially available on various MR scanner platforms (see more details in the section "Technical Considerations for Quantitative DCE-MRI"), conventional 3-dimensional spoiled gradient echo based sequences with Cartesian full k-space sampling are widely used for DCE-MRI data acquisition across institutions. Because high spatial resolution (sRes) in DCE-MRI is usually required for clear morphology interpretation, for example, the Breast Imaging-Reporting and Data System (BIRADS) standard[1] recommends an in-plane resolution $\leq$ 1 mm and slice thickness $\leq$ 3 mm for breast DCE-MRI in standard of care, the trade-off

[a] Advanced Imaging Research Center, Oregon Health & Science University, 3181 SW Sam Jackson Park Road, Portland, OR 97239, USA; [b] Radiology, Biomedical Engineering, and Holden Cancer Center, University of Iowa, 169 Newton Road, Iowa City, IA 52242, USA
* Corresponding author.
E-mail address: jim-holmes@uiowa.edu

Magn Reson Imaging Clin N Am 32 (2024) 47–61
https://doi.org/10.1016/j.mric.2023.09.001
1064-9689/24/© 2023 Elsevier Inc. All rights reserved.

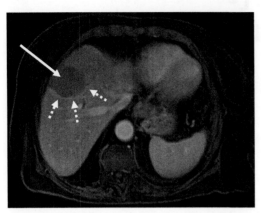

Fig. 1. For qualitative dynamic contrast-enhanced MRI (DCE-MRI) assessment of liver cancer, the contrasting agent (CA) passage is typically longer than sustainable breath-holds. Therefore, 3 separate time-phases are imaged during separate breath-holds to allow visualization of the arterial (25–30 s post-CA injection), portal-venous (65–70 s post-CA injection), and equilibrium phases (3–5 min post-CA injection). An example of the equilibrium time-phase is shown for an 81-year-old female patient with a classic hepatocellular carcinoma that was well depicted by signal drop-out in the center region (solid *arrow*) and rim enhancement (dashed *arrows*). (*Image Courtesy of* Francisco Donato, M.D., University of Iowa.)

between achievable sRes and temporal resolution (tRes) often results in low tRes (typically, > 45 s) time-course data that are not suitable for quantitative analysis with reasonable accuracy using pharmacokinetic (PK) models.[12–14] As a result, qualitative descriptions of the shape of signal intensity time-course curve or semi-quantitative parameters derived from the curve are often used to characterize CA kinetics from a DCE-MRI study.

Fig. 2 shows a diagram for the common descriptors in qualitative analysis of DCE-MRI signal (S) time-course data. Two temporal phases are generally included in qualitative assessment of the curve shape: the initial CA uptake phase and the delayed phase. The uptake phase usually starts from the pre-CA injection baseline data point and ends at a data point 1 to 2 min after CA injection depending on the actual data acquisition protocol. The uptake phase can be described as fast, medium, and slow uptake. The delayed phase starts at the end of the uptake phase and ends at the last data point of the DCE-MRI acquisition, and can be described as persistent, plateau, and wash-out curve shapes. One important application of qualitative curve shape description is for breast cancer diagnosis.[1] The wash-out and plateau patterns in the delayed phase are more likely to be associated with malignancy.[15] In a study of 266 breast lesions, Kuhl and

colleagues[3] showed 87% prevalence of malignancy in lesions exhibiting the wash-out pattern. In addition, signal time-course curve shape has been used for prediction of breast cancer response to neoadjuvant chemotherapy. Woolf and colleagues[4] demonstrated that changes in the primary breast tumor DCE-MRI curve shape after the first 2 cycles of chemotherapy were significantly correlated with pathologic response outcome and overall survival.

Many semi-quantitative metrics can be derived from DCE-MRI signal time-course data, including uptake slope, wash-out slope, percent signal change, time to peak, signal enhancement ratio (SER), and area under the signal intensity–time curve. **Fig. 3** depicts some of these metrics from a simulated noiseless DCE-MRI signal time-course with a wash-out pattern in the delayed phase. Like the qualitative descriptors, the semi-quantitative metrics are often used for cancer diagnosis and therapeutic monitoring. Noworolski and colleagues[16] found that the uptake and wash-out slopes provided accurate discrimination of cancerous and benign prostate tissue. Zhang and colleagues[17] showed that uptake slope, percent signal change, and time to peak could distinguish rectal cancer from normal rectal wall and gluteal muscle. In assessment of response to radiotherapy, Donaldson and colleagues[18] showed that percent of tumor voxels calculated based on a cut-off value in percent signal change from pre-treatment DCE-MRI was predictive of cervical cancer disease-free survival. Hylton and colleagues[5] demonstrated that DCE-MRI SER–based functional tumor volume after only the first cycle of neoadjuvant chemotherapy was predictive of breast cancer pathologic response to the entire therapy regimen that usually consists of 6 or more cycles of treatment. Combining both the qualitative descriptors and semi-quantitative metrics, Abramson and colleagues[6] showed that change in percent of tumor voxels with ≥ 100% signal change and wash-out curve pattern from DCE-MRI performed after the first chemotherapy cycle were predictive of breast cancer pathologic response to neoadjuvant chemotherapy.

Both qualitative and semi-quantitative approaches in analysis of DCE-MRI time-course data have the advantages of being simple and straightforward, and readily implementable in clinical settings. However, there are clear disadvantages. Although reflective of tissue biological conditions, both qualitative descriptors and semi-quantitative metrics are confounded due to their dependence on data acquisition details and scanner platforms and settings, making it difficult to compare study results across institutions.[19,20]

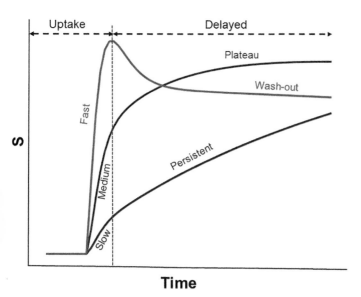

Fig. 2. A diagram of DCE-MRI signal (*S*) time-course data. The vertical dashed red line is usually at 1 to 2 min after the injection of contrast agent (CA), separating the time course between the initial CA uptake phase and the delayed phase. In qualitative interpretation of the *S* time-course data, the uptake phase is generally described as fast, medium, or slow; while the delayed phase as persistent, plateau, or wash-out.

In contrast, quantitative PK modeling of DCE-MRI time-course data allows estimation of parameters such as K^{trans} (volume transfer rate constant; **Table 1**) and v_e (extravascular, extracellular volume fraction; see **Table 1**) that are direct measures of tissue biological properties and in principle independent of data acquisition details and MRI scanner platforms and settings. Extracting quantitative parameters through PK modeling of time-course data, therefore, is the more desirable approach for DCE-MRI data analysis if sufficient tRes can be achieved in data acquisition (see more details in the section "Technical Considerations for Quantitative DCE-MRI").

In recent years, quantitative PK analysis of DCE-MRI data has been increasingly used in research, including in early-phase clinical trial settings, for cancer detection and evaluation of response to treatment.[12,19,21,22] For the latter application, DCE-MRI PK parameters generally outperform the standard approach of tumor size measurement in early prediction of therapy response, as changes in tumor size in response to therapy, especially targeted therapy, are often found to manifest later than changes in underlying biological properties[12,19,21,22] such as perfusion and permeability, which can be measured noninvasively with DCE-MRI. In a DCE-MRI study of brain

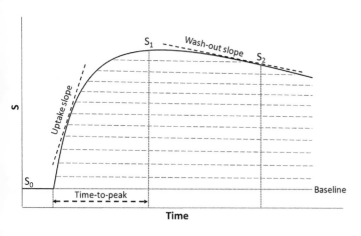

Fig. 3. Semi-quantitative metrics that are commonly derived from DCE-MRI signal (*S*) time-course data include uptake slope, wash-out slope, percent signal change, time-to-peak, signal enhancement ratio (SER), and area under the signal intensity–time curve (AUC). These metrics are shown using a simulated noiseless *S vs.* Time curve as an example, with S_0 representing the baseline (pre-CA injection) signal intensity, S_1 the peak intensity, and S_2 the delayed intensity. The 3 vertical red dashed lines indicate the times for when *S* starts to rise, and for S_1 and S_2, respectively. The 2 slopes and time-to-peak are shown with the black dashed lines and double-ended arrow, respectively. The slopes illustrated here are the maximum uptake and wash-out slopes based on the *S vs.* Time curve in the uptake and wash-out phase, respectively. The AUC is the area covered by the blue dashed lines, with the area between the first 2 red dashed lines called initial AUC (iAUC). Percent signal change, $[(S_1 - S_0)/S_0] \times 100\%$; SER, $(S_1 - S_0)/(S_2 - S_0)$.

Table 1
Definition of pharmacokinetic modeling parameters

Parameter	Description	Units
K^{trans}	volume transfer rate constant between blood plasma and extravascular, extracellular space (EES)	min^{-1}
k_{ep}	rate constant between EES and blood plasma, $= K^{trans}/v_e$	min^{-1}
k_{io}	unidirectional cellular water efflux rate constant	s^{-1}
k_{po}	unidirectional rate constant for water extravasation	s^{-1}
$v_b{}^a$	blood volume fraction, volume of blood space per unit volume of tissue	none
$v_e{}^a$	EES volume fraction, volume of EES per unit volume of tissue	none
$v_i{}^a$	extravascular, intracellular volume fraction, volume of intracellular space per unit volume of tissue	none

[a] $v_b + v_e + v_i = 1.0$; if blood volume is ignored, as in the TK model, $v_e + v_i = 1.0$.

tumors, Bergamino and colleagues[23] demonstrated strong correlations between K^{trans} value and tumor grade. **Fig. 4** shows an example of discriminating a malignant and a benign breast lesion using the K^{trans} parameter derived using the TK model, with both lesions found suspicious in standard of care mammography examinations and referred for biopsies. Based on the skewness of voxel-wise K^{trans} distribution within a tumor, Shukla-Dave and colleagues[24] showed that pre-therapy DCE-MRI could predict overall survival in a cohort of 62 head and neck cancer patients. Lavini and colleagues[25] demonstrated superiority of the K^{trans} parameter over tumor size measurement in assessing brain tumor response to Avastin, an antiangiogenic agent. **Fig. 5** illustrates an example of the advantage of K^{trans} over tumor size in early prediction of soft-tissue sarcoma response to preoperative chemoradiotherapy. A recent study by Thawani and colleagues[26] showed that quantitative parameters derived from post-neoadjuvant chemotherapy DCE-MRI data provided added value and improved accuracy in prediction of breast cancer recurrence when combined with clinicopathological information.

With the entire field of biomedical MRI moving toward quantitative imaging in the future, the rest of this article is devoted to review of quantitative DCE-MRI with PK modeling of the time-course data, including the major technical aspects that need to be taken into consideration when an investigator performs a quantitative DCE-MRI study.

QUANTITATIVE DCE-MRI
A. Background and General Approaches

PK modeling extracts model parameters that can be directly tied to physiologic and biological

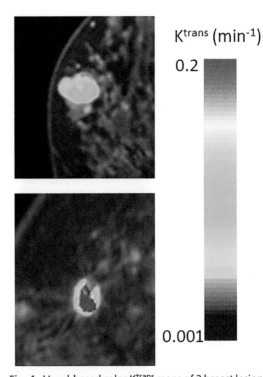

K^{trans} (min^{-1})

0.2

0.001

Fig. 4. Voxel-based color K^{trans} maps of 2 breast lesions are overlaid onto post-contrast DCE-MRI images (cropped), respectively. Both lesions had suspicious mammographic findings and the follow-up biopsies revealed that 1 was a benign fibroadenoma (top) and the other was a grade 2 invasive ductal carcinoma (bottom). The K^{trans} maps were generated from pharmacokinetic (PK) modeling using the TK model, of DCE-MRI data obtained before biopsies. The K^{trans} color scale is kept the same for the 2 lesions, demonstrating substantially higher K^{trans} values in the malignant lesion compared to the benign lesion. (Unpublished data from Oregon Health & Science University.)

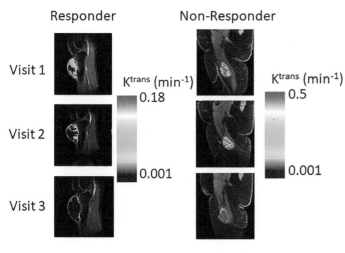

Responder   **Non-Responder**

Visit 1

K^{trans} (min^{-1}) 0.18 K^{trans} (min^{-1}) 0.5

Visit 2

0.001   0.001

Visit 3

Fig. 5. Voxel-based color K^{trans} maps (derived with the TK model) of 2 soft-tissue sarcomas are overlaid onto post-contrast DCE-MRI images (cropped), respectively. The tumor shown in the left column was located in the right thigh of a patient, while the tumor shown in the right column was located in the left thigh of another patient. Both patients underwent preoperative chemoradiotherapy including 3 cycles of chemotherapy plus 1 session of radiation. Quantitative DCE-MRI was performed pre-therapy (Visit 1), after the first cycle of chemotherapy (Visit 2), and after completion of chemoradiotherapy but before surgery (Visit 3). Pathologic review of tumor surgical specimens revealed that the patient on the left was a responder to preoperative chemoradiotherapy with 98% necrosis in the tumor, while the patient on the right was a non-responder with 5% necrosis in the tumor. It can be clearly observed that changes in K^{trans} after only 1 cycle of chemotherapy (at Visit 2) were predictive of response to treatment with K^{trans} showing substantial decrease in the responding sarcoma, while nearly stable in the non-responding sarcoma. On the other hand, the tumor sizes exhibited minimal changes throughout the treatment for both tumors. The K^{trans} color scales were kept the same for each patient, respectively, to illustrate changes in the K^{trans} value over the 3 DCE-MRI studies. (Unpublished data from Oregon Health & Science University.)

properties of the in vivo system under investigation, providing potentially more meaningful quantities for aforementioned clinical applications. All PK modeling approaches attempt to characterize the in vivo system with a small number of model parameters and often even fewer adjustable parameters during model fitting of the DCE-MRI time-course data. In practice, PK models can be divided into compartmental and spatially-distributed model categories. Compartmental models[27–32] assume that the CA concentration ([CA]) within a compartment is well-mixed (ie, the [CA] within a compartment is spatially uniform at any given time) and focus on temporal features only. Alternatively, the more realistic spatially distributed models account for both spatial and temporal variations of the [CA]. In terms of model parameter performance, the compartment models generally trade model parameter accuracy for precision when compared to spatially distributed models. For large multi-center trials, compartmental models have been used almost exclusively thus far. We will therefore focus on compartment models here. Interested readers can refer to the original works and a recent review[19] for more details on spatially distributed modeling approaches.

B. Compartmental Model Characteristics and Model Parameter Definition

PK modeling quantifies tracer kinetics after CA's administration to the body. Based on different model assumptions, slightly different differential equations[19] are used to model [CA] change in the tissue of interest throughout CA passage. While the tracer molecule in DCE MRI is often the gadolinium-based contrast agent (GBCA), the signal molecule is water. This is unlike many nuclear medicine imaging modalities such as PET where the tracer and signal molecule are the same. Therefore, a pulse-sequence-dependent signal to [CA] conversion needs to be established as part of all PK modeling. The most common approach is to use the spoiled gradient echo sequence (FLASH on Siemens, SPGR on GE, and FFE on Philips). Eq. (1) shows the T_1-weighted DCE-MRI signal to R_1 (= $1/T_1$) relationship when ignoring the T_2^* effect, which is usually very small when the echo time (TE, ~ 1.0 ms) is minimized on modern clinical scanners (simulation results not shown):

$$S(t) = S_0 \frac{(1 - e^{-(TR \cdot R_1(t))})\sin(\alpha)}{1 - \cos(\alpha)e^{-(TR \cdot R_1(t))}}$$

(Equation 1)

where S_0 is a scaling factor proportional to proton density and scanner receiver gain; α is the flip angle (FA); TR is the repetition time (s); $R_1(t)$ (s^{-1}) is the longitudinal relaxation rate constant at time t, and S(t) is the measured signal intensity at time t. For well-mixed compartments or systems, like whole blood, where cross-cell membrane water exchange satisfies the fast-exchange-limit (FXL) condition,[33] research studies[34,35] have shown that R_1 and [CA] generally obey a linear relationship as shown in Eq. (2),

$$R_1 = R_{1,0} + r1 \, [CA] \qquad \textbf{(Equation 2)}$$

where $R_{1,0}$ is the intrinsic tissue R_1 value before CA arrival and $r_1(s^{-1}mM^{-1})$ is the CA relaxivity. The proportional constant, r_1, describes the potency of the GBCA in accelerating the water proton T_1 relaxation ($\propto \Delta R_1 = R_1 - R_{1,0}$). PK modeling of the DCE-MRI time-course data generally proceeds following signal-to-[CA] conversion using Eqs. (1) and (2). Eq. (3) gives the formulation for the most commonly used Tofts and Kermode (TK) model[28,36]:

$$\frac{dC_t}{dt} = K^{trans} C_p(t) - k_{ep} C_t(t)$$
$$= K^{trans} \left(C_p(t) - \frac{C_t(t)}{v_e} \right) \qquad \textbf{(Equation 3)}$$

where $C_t(t)$ and $C_p(t)$ are the tissue and blood plasma [CA] at time t, respectively. The PK modeling parameters of Eq. (3) and others described below are listed in **Table 1**. **Fig. 6** is a cartoon illustrating some of the common model parameters.

Fig. 7 shows an example of prostate multiparametric MRI with the TK modeling results of the DCE-MRI data.

C. Technical Considerations for Quantitative DCE-MRI

a. Data Acquisition

i. Overall signal-to-noise ratio consideration PK modeling of noisy DCE-MRI data results in low accuracy and precision of the estimated PK parameters. Therefore, one is motivated to optimize a DCE-MRI protocol for the highest achievable signal-to-noise ratio (SNR) in order to produce the best data quality for PK modeling under a desired combination of sRes and tRes. For sequences like gradient echo, the optimal SNR for a given TR, α, and R_1 combination is governed by the Ernst angle. However, since the R_1 is [CA] dependent during a DCE-MRI study, the predicted Ernst angle is generally different for post-CA temporal frames. Therefore, a unique DCE-MRI protocol that is SNR-optimal for all study subjects generally does not exist and standardizing data acquisition for a specific application is important. **Fig. 8** illustrates the Ernst angle dependence on [CA] using typical DCE-MRI sequence parameters recommended by Quantitative Imaging Biomarkers Alliance (QIBA).[37] Using K^{trans} as a quantitative measure for capillary leakage, the 2 curves with different K^{trans} values show drastically

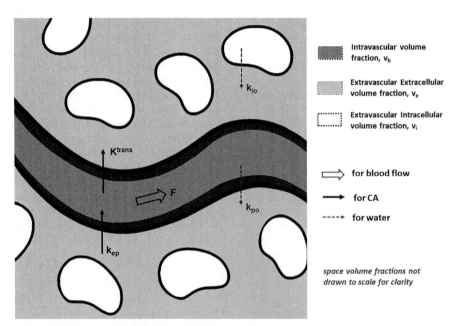

Fig. 6. A cartoon shows the most commonly modeled tissue compartments, blood volume fraction (v_b), extravascular extracellular space volume fraction (v_e), and extravascular intracellular volume fraction (v_i). The solid arrows illustrate the PK rate constants for CA tracer molecules, while the dashed arrows show the unidirectional efflux rate constants for equilibrium exchange of the MRI signal molecule, water. Only k_{io} and k_{po} are shown in the cartoon and the remaining rate constants necessary for defining the equilibrium water exchange can be derived. Most DCE-MRI PK models assume the fast-exchange-limit (FXL) condition for water exchange, such that the CA kinetics can be modeled similarly to that of nuclear medicine tracers. Although not described in detail in the main text, blood flow (F), shown as the open arrow, can also be modeled with DCE-MRI data, such as in modeling brain hemodynamics. See **Table 1** for parameter definitions.

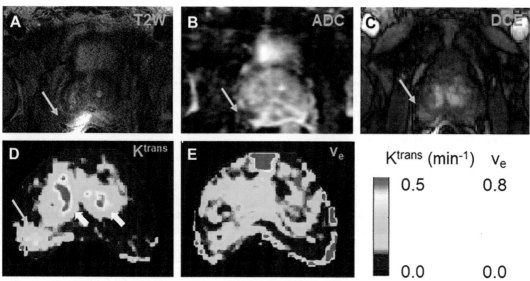

Fig. 7. Axial T_2-weighted image (*A*), apparent diffusion coefficient (ADC) map (*B*), and post-contrast DCE image (*C*) zoomed to include the prostate (top row). The biopsy-confirmed malignant lesion (orange *arrows*) demonstrated classic early and fast CA uptake in the DCE data, as well as reduced ADC values and lower signal intensity on T_2-weighted imaging. With color DCE parametric maps further masked to show only the prostate, elevated K^{trans} (derived with the TK model) (*D*) in the lesion area was evident when compared to the contralateral area of the peripheral zone, while the difference in v_e (*E*) was less specific. A region of fast enhancement (*white arrows* in D, center of the gland) associated with benign prostatic hyperplasia was not accompanied by reduced ADC and T2 signal. (Unpublished data from Oregon Health & Science University.)

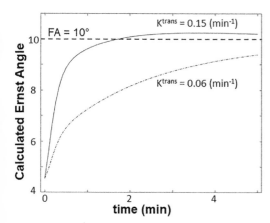

Fig. 8. A simulation showing the estimated CA concentration ([CA]) dependence of Ernst angles over the DCE-MRI acquisition period under 2 CA uptake conditions represented with K^{trans} values of 0.15 min^{-1} and 0.06 min^{-1}, respectively. The pulse sequence parameters used in simulation include repetition time (TR) = 5 ms and flip angle (FA) = 10° (dashed horizontal *line*). As CA passes through the in vivo system, [CA] is a functional of time and the function is largely characterized by K^{trans}. This makes the optimal signal-to-noise ratio (SNR) for each individual DCE-MRI frame dependent on K^{trans} as well.

different SNR optimization strategies for DCE-MRI data acquisition. For the higher K^{trans} value situation, the selected FA (= 10°) is close to the Ernst angle for the majority of the post-CA temporal frames, suggesting the acquisition protocol is optimized for good SNR overall. On the other hand, for the lower K^{trans} value situation the 10° FA is not suited for optimal SNR throughout the DCE temporal frames. This example highlights the importance of selecting an appropriate FA for SNR consideration when standardizing DCE-MRI acquisition with the same pulse-sequence parameters in a multi-center trial study. Recent developments in data acquisition[38] and automated data post-processing[39] have made quantitative DCE-MRI with high SNR feasible in clinical settings.

ii. sRes vs. tRes Conventional fully encoded Cartesian acquisitions place significant limitations on the achievable tRes for dynamic imaging scenarios. The well-known calculation for total acquisition time assuming readout in the x direction is given in Eq. (4):

$$Acquisition\ time\ =\ TR \bullet ny \bullet nz$$

(Equation 4)

where ny and nz are the number of phase-encode steps in the y and z directions, respectively. The ny and nz numbers are directly related to in-plane sRes and spatial coverage, respectively. In the setting of clinical breast DCE-MRI, sRes is typically prioritized and common protocols are on the order of TR = 4.7 ms, ny = 448, and nz = 142 yielding an acquisition time for a single DCE-MRI frame, or tRes, of 120 s for full k-space sampling. For liver DCE-MRI, tRes is prioritized due to respiratory motion and typically protocols are on the order of TR = 4 ms, ny = 200, and nz = 56 yielding a tRes of 44.8 s/time frame. In either case, the acquisition protocol utilizing full k-space sampling limits temporal sampling of signal change from the CA passage through the tissue of interest, resulting in low tRes data unsuited for PK modeling. Therefore, undersampled k-space acquisition strategies are being explored to resolve the trade-off between sRes and tRes in DCE-MRI acquisition. These strategies are often combined with advanced image reconstruction algorithms to mitigate the artifacts due to k-space undersampling.

iii. Simultaneous high sRes and tRes Accelerated data acquisition approaches combined with advanced image reconstruction algorithms have been proposed for fast dynamic imaging while retaining sufficient sRes and spatial coverage, such as parallel imaging,[40,41] non-Cartesian methods,[38,42–45] view-sharing techniques,[46–50] and advanced reconstruction methods.[38,51–55] It should be noted that although the acquisition and reconstruction strategies are closely related, there is still active research in the field to find the optimal combinations of acquisition and reconstruction methods for a given imaging scenario and to validate the performance of these advanced methods.[56] Alternative approaches have looked to combine separate acquisition approaches that independently provide high sRes or high tRes either using book-ended methods[57,58] or by interleaving these acquisitions[59] to allow fast imaging over the duration of full CA passage. Currently, most routine clinical and multi-site research protocols rely on parallel imaging with Cartesian-based view-sharing approaches[46–50] to improve imaging speed although the more advanced emerging techniques may provide further improved simultaneous high tRes and sRes.

b. Data Analysis
i. tRes and PK modeling DCE-MRI commonly employs a single inter-sample interval, known as tRes, to digitize the continuous and usually slow-varying [CA] via water proton signal changes. High tRes (short interval) in DCE-MRI data acquisition is advantageous as it allows for accurately capturing

temporal [CA] changes and results in more accurate estimations of modeling parameters. Using the TK model, Heisen and colleagues have shown that as tRes decreases, K^{trans} is progressively underestimated and v_e is progressively overestimated.[13] This trend is expected to hold for all PK models having similar model parameters. However, the kinetic analysis of the [CA] time-course is highly application dependent and the prioritization of acquisition characteristics such as tissue coverage, sRes, and tRes can be very much study specific. For example, early breast DCE-MRI work has demonstrated that higher sRes achieves better diagnostic confidence and accuracy even at the expense of lower tRes and losing quantitative kinetic information as long as the general time-course pattern of the lesion is preserved at lower tRes.[60] In other words, as long as the DCE-MRI data capture the slow varying time-course pattern, the precision and accuracy of the estimated PK modeling parameters may not be as crucial in breast cancer diagnosis. Imaging tRes is often insufficient to directly sample the arterial input function (AIF) and alternative strategies are typically needed as will be discussed in the next section. For example, a typical clinical breast DCE-MRI protocol with low tRes is not suitable for accurate sampling of the AIF or $C_p(t)$ [Eq. (3)], which is essential in PK modeling. Thus, a generic AIF, such as a population-based AIF derived from separate studies,[61] is often implemented for modeling of low tRes DCE-MRI data. On the other hand, to quantify the hemodynamics in brain tissue with intact blood–brain barrier using DCE-MRI, a tRes of less than 1.25 s is desired,[62] as blood flow quantification is directly related to the initial height of the scaled tissue response curve. Furthermore, Kershaw and colleagues have reported that high tRes as well as high SNR are required for accurate model parameter extraction when the more complicated adiabatic approximation to the tissue homogeneity model is used to model DCE-MRI data.[63] Since the contrast-to-noise ratio (CNR) and SNR may decrease with increased tRes (decreased sampling interval), protocol optimization with regard to tRes must also take these factors into account.[33]

ii. Arterial input function and PK modeling Uncertainties in the AIF estimation can lead to significant errors in the estimated PK parameters from DCE-MRI. Several approaches have been proposed to estimate the AIF and have been covered in prior literature reviews.[19] The authors briefly summarize these methods here. The gold standard approach of directly sampling blood during a DCE-MRI experiment was demonstrated by Larsson and colleagues[31,64] However, the technique has limitations in terms of clinical workflow and the invasive nature of the procedure. Population-based AIFs have been demonstrated and provide an estimate in experimental settings where tRes and technical challenges prevent direct measurement.[28,61] Reference tissue-based methods have been used by either estimating the signal change in an individual tissue region,[65] or in multiple tissue regions,[66] and using a calibration factor to relate the measured signal to the expected AIF signal. This approach places limitations on the achievable sRes and imaging field of view (FOV) in order to achieve sufficient tRes for measuring the rapidly changing AIF curve as discussed previously, in the tRes and PK modeling section. The next approach is to estimate the AIF using a specific enhancing vessel that is visible in the DCE imaging volume such as an incoming artery. However, known[67,68] confounders for this method include limited sRes,[69] SNR,[70] pulse sequence factors,[71] and inflow[72] effects. This approach is similarly limited by the imaging tRes. Finally, recent work has been proposed to simultaneously solve for both the AIF and the desired PK parameters using joint estimation algorithms.[73] Currently, the most practical and commonly used approach is the use of population-based estimates, although image-based methods and joint fitting[73] show promise for the future.

iii. Impact of native tissue T_1 measurement on PK modeling

Accurate measurement of the pre-contrast native tissue T_1 value, $T_{1,0}$, has been shown to improve accuracies of the derived PK parameters.[14,74] Voxel-based T_1 maps can be generated from a variety of techniques with the most common including Inversion Recovery-Spin echo, variable TR , and variable flip angle (VFA).[75] It should be noted that VFA is the most widely used method in multi-center studies due to shorter imaging protocol times, as a series of image volumes can be collected with different FAs in a short duration. $T_{1,0}$, given as $1/R_{1,0}$, is then calculated on a voxel-by-voxel basis by fitting for R_1 using the spoiled gradient echo equation [Eq. (1)]. Bane and colleagues recently presented a multi-site study conducted through the Data Acquisition Working Group of the National Cancer Institute (NCI)-sponsored Quantitative Imaging Network (QIN)[76,77] initiative to assess error sources for T_1 mapping,[78] concluding that a T_1 mapping VFA protocol consisting of 3 optimized FAs could provide errors of <15% while balancing limitations due to scan time and volume coverage.

A fundamental assumption of these pre-contrast T_1 mapping approaches is that the voxel-wise imaging FA or B1 is known. However, since the regional B1 is known to vary spatially due to perturbations in the transmit field caused by the object that is being imaged, corrections using B1 mapping are frequently utilized. This effect is worsened at higher field strength including 3T and higher and it is recommended that imaging protocols use hardware solutions such as multi-channel transmit RF coils and apply a voxel-wise correction based on a B1 map when possible.[79]

iv. Model selection for PK analysis

DCE-MRI has been used to study in vivo systems from normal brain tissue to malignant tumors. It is well recognized that DCE-MRI data acquisition and the associated PK modeling are highly dependent on the individual application. Extensive research efforts have been devoted to PK model selection for quantitative data analysis. Parameters like K^{trans} obtained from simple models such as the TK model often perform better for cancer applications. This is likely because, compared to more complicated models, the simpler models are more suitable for capturing the most noticeable parameter changes and less susceptible to various technical and biological confounding factors.

Foremost, model selection is application driven. The anticipated tissue-enhancement pattern can be used for acquisition protocol optimization as well as evaluating whether the system under investigation is permeability-limited or flow-limited.[36] The latter can limit the possible number of PK models suitable for data analysis. Starting by removing unsuitable PK models improves overall performance by simplifying DCE-MRI data quantification while cutting down unnecessary computation time. If more than one model remains as a potential candidate, a standard approach for model selection such as the Akaike information criterion (AIC) can be used to select the best model.[80] Often, nested family models with increased complexity are likely candidates for an application, and data-driven F-test[81] and, more recently, the adaptive model approach[82] can be used for systematic model selection. Using Bayesian-based model selection, Duan and colleagues[83] further showed that distinct optimal models can be selected for different individual voxels within the same cervical tumor, demonstrating that proper model selection on the voxel basis could improve PK modeling's capability in characterizing cervical tumor heterogeneity. In addition, the authors also observed transition of optimal PK models for a lesion in response to therapy. The ramifications of these discoveries need to be further investigated before being widely adopted for voxel-based optimal model selection.

All model selection approaches also inherently take into account details on data quality, like tRes, sRes, SNR, and CNR. That is, proper model selection strikes a balance between model complexity and data quality.[80–83] For example, for most cancer DCE-MRI studies with suboptimal tRes, the simple TK model is often more reliable and its parameter changes in a longitudinal study more likely mitigate errors from confounding issues, such as AIF uncertainty,[84] in data modeling.

Since [CA] is measured indirectly through water proton signal and the in vivo distributions of CA and water molecules are never the same (GBCA remains in the extracellular compartment), water exchange effect[30,85] is therefore fundamental to DCE-MRI measurement and modeling. The linear relationship between water proton R_1 and [CA] shown in Eq. (2) only works well for data acquired with the exchange effect minimized,[33] which can only be achieved with a substantial SNR penalty.[33] For most data acquisition schemes optimized for post-contrast SNR, the water exchange effect is embedded in the data, which can be modeled with water exchange-sensitized models.[30,86] It may also be necessary to investigate error propagation on modeling parameters in a 2-step modeling approach that employs Eq. (2), which only works well under the FXL condition, to obtain [CA] and then models [CA] change like a tracer. Alternatively, water exchange-sensitized models[30,86] can be used for PK modeling when the FXL condition is not met. Recent results show that cross-cell membrane water exchange kinetics reflect cellular metabolic activities,[87] making k_{io} (a unique parameter in water exchange-sensitized models, see **Table 1**) an attractive imaging biomarker. Previous promising results[88] of k_{io} in monitoring breast cancer treatment response indicate the need for further investigations. k_{po} (see **Table 1**) is another unique parameter accounting for cross-blood vessel wall water exchange when the water exchange-sensitized models include the blood compartment.

c. Importance of Standardization

A group of investigators from NCI QIN have recently called for wider incorporation of quantitative imaging biomarkers (QIBs) into clinical trials, and eventually, clinical practice for evaluation of cancer therapy response.[22] In the emerging era of precision medicine, QIBs that are obtained from noninvasive imaging studies can be potentially integrated with other quantitative biomarkers from genomics, transcriptomics, proteomics, and metabolomics to facilitate individualized treatment strategies and improve outcomes.[89] However, the variability in QIB quantification is a major obstacle

in translating QIBs into clinical trials and practice. Quantification of QIBs often involves multiple steps in data acquisition and analysis that can introduce variabilities in the estimated QIB values, for example, from differences in data acquisition methods associated with different vendor scanner platforms to different computer algorithms and software tools for data analysis, negatively impacting the accuracy and precision of derived QIBs. Increased QIB variability, or measurement error, results in decreased predictive performance[90] and consequently the need for larger sample size to achieve statistical significance in a clinical trial when QIBs are used as trial endpoints.[90,91] Therefore, it is of paramount importance to improve repeatability and reproducibility of QIBs.[37,90,91]

As discussed earlier, many factors in data acquisition and analysis can cause variabilities in estimated quantitative DCE-MRI parameters, including tRes,[13,92] AIF determination,[31,64,67–69] $T_{1,0}$ quantification,[76–78] PK model selection,[80–83] and even differences in software versions that are based on the same PK model.[93,94] One clear solution to this problem is to standardize data acquisition and analysis, especially for multicenter study settings where variations in both data acquisition and analysis protocols across sites could be problematic. Using the same pulse sequence and acquisition parameters for DCE-MRI can largely ensure the same tRes across sites. Likewise, $T_{1,0}$ quantification should be undertaken with the same pulse sequence and acquisition parameters: for example, the number of FAs and the FA values should be kept the same when the VFA method[95] is used to measure $T_{1,0}$. Alternatively, using a fixed population-averaged $T_{1,0}$[96] may also help reduce parameter variabilities due to errors in $T_{1,0}$ measurement. Periodic QA/QC (quality assurance/ quality control) scans using a phantom with ground-truth T_1 values are recommended to assure scanner performance in accurate T_1 measurement for quantitative DCE-MRI studies.[37] When determining the AIF to be employed in PK modeling, using a fixed population-averaged AIF[97–99] or using a reference tissue region to adjust the amplitude of AIF measured from DCE-MRI data[84,100] can reduce parameter variabilities caused by uncertainties in AIF determination. Finally, the same PK model should be used to ensure that the same mathematical formulas are used to fit the DCE-MRI time-course data; and the same software package should be used to ensure that the same scaling factors and fitting optimization algorithms are applied in data analysis. Furthermore, for longitudinal DCE-MRI studies to monitor disease progression or response to treatment, using percent changes of quantitative DCE-MRI parameters as imaging end-points has the advantage of partially canceling out systematic errors in parameter estimation caused by the aforementioned factors,[84,93,100] although this will not mitigate random errors incurred in data acquisition and analysis.

SUMMARY

Since its inception several decades ago, DCE-MRI is now a well-established imaging method for a variety of applications in both standard of care and research settings. Due to low tRes of acquired data and complexity of PK data modeling, qualitative or semi-quantitative analysis of DCE-MRI time-course data is the standard approach in current clinical practice. However, quantitative DCE-MRI is a more desirable imaging modality for precision medicine in the future. Quantitative parameters derived from PK data modeling are directly reflective of tissue biological and physiologic characteristics and can be compared across studies conducted at different institutions and scanner platforms. Simultaneous high sRes and tRes DCE-MRI acquisitions are currently feasible using commercially available sequences, which afford both accurate morphology assessment and PK modeling of time-course data. Therefore, DCE-MRI with quantitative PK modeling may become an important tool in future clinical practice. Investigators need to pay close attention to the technical aspects of DCE-MRI acquisition and analysis that can affect accuracy and precision of the estimated PK parameters, such as tRes, SNR, AIF, and $T_{1,0}$ quantifications as well as PK model and software selection. Finally, standardization of DCE-MRI data acquisition and PK modeling protocols, as well as implementing QA/QC procedures, is of paramount importance in reducing PK parameter variabilities, especially for multi-site studies.

CLINICS CARE POINTS

- Non-invasive DCE-MRI can be used as a qualitative, semi-quantitative, or quantitative technique in a wide range of clinical applications, from tumor characterization to brain hemodynamics.
- Current clinical DCE-MRI protocols using conventional pulse sequences frequently compromise temporal resolution (tRes) for high spatial resolution (sRes), rendering the DCE-MRI time-course data unsuitable for quantitative PK modeling.

- Recent advances in MRI technology allow for simultaneous high sRes and tRes in DCE-MRI data acquisition, thus facilitating quantitative PK modeling of time-course data.
- Many technical aspects in acquisition and analysis including SNR, tRes, AIF and $T_{1,0}$ quantifications, as well as PK model selection, need to be taken into account when performing quantitative DCE-MRI. Standardization in data acquisition and analysis protocols is the key to reducing variabilities in estimated PK parameters.

ACKNOWLEDGMENTS

Grant support: NIH, United States grant R01 CA248192. Clinical example for liver MRI provided by Francisco Donato M.D.

DISCLOSURES

The University of Iowa receives research support from GE Healthcare, United States.

REFERENCES

1. American College of Radiology, Breast Imaging Reporting and Data System (BI-RADS). https://www.acr.org/-/media/ACR/Files/RADS/BI-RADS/MRI-Reporting.pdf. Accessed August 28, 2023.
2. American College of Radiology, Prostate Imaging – Reporting and Data System (PI-RADS-V2.1). https://www.acr.org/-/media/ACR/Files/RADS/PI-RADS/PI-RADS-V2-1.pdf. Accessed August 28,2023.
3. Kuhl CK, Mielcareck P, Klaschik S, et al. Dynamic breast MR imaging: are signal intensity time course data useful for differential diagnosis of enhancing lesions? Radiology 1999;211(1):101–10.
4. Woolf DK, Padhani AR, Taylor NJ, et al. Assessing response in breast cancer with dynamic contrast-enhanced magnetic resonance imaging: are signal intensity-time curves adequate? Breast Cancer Res Treat 2014;147(2):335–43.
5. Hylton NM, Blume JD, Bernreuter WK, et al. Locally advanced breast cancer: MR imaging for prediction of response to neoadjuvant chemotherapy–results from ACRIN 6657/I-SPY TRIAL. Radiology 2012;263(3):663–72.
6. Abramson RG, Li X, Hoyt TL, et al. Early assessment of breast cancer response to neoadjuvant chemotherapy by semi-quantitative analysis of high-temporal resolution DCE-MRI: preliminary results. Magn Reson Imaging 2013;31(9):1457–64.
7. Wu C, Pineda F, Hormuth DA 2nd, et al. Quantitative analysis of vascular properties derived from ultrafast DCE-MRI to discriminate malignant and

benign breast tumors. Magn Reson Med 2019; 81(3):2147–60.

8. Huang W, Tudorica LA, Li X, et al. Discrimination of benign and malignant breast lesions by using shutter-speed dynamic contrast-enhanced MR imaging 1. Radiology 2011;261(2):394–403.

9. Li X, Priest RA, Woodward WJ, et al. Feasibility of shutter-speed DCE-MRI for improved prostate cancer detection. Magn Reson Med 2013;69(1):171–8.

10. Tudorica A, Oh KY, Chui SY, et al. Early prediction and evaluation of breast cancer response to neoadjuvant chemotherapy using quantitative DCE-MRI. Transl Oncol 2016;9(1):8–17.

11. Jajamovich GH, Huang W, Besa C, et al. DCE-MRI of hepatocellular carcinoma: perfusion quantification with Tofts model versus shutter-speed model–initial experience. Magma 2016;29(1):49–58.

12. Leach MO, Morgan B, Tofts PS, et al. Imaging vascular function for early stage clinical trials using dynamic contrast-enhanced magnetic resonance imaging. Eur Radiol 2012;22(7):1451–64.

13. Heisen M, Fan X, Buurman J, et al. The influence of temporal resolution in determining pharmacokinetic parameters from DCE-MRI data. Magn Reson Med 2010;63(3):811–6.

14. Di Giovanni P, Azlan CA, Ahearn TS, et al. The accuracy of pharmacokinetic parameter measurement in DCE-MRI of the breast at 3 T. Phys Med Biol 2010;55(1):121–32.

15. Erguvan-Dogan B, Whitman GJ, Kushwaha AC, et al. BI-RADS-MRI: a primer. AJR Am J Roentgenol 2006;187(2):W152–60.

16. Noworolski SM, Henry RG, Vigneron DB, et al. Dynamic contrast-enhanced MRI in normal and abnormal prostate tissues as defined by biopsy, MRI, and 3D MRSI. Magn Reson Med 2005;53(2): 249–55.

17. Zhang XM, Yu D, Zhang HL, et al. 3D dynamic contrast-enhanced MRI of rectal carcinoma at 3T: correlation with microvascular density and vascular endothelial growth factor markers of tumor angiogenesis. J Magn Reson Imaging 2008;27(6): 1309–16.

18. Donaldson SB, Buckley DL, O'Connor JP, et al. Enhancing fraction measured using dynamic contrast-enhanced MRI predicts disease-free survival in patients with carcinoma of the cervix. Br J Cancer 2010;102(1):23–6.

19. Khalifa F, Soliman A, El-Baz A, et al. Models and methods for analyzing DCE-MRI: a review. Med Phys 2014;41(12):124301.

20. Jansen SA, Shimauchi A, Zak L, et al. Kinetic curves of malignant lesions are not consistent across MRI systems: need for improved standardization of breast dynamic contrast-enhanced MRI acquisition. AJRAmerican journal of roentgenology 2009;193(3):832–9.

21. O'Connor JP, Jackson A, Parker GJ, et al. Dynamic contrast-enhanced MRI in clinical trials of antivascular therapies. Nat Rev Clin Oncol 2012;9(3): 167–77.

22. Yankeelov TE, Mankoff DA, Schwartz LH, et al. Quantitative imaging in cancer clinical trials. Clin Cancer Res 2016;22(2):284–90.

23. Bergamino M, Saitta L, Barletta L, et al. Measurement of blood-brain barrier permeability with T1-weighted dynamic contrast-enhanced MRI in brain tumors: a comparative study with two different algorithms. ISRN Neurosci 2013;2013:905279.

24. Shukla-Dave A, Lee NY, Jansen JF, et al. Dynamic contrast-enhanced magnetic resonance imaging as a predictor of outcome in head-and-neck squamous cell carcinoma patients with nodal metastases. Int J Radiat Oncol Biol Phys 2012;82(5):1837–44.

25. Lavini C, Verhoeff JJ, Majoie CB, et al. Model-based, semiquantitative and time intensity curve shape analysis of dynamic contrast-enhanced MRI: a comparison in patients undergoing antiangiogenic treatment for recurrent glioma. J Magn Reson Imaging 2011;34(6):1303–12.

26. Thawani R, Gao L, Mohinani A, et al. Quantitative DCE-MRI prediction of breast cancer recurrence following neoadjuvant chemotherapy: a preliminary study. BMC Med Imaging 2022;22(1):182.

27. Brix G, Semmler W, Port R, et al. Pharmacokinetic parameters in CNS Gd-DTPA enhanced MR imaging. J Comput Assist Tomogr 1991;15(4):621–8.

28. Tofts PS, Kermode AG. Measurement of the blood-brain barrier permeability and leakage space using dynamic MR imaging. 1. Fundamental concepts. Magn Reson Med 1991;17(2):357–67.

29. Tofts PS. Modeling tracer kinetics in dynamic Gd-DTPA MR imaging. J Magn Reson Imag : JMRI. 1997;7(1):91–101.

30. Li X, Rooney WD, Springer CS Jr. A unified magnetic resonance imaging pharmacokinetic theory: intravascular and extracellular contrast reagents. Magn Reson Med 2005;54(6):1351–9.

31. Larsson HB, Stubgaard M, Frederiksen JL, et al. Quantitation of blood-brain barrier defect by magnetic resonance imaging and gadolinium-DTPA in patients with multiple sclerosis and brain tumors. Magn Reson Med 1990;16(1):117–31.

32. Brix G, Kiessling F, Lucht R, et al. Microcirculation and microvasculature in breast tumors: pharmacokinetic analysis of dynamic MR image series. Magn Reson Med 2004;52(2):420–9.

33. Li X, Huang W, Rooney WD. Signal-to-noise ratio, contrast-to-noise ratio and pharmacokinetic modeling considerations in dynamic contrast-enhanced magnetic resonance imaging. Magn Reson Imag 2012;30(9):1313–22.

34. Rohrer M, Bauer H, Mintorovitch J, et al. Comparison of magnetic properties of MRI contrast media

solutions at different magnetic field strengths. Invest Radiol 2005;40(11):715–24.

35. Shen Y, Goerner FL, Snyder C, et al. T1 relaxivities of gadolinium-based magnetic resonance contrast agents in human whole blood at 1.5, 3, and 7 T. Invest Radiol 2015;50(5):330–8.

36. Tofts PS, Brix G, Buckley DL, et al. Estimating kinetic parameters from dynamic contrast-enhanced T(1)-weighted MRI of a diffusable tracer: standardized quantities and symbols. J Magn Reson Imag : JMRI. 1999;10(3):223–32.

37. Shukla-Dave A, Obuchowski NA, Chenevert TL, et al. Quantitative imaging biomarkers alliance (QIBA) recommendations for improved precision of DWI and DCE-MRI derived biomarkers in multicenter oncology trials. J Magn Reson Imaging 2019;49(7):e101–21.

38. Feng L, Grimm R, Block KT, et al. Golden-angle radial sparse parallel MRI: combination of compressed sensing, parallel imaging, and golden-angle radial sampling for fast and flexible dynamic volumetric MRI. Magn Reson Med 2014;72(3):707–17.

39. Nalepa J, Ribalta Lorenzo P, Marcinkiewicz M, et al. Fully-automated deep learning-powered system for DCE-MRI analysis of brain tumors. Artif Intell Med 2020;102:101769.

40. Griswold MA, Jakob PM, Heidemann RM, et al. Generalized autocalibrating partially parallel acquisitions (GRAPPA). Magn Reson Med 2002;47(6):1202–10.

41. Pruessmann KP, Weiger M, Scheidegger MB, et al. SENSE: sensitivity encoding for fast MRI. Magn Reson Med 1999;42(5):952–62.

42. Lin W, Guo J, Rosen MA, et al. Respiratory motion-compensated radial dynamic contrast-enhanced (DCE)-MRI of chest and abdominal lesions. Magn Reson Med 2008;60(5):1135–46.

43. Lee JH, Hargreaves BA, Hu BS, et al. Fast 3D imaging using variable-density spiral trajectories with applications to limb perfusion. Magn Reson Med 2003;50(6):1276–85.

44. Chen Y, Lee GR, Wright KL, et al. Free-breathing liver perfusion imaging using 3-dimensional through-time spiral generalized autocalibrating partially parallel acquisition acceleration. Invest Radiol 2015;50(6):367–75.

45. Xu B, Spincemaille P, Chen G, et al. Fast 3D contrast enhanced MRI of the liver using temporal resolution acceleration with constrained evolution reconstruction. Magn Reson Med 2013;69(2):370–81.

46. Mann RM, Mus RD, van Zelst J, et al. A novel approach to contrast-enhanced breast magnetic resonance imaging for screening: high-resolution ultrafast dynamic imaging. Invest Radiol 2014;49(9):579–85.

47. van Vaals JJ, Brummer ME, Dixon WT, et al. "Keyhole" method for accelerating imaging of contrast agent uptake. J Magn Reson Imaging 1993;3(4):671–5.

48. Jones RA, Haraldseth O, Muller TB, et al. K-space substitution: a novel dynamic imaging technique. Magn Reson Med 1993;29(6):830–4.

49. Saranathan M, Rettmann DW, Hargreaves BA, et al. DIfferential subsampling with cartesian ordering (DISCO): a high spatio-temporal resolution Dixon imaging sequence for multiphasic contrast enhanced abdominal imaging. J Magn Reson Imaging 2012;35(6):1484–92.

50. Song HK, Dougherty L. Dynamic MRI with projection reconstruction and KWIC processing for simultaneous high spatial and temporal resolution. Magn Reson Med 2004;52(4):815–24.

51. Liang Z. Spatiotemporal imagingwith partially separable functions. In: 2007 4th IEEE International Symposium on Biomedical Imaging: From Nano to Macro. ; 2007:988-991. doi:10.1109/ISBI.2007.357020.

52. Lustig M, Donoho D, Pauly JM. Sparse MRI: The application of compressed sensing for rapid MR imaging. Magn Reson Med 2007;58(6):1182–95.

53. Chan RW, Ramsay EA, Cheung EY, et al. The influence of radial undersampling schemes on compressed sensing reconstruction in breast MRI. Magn Reson Med 2012;67(2):363–77.

54. Block KT, Uecker M, Frahm J. Undersampled radial MRI with multiple coils. iterative image reconstruction using a total variation constraint. Magn Reson Med 2007;57(6):1086–98.

55. Velikina JV, Alexander AL, Samsonov A. Accelerating MR parameter mapping using sparsity-promoting regularization in parametric dimension. Magn Reson Med 2013;70(5):1263–73.

56. Wang PN, Velikina JV, Strigel RM, et al. Comparison of data-driven and general temporal constraints on compressed sensing for breast DCE MRI. Magn Reson Med 2021;85(6):3071–84.

57. Pineda FD, Medved M, Wang S, et al. Ultrafast bilateral DCE-MRI of the breast with conventional fourier sampling: preliminary evaluation of semi-quantitative analysis. Acad Radiol 2016;23(9):1137–44.

58. Abe H, Mori N, Tsuchiya K, et al. Kinetic analysis of benign and malignant breast lesions with ultrafast dynamic contrast-enhanced mri: comparison with standard kinetic assessment. AJR Am J Roentgenol 2016;207(5):1159–66.

59. Georgiou L, Sharma N, Broadbent DA, et al. Estimating breast tumor blood flow during neoadjuvant chemotherapy using interleaved high temporal and high spatial resolution MRI. Magn Reson Med 2018;79(1):317–26.

60. Kuhl CK, Schild HH, Morakkabati N. Dynamic bilateral contrast-enhanced MR imaging of the breast: trade-off between spatial and temporal resolution. Radiology 2005;236(3):789–800.

61. Weinmann HJ, Laniado M, Mutzel W. Pharmacokinetics of GdDTPA/dimeglumine after intravenous

injection into healthy volunteers. Physiol Chem Phys Med NMR 1984;16(2):167–72.

62. Larsson HBW, Vestergaard MB, Lindberg U, et al. Brain capillary transit time heterogeneity in healthy volunteers measured by dynamic contrast-enhanced T(1) -weighted perfusion MRI. J Magn Reson Imaging 2017;45(6):1809–20.

63. Kershaw LE, Cheng HL. Temporal resolution and SNR requirements for accurate DCE-MRI data analysis using the AATH model. Magn Reson Med 2010;64(6):1772–80.

64. Larsson HB, Tofts PS. Measurement of blood-brain barrier permeability using dynamic Gd-DTPA scanning–a comparison of methods. Magn Reson Med 1992;24(1):174–6.

65. Kovar DA, Lewis M, Karczmar GS. A new method for imaging perfusion and contrast extraction fraction: input functions derived from reference tissues. J Magn Reson Imag : JMRI. 1998;8(5):1126–34.

66. Yang C, Karczmar GS, Medved M, et al. Estimating the arterial input function using two reference tissues in dynamic contrast-enhanced MRI studies: fundamental concepts and simulations. Magn Reson Med 2004;52(5):1110–7.

67. Fritz-Hansen T, Rostrup E, Larsson HB, et al. Measurement of the arterial concentration of Gd-DTPA using MRI: a step toward quantitative perfusion imaging. Magn Reson Med 1996;36(2):225–31.

68. Port RE, Knopp MV, Hoffmann U, et al. Multicompartment analysis of gadolinium chelate kinetics: blood-tissue exchange in mammary tumors as monitored by dynamic MR imaging. J Magn Reson Imaging 1999;10(3):233–41.

69. van der Schaaf I, Vonken EJ, Waaijer A, et al. Influence of partial volume on venous output and arterial input function. AJNR Am J Neuroradiol 2006;27(1):46–50.

70. Naeyer DD. Algorithm development and protocol optimization for pharmacokinetic modeling of dynamic contrast-enhanced magnetic resonance imaging. Ghent, Belgium: Ph.D. dissertation,Ghent University; 2011.

71. Cron GO, Foottit C, Yankeelov TE, et al. Arterial input functions determined from MR signal magnitude and phase for quantitative dynamic contrast-enhanced MRI in the human pelvis. Magn Reson Med 2011;66(2):498–504.

72. Ivancevic MK, Zimine I, Montet X, et al. Inflow effect correction in fast gradient-echo perfusion imaging. Magn Reson Med 2003;50(5):885–91.

73. Fluckiger JU, Schabel MC, Dibella EV. Model-based blind estimation of kinetic parameters in dynamic contrast enhanced (DCE)-MRI. Magn Reson Med 2009;62(6):1477–86.

74. Tofts PS, Berkowitz B, Schnall MD. Quantitative analysis of dynamic Gd-DTPA enhancement in breast tumors using a permeability model. Magn Reson Med 1995;33(4):564–8.

75. Yankeelov TE, Gore JC. Dynamic contrast enhanced magnetic resonance imaging in oncology: theory, data acquisition, analysis, and examples. Curr Med Imaging Rev 2009;3(2):91–107.

76. National Cancer Institute, Cancer imaging program, 2012, QIN Network Organization website, Available at: https://imaging.cancer.gov/programs_resources/specialized_initiatives/qin.htm. Accessed August 01, 2023.

77. Kurland BF, Gerstner ER, Mountz JM, et al. Promise and pitfalls of quantitative imaging in oncology clinical trials. Magn Reson Imaging 2012;30(9):1301–12.

78. Bane O, Hectors SJ, Wagner M, et al. Accuracy, repeatability, and interplatform reproducibility of T(1) quantification methods used for DCE-MRI: Results from a multicenter phantom study. Magn Reson Med 2018;79(5):2564–75.

79. Kim H. Variability in quantitative DCE-MRI: sources and solutions. J Nat Sci 2018;4(1).

80. Naish JH, Kershaw LE, Buckley DL, et al. Modeling of contrast agent kinetics in the lung using T1-weighted dynamic contrast-enhanced MRI. Magn Reson Med 2009;61(6):1507–14.

81. Ewing JR, Bagher-Ebadian H. Model selection in measures of vascular parameters using dynamic contrast-enhanced MRI: experimental and clinical applications. NMR in biomedicine 2013;26(8):1028–41.

82. Bagher-Ebadian H, Brown SL, Ghassemi MM, et al. Dynamic contrast enhanced (DCE) MRI estimation of vascular parameters using knowledge-based adaptive models. Sci Rep 2023;13(1):9672.

83. Duan C, Kallehauge JF, Bretthorst GL, et al. Are complex DCE-MRI models supported by clinical data? Magn Reson Med 2017;77(3):1329–39.

84. Huang W, Chen Y, Fedorov A, et al. The impact of arterial input function determination variations on prostate dynamic contrast-enhanced magnetic resonance imaging pharmacokinetic modeling: a multicenter data analysis challenge. Tomography 2016;2(1):56–66.

85. Li X, Mangia S, Lee JH, et al. NMR shutter-speed elucidates apparent population inversion of (1) H2 O signals due to active transmembrane water cycling. Magn Reson Med 2019;82(1):411–24.

86. Yankeelov TE, Rooney WD, Li X, et al. Variation of the relaxographic "shutter-speed" for transcytolemmal water exchange affects the cr bolus-tracking curve shape. Magn Reson Med 2003;50(6):1151–69.

87. Zhang Y, Poirier-Quinot M, Springer CS Jr, et al. Active trans-plasma membrane water cycling in yeast is revealed by NMR. Biophys J 2011;101(11):2833–42.

88. Springer CS, Li X, Tudorica LA, et al. Intratumor mapping of intracellular water lifetime: Metabolic images of breast cancer? NMR Biomed 2014; 27(7):760–73.

89. Pinker K, Chin J, Melsaether AN, et al. Precision medicine and radiogenomics in breast cancer: new approaches toward diagnosis and treatment. Radiology 2018;287(3):732–47.

90. Ye S, Lim JY, Huang W. Statistical considerations for repeatability and reproducibility of quantitative imaging biomarkers. BJR Open 2022;4(1): 20210083.

91. Obuchowski NA, Mozley PD, Matthews D, et al. Statistical considerations for planning clinical trials with quantitative imaging biomarkers. J Natl Cancer Inst 2019;111(1):19–26.

92. Crombe A, Saut O, Guigui J, et al. Influence of temporal parameters of DCE-MRI on the quantification of heterogeneity in tumor vascularization. J Magn Reson Imaging 2019;50(6):1773–88.

93. Huang W, Li X, Chen Y, et al. Variations of dynamic contrast-enhanced magnetic resonance imaging in evaluation of breast cancer therapy response: a multicenter data analysis challenge. Translational oncology 2014;7(1):153–66.

94. Heye T, Davenport MS, Horvath JJ, et al. Reproducibility of dynamic contrast-enhanced MR imaging. Part I. Perfusion characteristics in the female pelvis by using multiple computer-aided diagnosis perfusion analysis solutions. Radiology 2013; 266(3):801–11.

95. Deoni SC, Rutt BK, Peters TM. Rapid combined T1 and T2 mapping using gradient recalled acquisition in the steady state. Magn Reson Med 2003; 49(3):515–26.

96. Huang W, Wang Y, Panicek DM, et al. Feasibility of using limited-population-based average R10 for pharmacokinetic modeling of osteosarcoma dynamic contrast-enhanced magnetic resonance imaging data. Magn Reson Imaging 2009;27(6): 852–8.

97. Parker GJ, Roberts C, Macdonald A, et al. Experimentally-derived functional form for a population-averaged high-temporal-resolution arterial input function for dynamic contrast-enhanced MRI. Magn Reson Med 2006;56(5):993–1000.

98. Wang Y, Huang W, Panicek DM, et al. Feasibility of using limited-population-based arterial input function for pharmacokinetic modeling of osteosarcoma dynamic contrast-enhanced MRI data. Magn Reson Med 2008;59(5):1183–9.

99. Rata M, Collins DJ, Darcy J, et al. Assessment of repeatability and treatment response in early phase clinical trials using DCE-MRI: comparison of parametric analysis using MR- and CT-derived arterial input functions. Eur Radiol 2016;26(7): 1991–8.

100. Huang W, Chen Y, Fedorov A, et al. The impact of arterial input function determination variations on prostate dynamic contrast-enhanced magnetic resonance imaging pharmacokinetic modeling: a multicenter data analysis challenge, part II. Tomography 2019;5(1):99–109.

Arterial Spin Labeling Perfusion Imaging

Manuel Taso, PhD, David C. Alsop, PhD*

KEYWORDS

• Perfusion • Arterial spin labeling • Blood flow • MR imaging

KEY POINTS

- Arterial spin labeling (ASL) is a noninvasive, contrast administration free perfusion MR imaging method using radiofrequency (RF) and gradient fields to label arterial blood.
- ASL can be used to quantify absolute blood flow in physiologic units.
- ASL has been widely used to study cerebral blood flow and its modifications in a variety of neurodegenerative, inflammatory, vascular, and oncological applications.
- Although more challenging because of motion and main magnetic field and RF inhomogeneities, appropriate implementations of ASL can also be used for perfusion imaging outside of the brain.

INTRODUCTION

The excellent soft tissue contrast and spatial resolution of MR imaging is often insufficient to detect and characterize pathology. Adding sensitivity to vascular transport characteristics of tissue can be a powerful approach to enhancing diagnostic power. The most standard clinical approach to adding such sensitivity is by the injection of gadolinium chelated within a molecule of substantial size in order to minimize toxicity.[1] Such chelated gadolinium contrast agents alter T1 and potentially T2 of tissues they enter. The effect of contrast injection on tissue signal in MR imaging depends primarily on vascular permeability to the contrast agent, interstitial volume fraction, and tissue perfusion.[2] The perfusion sensitivity of contrast MR imaging can be at least partially isolated with high temporal resolution imaging and quantitative analysis[3] but these methods can be challenging. Additionally, the injection of contrast agent adds complication, cost, and potential risks.[4,5] These issues with contrast-based perfusion imaging have helped motivate interest in a contrast-free perfusion imaging method known as arterial spin labeling[6] (ASL).

ASL MR imaging uses the magnetic field gradients and radiofrequency (RF) pulses of the MR imaging scanner to modify, or label, the spins of inflowing arterial blood. Most commonly, the spatial selectivity of RF pulses and gradients are used to change the sign, or invert, the spins of water in blood. After some time, the labeled blood water enters the tissue and slightly reduces the signal of images. Unlike contrast methods, ASL has low sensitivity to vascular permeability, because vascular permeability to small water molecules is high, and almost no sensitivity to interstitial volume fraction, because water easily moves between interstitial and intercellular space. This means ASL is not a direct alternative to contrast MR imaging. However, ASL can be superior to, or at least highly competitive with, contrast-based methods for perfusion imaging in many applications.[7] Here, we review ASL methods and terminology and highlight some applications of ASL MR imaging.

ARTERIAL SPIN LABELING BASICS

The basic ASL experiment uses 2 separate acquisitions.[8,9] In a first experiment, a bolus is formed by using RF magnetic field gradient saturation or

Division of MRI Research, Department of Radiology, Beth Israel Deaconess Medical Center and Harvard Medical School, Boston, MA, USA
* Corresponding author. Department of Radiology, Ansin 226, Beth Israel Deaconess Medical Center, 330 Brookline Avenue, Boston, MA 02215.
E-mail address: dalsop@bidmc.harvard.edu

Magn Reson Imaging Clin N Am 32 (2024) 63–72
https://doi.org/10.1016/j.mric.2023.08.005
1064-9689/24/© 2023 Elsevier Inc. All rights reserved.

inversion pulses to label upstream arterial blood water, followed by a wait time (referred to as post-labeling delay, or PLD) before image acquisition, creating what is referred to as a "labeled" image. This wait time, or PLD, is required to let labeled blood reach and exchange within the tissue of interest. The experiment is then repeated without labeling, creating a control image. By subtracting both images (dM = Mcontrol − Mlabel), static tissues will be suppressed leaving only perfusion-related signal. This process is highlighted in **Fig. 1**. Because the ASL signal labels the longitudinal magnetization of blood that recovers back to equilibrium with the time constant T1, approximately 1.6 seconds at 3T,[10] this labeled magnetization has a short lifetime of a few seconds, which has to be considered for imaging and quantification.

Labeling Strategies

Spin labeling can be achieved based on spatial or velocity selectivity. Both of these strategies will be briefly described in this section.

Spatially selective ASL, which has been the most widely used during the past 20 years, uses spatially selective pulses to label blood outside of the region being imaged. This form of ASL labeling can again be subdivided into 2 main categories referred to as pulsed arterial spin labeling (PASL) and continuous/pseudocontinuous arterial spin labeling (CASL/PCASL) methods.

PASL relies on a discrete inversion (ie, at a single time-point) of a large volume to ensure that sufficient blood is labeled. In **Fig. 2**, we illustrate one of the earliest PASL implementations named flow-sensitive alternating inversion recovery (FAIR),[11,12] in which the labeled image is formed by a nonselective inversion inverting all spins within the volume of the transmitting RF coil. For the control condition, a selective inversion is used to invert only the slice of interest, hence effectively labeling blood in a large volume determined by the subtraction of the nonselective to the selective experiment. With the use of robust adiabatic inversion pulses, PASL methods are easy to implement on a clinical scanner, achieve high-labeling efficiency (>90%), and deposit modest radiofrequency power (eg, SAR), which can be highly beneficial, especially at ultra-high-field (ie, > 3T). Achieving large volume coverage can be difficult with FAIR, and blood-flow quantification can be compromised by the inflow of unlabeled blood from outside the region where the radiofrequency and gradient coils are effective. To address this issue, postinversion saturation pulses are commonly used to suppress late arriving blood, using strategies such as Q2TIPS or QUIPSS II.[13,14] Although FAIR is the method illustrated here, multiple other strategies have been proposed as described in the ASL white paper.[6]

In contrast to pulsed labeling, continuous labeling aims to label the inflowing blood continuously, much like a continuous infusion. Continuous labeling strategies hold promise for easier quantification, higher signal compared with PASL and better compatibility with short bore equipment. Continuous ASL was originally proposed in 1992[9] based on the principle of flow-driven adiabatic inversion suggested originally for angiography.[15] Although the signal-to-noise ratio (SNR) advantage compared with PASL has been experimentally demonstrated,[16] the original implementation of CASL suffered from significant shortcomings that not only limited potential for widespread use, such as hardware incompatibility with modern

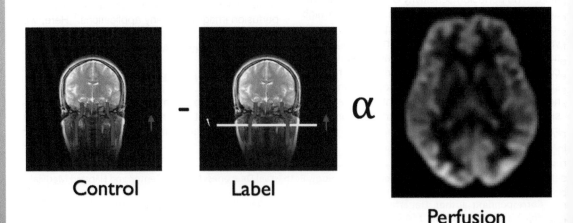

Control   −   Label α

Perfusion

Fig. 1. The basic ASL experiment. An image acquired after labeling arterial blood (Label) is subtracted from one without labeling (Control) to produce a perfusion-weighted image (right).

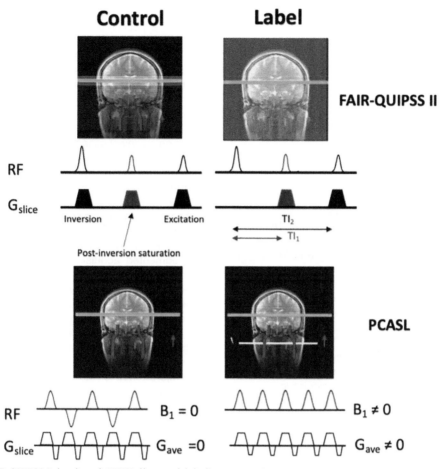

Fig. 2. FAIR-QUIPSS II (*top*) and PCASL (*bottom*) labeling strategies.

MR imagers (scanners with body transmit coils usually do not allow continuous operation of the RF power amplifiers) but also limited multislice capabilities because of magnetization transfer effects. This specific point was addressed using either hardware modifications, such as a dedicated local surface coil for labeling,[17] or modified sequences with amplitude modulation of the control condition[18] to leave inflowing magnetization unaffected while having the same MT as the label experiment. This was successfully used for multislice CASL, at the cost of higher power deposition and reduced labeling efficiency.

More recently, a modification of CASL was proposed to overcome those limitations.[19] By replacing a continuous RF waveform with short, repeated RF pulses in the presence of a slice-selective gradient, **Fig. 2**, pseudocontinuous labeling (eg, PCASL) achieved the benefits of CASL, while enabling multislice and/or 3D acquisitions on clinical scanners equipped with body coil transmit and phased-array coils. PCASL is now widely used and is recommended by a consensus

white paper.[6] By applying additional slice-selective gradients to restrict the labeling plane to individual vessels or modulate the signal in different feeding arteries, vessel-selective labeling is also feasible with PCASL[20,21] enabling perfusion territory mapping.

A disadvantage of spatially selective labeling strategies, such as FAIR and PCASL, is the label can take a substantial time, relative to T1, to move from where it is labeled to the imaged region. Velocity-selective labeling overcomes this limitation by labeling blood based on its motion, rather than its location.[22,23] The basic velocity-selective ASL (VS-ASL) experiment relies on the use of motion-sensitizing gradients that lead to spin dephasing and signal attenuation above a cutoff velocity[22] determined by gradient timing and amplitude. Although velocity-selective labeling has shown promise for some time, several implementation challenges including reduced labeling efficiency when saturation is used, contamination by labeling of other moving fluids, such as cerebrospinal fluid, and systematic labeling errors from gradient eddy current imperfections have impeded widespread use.

Recent developments including improved velocity-selective saturation schemes using advanced RF pulse design,[24] and development of velocity-selective inversion based methods,[25] have reinvigorated interest in VS-ASL as highlighted in a recent review by the International Society for Magnetic Resonance in Medicine Perfusion study group.[26]

Imaging Sequences

ASL can be used in conjunction with more or less any imaging readout amenable to magnetization preparation. Early experiments usually combined ASL with two-dimensional (2D) single-shot echo-planar-imaging (EPI) because of its speed and freezing of motion. More recently, simultaneous-multi-slice excitation has enabled the acquisition of a large number of EPI slices within a single repetition time, **Fig. 3**.[27,28] Other popular options for single-slice or 2D multislice imaging have used gradient-echo variants such as balanced SSFP[29] or single-shot fast spin echo.[30] This has particularly been helpful to develop body applications in which motion during long-segmented readouts is a major issue.

Three-dimensional (3D) acquisitions, however, have significant advantages such as higher SNR, greater spatial coverage, and excellent compatibility with background suppression (described in the next paragraph), **Fig. 3**. These benefits come at the cost of prolonged acquisition times due to the segmented nature of 3D readouts. Most popular among 3D readouts is Gradient-Spin Echo (GRASE) or non-Cartesian turbo spin echo/fast spin echo (TSE/FSE) using stack-of-spirals as recommended in the original ASL white paper, providing optimal balance between speed, resolution, and image quality.[6,31] Other strategies have

been proposed using, for example, Cartesian FSE/TSE especially combined with acceleration techniques such as parallel imaging or more recently compressed-sensing and/or deep-learning for image reconstruction, allowing high-quality whole organ imaging with minimal blurring and/or signal losses. A few applications have shown the potential for whole kidneys imaging[32–34] or brain imaging at an unprecedented resolution on a clinical scanner.[35]

One potential problem with slower 3D acquisition techniques is that the change in image intensity from labeling represents a small fraction of the fully relaxed magnetization ($\approx 1\%$–2%), making it sensitive to various sources of signal fluctuations such as hardware instabilities or bulk/physiologic motion, degrading image quality in long/segmented acquisitions. Fortunately, background suppression strategies[36] have been proposed and are now widely used to reduce static tissue signal up to 100-fold, although at a small loss of labeling efficiency due to imperfect inversion. Background suppression is usually achieved using a combination of saturation and inversion pulses, typically from 2 to 5, at optimized timings to enable attenuation of a wide-range of tissues based on their T1.[37] This has particularly been beneficial not only for combining with segmented 3D imaging techniques but also for imaging challenging areas such as outside of the brain.

QUANTIFICATION

Quantification in MR imaging, rather than using images with strong sensitivity to desired parameters (often referred to as "weighted" images), is of increasing interest to improve the consistency of imaging across scanners and sites and potentially to increase diagnostic sensitivity.[38] In ASL perfusion imaging, quantification can help remove

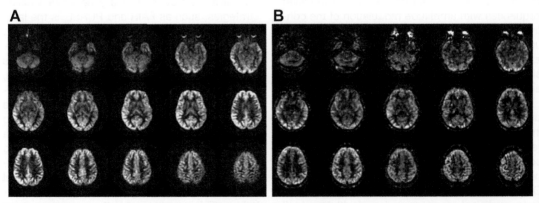

Fig. 3. Whole-brain perfusion-weighted images collected in a healthy volunteer using unbalanced PCASL at 3T with (*A*) a 3D, background suppressed stack-of-spirals FSE readout and (*B*) a 2D, unsuppressed gradient-echo EPI with simultaneous multislice excitation.

sensitivity to undesired parameters, such as the arterial transit time from the labeling location to the imaged tissue. In addition, because perfusion is a physiologic quantity that can be estimated by many experimental and clinical methods other than MR imaging, quantification of perfusion with ASL is particularly desirable. Fortunately, a quantitative estimate of perfusion from ASL images is relatively simple and need not require additional acquisitions or complicated mathematical fitting.[6] Improving on the accuracy of simpler estimates is an active area of research but whether the benefits of improved accuracy outweigh the great complexity of acquisition and analysis remains to be demonstrated.

The ASL effect essentially represents a competition between perfusion carrying labeled blood water into tissue and T1 decay of the accumulating label.[9,39,40] Quantification begins with a model for how labeling affects the spins in arterial blood water and tissue. Fortunately, labeling methods are sufficiently robust that measured inversion or saturation efficiencies from other studies can be used as good estimates of the effect of labeling on blood. T1 of blood is also often assumed from earlier measurements, although this may contribute to errors in anemic populations. T1 of tissue can be measured but often an assumed value is also used. If acquired with appropriate timing parameters to minimize sensitivity to arterial transit time, such as a sufficiently long PLD[39] for PCASL, an assumed arterial transit time can be used. Dividing by a reference proton density-weighted image acquired with the same imaging method removes coil and scanner sensitivity effects and essentially calibrates the imaging sensitivity to labeled water. Operationally, quantification can thus be as easy as subtracting label and control images, dividing by the reference image, and multiplying by a calibration constant determined from the model and the assumed parameters. The simplicity of this approach has enabled automatic quantification on the scanner in several vendor and research implementations.

APPLICATIONS
Arterial Spin Labeling for Cerebral Blood-Flow Imaging

The capability for noninvasive quantitative perfusion imaging has led to an explosion in research and clinical applications that are too broad to adequately review here. Instead, we give some examples that highlight advantages of ASL and illustrate the breadth of uses.

Arguably the largest category of ASL studies is in the study of normal brain function. Because ASL can provide a quantitative measure of brain function in just a few minutes, it can readily be included in population-based studies or in studies of function modulation by drugs or other interventions. ASL sequences have been added to population studies such as the Human Connectome Project-Aging[41] and the UK Biobank[42] where the correlates of age and other health-related factors have been probed. ASL has been used to study the brain effects of therapeutic drugs[43] and their relationship to neurotransmitter changes. The effects of mood,[44] exercise,[45] and electrical[46] interventions have been probed and reported. In all these cases, the temporal stability and absolute quantification of ASL simplify cross subject and cross scan designs that are more challenging for some other brain function measures, such as blood oxygenation level-dependent fMR imaging.[47]

Some of the clearest clinical applications of ASL MR imaging are in neuro pathologic conditions where perfusion can be elevated. Very high flow has been observed with ASL in high-grade gliomas[48,49] and ASL can be used to monitor recurrence, **Fig. 4**, and differentiate it from radiation necrosis.[50] Some of the high flow in glioblastoma may represent shunted flow through inefficient vascular networks.[51] Such shunted flow also contributes to high signal in arterial venous malformations. Residual signal after arteriovenous malformation (AVM) embolization has been used as an indicator of residual AVM after therapy.[52] Active infections often present with elevated flow[53] including progressive multifocal leukoencephalopathy[54] and herpes simplex encephalitis.[55] In suspected acute stroke, normal or elevated ASL perfusion may indicate spontaneous reperfusion or misdiagnosis.[56,57]

Many cerebral pathologic conditions can lead to decreased perfusion on MR imaging. Although ASL can provide valuable information in many cases, care must be taken in interpretation since aging, vascular disease, and even technical failures can lead to reduced perfusion unrelated to the pathology of interest. In severe cases of cerebrovascular disease, such as carotid occlusion or stroke, long arterial transit times can lead to underestimation of flow.[58] Still, ASL has been used to assess the hemodynamic impact of stenosis and to estimate the volume of tissue at risk in stroke.[59] The absolute quantification of ASL allows for repeated scans before and after acetazolamide administration or elevated respiratory CO_2 inhalation that can be used to assess reserve capacity to increase flow in patients with chronic stenotic disease.[60] Reduced perfusion in the posterior cingulate and the temporal, parietal, and frontal

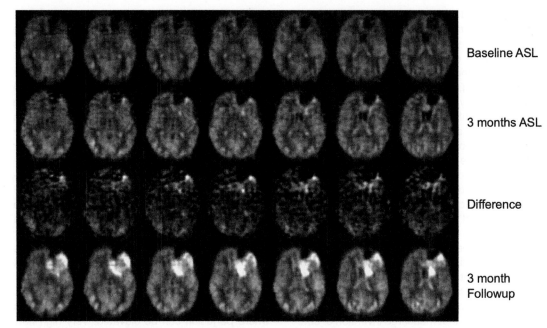

Fig. 4. Example of longitudinal ASL in a patient with a high-grade glioma following resection and radiation, highlighting the high perfusion of recurrent high-grade glioma and the potential of ASL for monitoring tumor recurrence.

association cortices has been shown in Alzheimer disease.[61] Distinct spatial patterns of hypoperfusion have also been reported for Parkinson disease.[62] Interictal epilepsy usually presents with asymmetric hypoperfusion that can be useful in lateralizing temporal lobe epilepsy[63] and identifying foci in atypical epilepsies.[64]

Arterial Spin Labeling Outside of the Brain

The promise of a noninvasive, quantitative perfusion imaging technique creates tremendous possibilities for a wide variety of research and clinical applications outside of the brain. As with most MR imaging methods, greater motion, magnetic

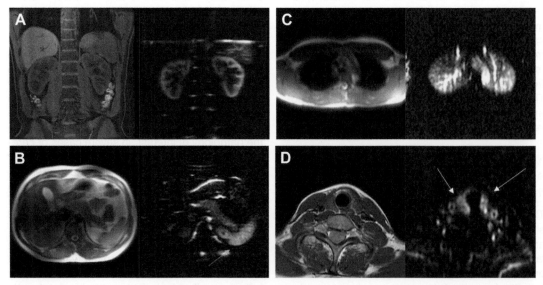

Fig. 5. ASL images, along with anatomic images to their left, acquired in various anatomic locations including (*A*) kidneys, (*B*) pancreas (*red arrow*) and spleen (*green arrow*), (*C*) lungs, and (*D*) thyroid (*yellow arrows*). All data were acquired at 3T using a PCASL-prepared single-shot FSE sequence.

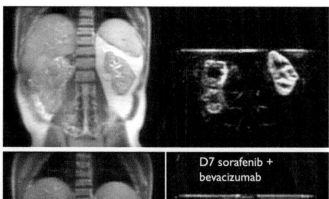
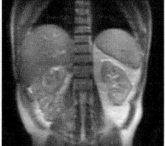
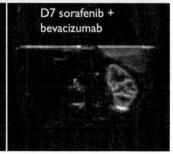

D7 sorafenib + bevacizumab

Fig. 6. ASL evaluation of therapeutic response in a case of recurrent renal cell carcinoma in the nephrectomy bed treated with a combination of antiangiogenic drugs. Images 7 days after therapy (*bottom*) show dramatic decrease relative to the pretreatment scan. (*From* Pedrosa I, Alsop DC, Rofsky NM. Magnetic resonance imaging as a biomarker in renal cell carcinoma. Cancer. 2009;115(S10):2334-2345. doi:10.1002/cncr.24237.)

field inhomogeneities, and radiofrequency transmit field imperfections make ASL more challenging in the body. Fortunately, it was shown as early as 1995[65] that ASL could be successfully used outside of the brain, in that case for renal imaging. Since then, ASL has been used to measure and quantify blood flow in a variety of anatomic locations and conditions, including, nonexhaustively, to measure myocardial, pulmonary, renal, pancreatic, hepatic, placental, and musculoskeletal blood flow. For more details, the reader is referred to a recent review from the ISMRM perfusion study group covering extensively extracranial ASL applications and state-of-the-art methods of body ASL.[66] An illustration of various possibilities is shown in **Fig. 5**.

Renal perfusion imaging has been particularly active, leading to the proposal of a dedicated set of recommendations for clinical renal perfusion imaging.[67] Imaging renal function in native and transplanted kidneys has been successfully achieved with ASL.[68,69] ASL has also been used successfully for characterizing renal cancer, allowing discrimination between histologic subtypes[70] or to assess treatment response to novel therapies such as antiangiogenics, **Fig. 6**.[71,72]

SUMMARY AND PERSPECTIVES

During the past 30 years, ASL has evolved from a novel idea for noninvasive blood flow measurement to a robust, versatile technique usable both in clinical routine and basic research. The promise of a quantitative, repeatable technique allowing the

noninvasive study of human physiology in normal and diseased conditions has triggered extensive research activity both in improved methods and in medical applications as seen in this brief and nonexhaustive review of ASL possibilities.

CLINICS CARE POINTS

- ASL is a noncontrast method to image perfusion.

- ASL signal and MR imaging contrast agent signal enhancement are affected by different physics and physiologic factors. ASL is relatively unaffected by vascular permeability and tissue interstitial space fraction that strongly affect contrast enhancement.

- ASL has been widely used in the brain for study and diagnosis of tumors, dementia, ischemic disease, epilepsy, and other applications.

- Interest in ASL perfusion imaging in high flow tissues outside the brain has led to improved methods that are undergoing evaluation for clinical use.

DISCLOSURES

M. Taso is now an employee of Siemens Medical Solutions USA. D.C. Alsop receives royalties through his institution from GE, Siemens, Philips, Hitachi, and UIH America for patents related to pseudocontinuous ASL methods.

REFERENCES

1. Carr D, Brown J, Bydder G, et al. Gadolinium-DTPA as a contrast agent in MRI: initial clinical experience in 20 patients. Am J Roentgenol 1984;143(2): 215–24.

2. Tofts PS, Kermode AG. Measurement of the blood-brain barrier permeability and leakage space using dynamic MR imaging. 1. Fundamental concepts. Magn Reson Med 1991;17(2):357–67.

3. Ostergaard L, Weisskoff RM, Chesler DA, et al. High resolution measurement of cerebral blood flow using intravascular tracer bolus passages. Part I: Mathematical approach and statistical analysis. Magn Reson Med 1996;36(5):715–25.

4. Fraum TJ, Ludwig DR, Bashir MR, et al. Gadolinium-based contrast agents: A comprehensive risk assessment. J Magn Reson Imaging JMRI 2017; 46(2):338–53.

5. Gulani V, Calamante F, Shellock FG, et al. International Society for Magnetic Resonance in Medicine. Gadolinium deposition in the brain: summary of evidence and recommendations. Lancet Neurol 2017; 16(7):564–70.

6. Alsop DC, Detre JA, Golay X, et al. Recommended implementation of arterial spin-labeled perfusion MRI for clinical applications: A consensus of the ISMRM perfusion study group and the European consortium for ASL in dementia. Magn Reson Med 2015;73(1):102–16.

7. Quattrocchi CC, Agarwal N, Taso M, et al. Report on the ISMRM-ESMRMB 2022 hot topic debate on the future of gadolinium as a contrast agent. Magma N Y N 2022;35(5):707–10.

8. Detre JA, Leigh JS, Williams DS, et al. Perfusion imaging. Magn Reson Med 1992;23(1):37–45.

9. Williams DS, Detre JA, Leigh JS, et al. Magnetic resonance imaging of perfusion using spin inversion of arterial water. Proc Natl Acad Sci USA 1992;89(1): 212–6.

10. Zhang X, Petersen ET, Ghariq E, et al. In vivo blood T1 measurements at 1.5 T, 3 T, and 7 T. Magn Reson Med 2013;70(4):1082–6.

11. Kwong KK, Chesler DA, Weisskoff RM, et al. Mr perfusion studies with t1-weighted echo planar imaging. Magn Reson Med 1995;34(6):878–87.

12. Kim SG, Tsekos NV. Perfusion imaging by a flow-sensitive alternating inversion recovery (FAIR) technique: application to functional brain imaging. Magn Reson Med 1997;37(3):425–35.

13. Luh WM, Wong EC, Bandettini PA, et al. QUIPSS II with thin-slice TI1 periodic saturation: A method for improving accuracy of quantitative perfusion imaging using pulsed arterial spin labeling. Magn Reson Med 1999;41(6):1246–54.

14. Wong EC, Buxton RB, Frank LR. Quantitative imaging of perfusion using a single subtraction (QUIPSS and QUIPSS II). Magn Reson Med 1998;39(5): 702–8.

15. Dixon WT, Du LN, Faul DD, et al. Projection angiograms of blood labeled by adiabatic fast passage. Magn Reson Med 1986;3(3):454–62.

16. Wang J, Alsop DC, Li L, et al. Comparison of quantitative perfusion imaging using arterial spin labeling at 1.5 and 4.0 Tesla. Magn Reson Med 2002;48(2): 242–54.

17. Zaharchuk G, Ledden PJ, Kwong KK, et al. Multislice perfusion and perfusion territory imaging in humans with separate label and image coils. Magn Reson Med 1999;41(6):1093–8.

18. Alsop DC, Detre JA. Multisection cerebral blood flow MR imaging with continuous arterial spin labeling. Radiology 1998;208(2):410–6.

19. Dai W, Garcia D, de Bazelaire C, et al. Continuous flow-driven inversion for arterial spin labeling using pulsed radio frequency and gradient fields. Magn Reson Med 2008;60(6):1488–97.

20. Dai W, Robson PM, Shankaranarayanan A, et al. Modified pulsed continuous arterial spin labeling for labeling of a single artery. Magn Reson Med 2010;64(4):975–82.

21. Wong EC. Vessel-encoded arterial spin-labeling using pseudocontinuous tagging. Magn Reson Med 2007;58(6):1086–91.

22. Duhamel G, de Bazelaire C, Alsop DC. Evaluation of systematic quantification errors in velocity-selective arterial spin labeling of the brain. Magn Reson Med 2003;50(1):145–53.

23. Wong EC, Cronin M, Wu WC, et al. Velocity-selective arterial spin labeling. Magn Reson Med 2006;55(6): 1334–41.

24. Guo J, Meakin JA, Jezzard P, et al. An optimized design to reduce eddy current sensitivity in velocity-selective arterial spin labeling using symmetric BIR-8 pulses. Magn Reson Med 2015;73(3): 1085–94.

25. Qin Q, van Zijl PCM. Velocity-selective-inversion prepared arterial spin labeling. Magn Reson Med 2016; 76(4):1136–48.

26. Qin Q, Alsop DC, Bolar DS, et al. Velocity-selective arterial spin labeling perfusion MRI: A review of the state of the art and recommendations for clinical implementation. Magn Reson Med 2022;88(4): 1528–47.

27. Feinberg DA, Beckett A, Chen L. Arterial spin labeling with simultaneous multi-slice echo planar imaging. Magn Reson Med 2013;70(6):1500–6.

28. Kim T, Shin W, Zhao T, et al. Whole brain perfusion measurements using arterial spin labeling with multiband acquisition. Magn Reson Med 2013;70(6): 1653–61.

29. Martirosian P, Klose U, Mader I, et al. FAIR true-FISP perfusion imaging of the kidneys. Magn Reson Med 2004;51(2):353–61.

30. Robson PM, Madhuranthakam AJ, Dai W, et al. Strategies for reducing respiratory motion artifacts in renal perfusion imaging with arterial spin labeling. Magn Reson Med 2009;61(6):1374–87.

31. Vidorreta M, Balteau E, Wang Z, et al. Evaluation of segmented 3D acquisition schemes for whole-brain high-resolution arterial spin labeling at 3 T. NMR Biomed 2014;27(11):1387–96.

32. Greer JS, Wang X, Wang Y, et al. Robust pCASL perfusion imaging using a 3D Cartesian acquisition with spiral profile reordering (CASPR). Magn Reson Med 2019;82(5):1713–24.

33. Robson PM, Madhuranthakam AJ, Smith MP, et al. Volumetric Arterial Spin-labeled Perfusion Imaging of the Kidneys with a Three-dimensional Fast Spin Echo Acquisition. Acad Radiol 2016;23(2):144–54.

34. Taso M, Zhao L, Guidon A, et al. Volumetric abdominal perfusion measurement using a pseudo-randomly sampled 3D fast-spin-echo (FSE) arterial spin labeling (ASL) sequence and compressed sensing reconstruction. Magn Reson Med 2019; 82(2):680–92.

35. Taso M, Munsch F, Zhao L, et al. Regional and depth-dependence of cortical blood-flow assessed with high-resolution Arterial Spin Labeling (ASL). J Cerebr Blood Flow Metabol 2021;41(8):1899–911.

36. Ye FQ, Frank JA, Weinberger DR, et al. Noise reduction in 3D perfusion imaging by attenuating the static signal in arterial spin tagging (ASSIST). Magn Reson Med 2000;44(1):92–100.

37. Maleki N, Dai W, Alsop DC. Optimization of background suppression for arterial spin labeling perfusion imaging. Magma N Y N 2012;25(2):127–33.

38. Jara H, Sakai O, Farrher E, et al. Primary Multiparametric Quantitative Brain MRI: State-of-the-Art Relaxometric and Proton Density Mapping Techniques. Radiology 2022;305(1):5–18.

39. Alsop DC, Detre JA. Reduced transit-time sensitivity in noninvasive magnetic resonance imaging of human cerebral blood flow. J Cereb Blood Flow Metab 1996;16(6):1236–49.

40. Buxton RB, Frank LR, Wong EC, et al. A general kinetic model for quantitative perfusion imaging with arterial spin labeling. Magn Reson Med 1998; 40(3):383–96.

41. Juttukonda MR, Li B, Almaktoum R, et al. Characterizing cerebral hemodynamics across the adult life-span with arterial spin labeling MRI data from the Human Connectome Project-Aging. Neuroimage 2021;230:117807.

42. Miller KL, Alfaro-Almagro F, Bangerter NK, et al. Multimodal population brain imaging in the UK Biobank prospective epidemiological study. Nat Neurosci 2016;19(11):1523.

43. Dukart J, Holiga Š, Chatham C, et al. Cerebral blood flow predicts differential neurotransmitter activity. Sci Rep 2018;8(1):4074.

44. Bratman GN, Hamilton JP, Hahn KS, et al. Nature experience reduces rumination and subgenual prefrontal cortex activation. Proc Natl Acad Sci USA 2015;112(28):8567–72.

45. MacIntosh BJ, Crane DE, Sage MD, et al. Impact of a Single Bout of Aerobic Exercise on Regional Brain Perfusion and Activation Responses in Healthy Young Adults. PLoS One 2014;9(1):e85163.

46. Shinde AB, Lerud KD, Munsch F, et al. Effects of tDCS dose and electrode montage on regional cerebral blood flow and motor behavior. Neuroimage 2021;237:118144.

47. Aguirre GK, Detre JA, Zarahn E, et al. Experimental design and the relative sensitivity of BOLD and perfusion fMRI. Neuroimage 2002;15(3):488–500.

48. Warmuth C, Gunther M, Zimmer C. Quantification of blood flow in brain tumors: comparison of arterial spin labeling and dynamic susceptibility-weighted contrast-enhanced MR imaging. Radiology 2003; 228(2):523–32.

49. Wolf RL, Wang J, Wang S, et al. Grading of CNS neoplasms using continuous arterial spin labeled perfusion MR imaging at 3 Tesla. J Magn Reson Imaging JMRI 2005;22(4):475–82.

50. Lai G, Mahadevan A, Hackney D, et al. Diagnostic Accuracy of PET, SPECT, and Arterial Spin-Labeling in Differentiating Tumor Recurrence from Necrosis in Cerebral Metastasis after Stereotactic Radiosurgery. AJNR Am J Neuroradiol 2015; 36(12):2250–5.

51. Nabavizadeh SA, Akbari H, Ware JB, et al. Arterial Spin Labeling and Dynamic Susceptibility Contrast-enhanced MR Imaging for evaluation of arteriovenous shunting and tumor hypoxia in glioblastoma. Sci Rep 2019;9(1):8747.

52. Heit JJ, Thakur NH, Iv M, et al. Arterial-spin labeling MRI identifies residual cerebral arteriovenous malformation following stereotactic radiosurgery treatment. J Neuroradiol J Neuroradiol 2020;47(1):13–9.

53. Noguchi T, Yakushiji Y, Nishihara M, et al. Arterial Spin-labeling in Central Nervous System Infection. Magn Reson Med Sci 2016;15(4):386–94.

54. Khoury MN, Gheuens S, Ngo L, et al. Hyperperfusion in progressive multifocal leukoencephalopathy is associated with disease progression and absence of immune reconstitution inflammatory syndrome. Brain J Neurol 2013;136(Pt 11):3441–50.

55. Li R, Shi PA, Liu TF, et al. Role of 3D Pseudocontinuous Arterial Spin-Labeling Perfusion in the Diagnosis and Follow-Up in Patients with Herpes Simplex Encephalitis. Am J Neuroradiol 2019; 40(11):1901–7.

56. Buch K, Hakimelahi R, Locascio JJ, et al. Clinical utility of arterial spin labeling perfusion images in the emergency department for the work-up of stroke-like symptoms. Neuroradiology 2022;64(5): 925–34.

57. Wang DJJ, Alger JR, Qiao JX, et al. The value of arterial spin-labeled perfusion imaging in acute ischemic stroke: comparison with dynamic susceptibility contrast-enhanced MRI. Stroke 2012;43(4): 1018–24.

58. Di Napoli A, Cheng SF, Gregson J, et al. Arterial Spin Labeling MRI in Carotid Stenosis: Arterial Transit Artifacts May Predict Symptoms. Radiology 2020; 297(3):652–60.

59. Niibo T, Ohta H, Yonenaga K, et al. Arterial spin-labeled perfusion imaging to predict mismatch in acute ischemic stroke. Stroke 2013;44(9):2601–3.

60. Detre JA, Samuels OB, Alsop DC, et al. Noninvasive magnetic resonance imaging evaluation of cerebral blood flow with acetazolamide challenge in patients with cerebrovascular stenosis. J Magn Reson Imaging JMRI 1999;10(5):870–5.

61. Alsop DC, Detre JA, Grossman M. Assessment of cerebral blood flow in Alzheimer's disease by spin-labeled magnetic resonance imaging. Ann Neurol 2000;47(1):93–100.

62. Melzer TR, Watts R, MacAskill MR, et al. Arterial spin labelling reveals an abnormal cerebral perfusion pattern in Parkinson's disease. Brain J Neurol 2011;134(Pt 3):845–55.

63. Wolf RL, Alsop DC, Levy-Reis I, et al. Detection of mesial temporal lobe hypoperfusion in patients with temporal lobe epilepsy by use of arterial spin labeled perfusion MR imaging. AJNR Am J Neuroradiol 2001;22(7):1334–41.

64. Lam J, Tomaszewski P, Gilbert G, et al. The utility of arterial spin labeling in the presurgical evaluation of poorly defined focal epilepsy in children. J Neurosurg Pediatr 2020;27(3):243–52.

65. Roberts DA, Detre JA, Bolinger L, et al. Renal perfusion in humans: MR imaging with spin tagging of arterial water. Radiology 1995;196(1):281–6.

66. Taso M, Aramendía-Vidaurreta V, Englund EK, et al. Update on state-of-the-art for arterial spin labeling (ASL) human perfusion imaging outside of the brain. Magn Reson Med 2023;89(5):1754–76.

67. Nery F, Buchanan CE, Harteveld AA, et al. Consensus-based technical recommendations for clinical translation of renal ASL MRI. Magn Reson Mater Phys Biol Med 2020;33(1):141–61.

68. Artz NS, Sadowski EA, Wentland AL, et al. Arterial spin labeling MRI for assessment of perfusion in native and transplanted kidneys. Magn Reson Imaging 2011;29(1):74–82.

69. Echeverria-Chasco R, Vidorreta M, Aramendía-Vidaurreta V, et al. Optimization of pseudo-continuous arterial spin labeling for renal perfusion imaging. Magn Reson Med 2021;85(3):1507–21.

70. Lanzman RS, Robson PM, Sun MR, et al. Arterial Spin-labeling MR Imaging of Renal Masses: Correlation with Histopathologic Findings. Radiology 2012; 265(3):799–808.

71. Pedrosa I, Alsop DC, Rofsky NM. Magnetic resonance imaging as a biomarker in renal cell carcinoma. Cancer 2009;115(S10):2334–45.

72. Tsai LL, Bhatt RS, Strob MF, et al. Arterial Spin labeled perfusion MRI for the evaluation of response to tyrosine kinase inhibition therapy in metastatic renal cell carcinoma. Radiology 2020;298(2): 332–40.

MR Perfusion Imaging for Gliomas

Jina Lee, MS[a], Melissa M. Chen, MD[a], Ho-Ling Liu, PhD[b], F. Eymen Ucisik, MD[a], Max Wintermark, MD[a], Vinodh A. Kumar, MD[a],*

KEYWORDS

- Perfusion • Dynamic contrast-enhanced • Dynamic susceptibility contrast • Arterial spin labeling
- Brain tumor • Glioma

KEY POINTS

- Multiparametric MR imaging can enhance the diagnostic accuracy of gliomas by distinguishing them from other neoplasms and nonneoplastic lesions.
- Multiparametric MR imaging can distinguish low-grade from high-grade gliomas, which can help guide treatment planning.
- Multiparametric MR imaging can help to distinguish radiation necrosis and pseudoprogression from glioma recurrence.

INTRODUCTION

Although central nervous system (CNS) tumors constitute only 1% of cancers, they are one of the leading causes of cancer deaths in young adults.[1] Nearly 30% of all brain tumors are malignant.[1] For example, glioblastoma prognosis is poor with a median survival of 6 to 10 months and 14.6 to 21 months in those treated with standard therapy.[2] Furthermore, correctly diagnosing gliomas from other CNS neoplasms and nonneoplastic etiologies is important for treatment planning. For example, the first-line treatment of high-grade glioma (HGG) would be maximal surgical resection followed by chemoradiotherapy,[3] whereas the recommended treatment of primary central nervous system lymphoma (PCNSL) would be chemotherapy without surgical resection.[4] Following glioma treatment, patients must continuously be monitored for tumor recurrence or tumor progression, which is difficult to distinguish from treatment-related changes such as pseudoprogression and radiation necrosis with conventional MR imaging[5,6]; in these instances MR perfusion imaging is beneficial.

Advanced MR perfusion techniques can improve the accuracy of diagnosis and monitoring of treatment of gliomas in patients.[7] Perfusion imaging can reveal physiologic features that could help classify gliomas, including their molecular signature,[8] and grading.[6] As a single perfusion parameter may not adequately assess the spatial heterogeneity of tumors, including more than one perfusion parameter has been shown to be valuable.[7,9–13] Our goal is to discuss the current updated use of MR perfusion imaging techniques in accurately diagnosing gliomas and monitoring them after standard-of-care chemoradiation therapy and other treatment regimens such as immunotherapy.

IMAGING TECHNIQUE

Three major methods of perfusion MR imaging include T2*-weighted dynamic susceptibility contrast (DSC), T1-weighted dynamic contrast-enhanced (DCE), and arterial spin labeling (ASL) imaging. The most commonly used imaging biomarkers obtained from these 3 perfusion imaging methods are relative cerebral blood volume (rCBV), volume transfer constant (K^{trans}), and relative cerebral blood flow (rCBF), respectively.

DSC imaging is the most widely used perfusion method.[5] rCBV is commonly normalized by

[a] Department of Neuroradiology, The University of Texas MD Anderson Cancer Center, 1400 Pressler Street, Houston, TX 77030, USA; [b] Department of Imaging Physics, The University of Texas MD Anderson Cancer Center, 1400 Pressler Street, Houston, TX 77030, USA
* Corresponding author.
E-mail address: vakumar@mdanderson.org

Magn Reson Imaging Clin N Am 32 (2024) 73–83
https://doi.org/10.1016/j.mric.2023.07.003
1064-9689/24/© 2023 Elsevier Inc. All rights reserved.

calculating the ratio of rCBV within the tumor or lesion divided by rCBV of the contralateral normal white matter. This imaging technique is a measure of neoangiogenesis, and it can characterize brain tumor hemodynamics.[7] The advantages of DSC imaging is its short acquisition time, wide availability,[5] easier to post-process relative to DCE and ASL,[7] and its sensitivity to T2* changes due to the gadolinium-based contrast agent.[7] However, DSC is prone to magnetic susceptibility artifacts,[5] such as from blood products or prior craniotomy changes.

DCE imaging measures the changes in MR signal over a specific time course during the administration of a gadolinium contrast agent in the form of a signal intensity curve.[5,7] This curve is a reflection of the perfusion, permeability,[5] and surface area of tumor vasculature.[14] Many tumors demonstrate increased vessel permeability in tumors, resulting in the leakage of intravascular contrast agents into the extracellular space. This leakage can be quantified using a parameter called K^{trans}, which reflects the efflux rate of contrast from plasma to the extravascular extracellular space.[5] DCE imaging is advantageous because it has a high spatial resolution, is less affected by susceptibility artifacts,[5] and is sensitive to capillaries, enabling the quantitative assessment of the blood–brain barrier (BBB). However, its more complex postprocessing steps and pharmacokinetic modeling may interfere with its widespread clinical use.[5]

ASL imaging uses magnetically labeled water molecules in arterial blood as endogenous tracers upstream of the volume of interest to quantitively measure the amount of CBF in the tumor.[5] A major advantage of ASL is that unlike DSC and DCE, ASL does not use contrast agents.[5] Thus, ASL may be the method of choice when avoidance of contrast agents is a priority for the patient's care, such as in children and for those who undergo frequent imaging. Additionally, no leakage correction is needed as the tracer is diffusible, unlike in DSC.[5] However, ASL does require a longer acquisition time with a lower signal-to-noise ratio and there is a higher risk of motion artifacts compared with DSC.[5]

At our institution, we use all 3 MR perfusion techniques in the evaluation of complex posttreatment glioma cases.

CLINICAL APPLICATIONS
Differential Diagnosis

In the following section, we will provide perfusion parameters that facilitate the differentiation of gliomas from other tumor types (**Table 1**).

HGGs have higher rCBV,[15–17] rCBF,[16,18,19] and K^{trans}[20,21] than brain metastases (BM) in the tumoral

and surrounding peritumoral region. Higher perfusion parameters may be seen in the peritumoral region in gliomas because gliomas are infiltrative into the surrounding white matter, as compared with BM, which are well circumscribed and without infiltrating cells.[15,16,22] Furthermore, the vasogenic edema surrounding BM could compress the microcirculation, resulting in lower peritumoral rCBV[15] compared with HGGs. Additionally, the central necrosis (if present) in HGG can lead to hypoxia and increased neovascularization.[23] Finally, HGGs have defects or pores in the vasculature that are 10 times larger than BM,[24] which could explain the greater leakage and permeability of blood vessels relative to BM. Although the threshold values vary across institutions, some of the reported median peritumoral rCBV and rCBF cutoff value range from 1.0 to 1.2[16,17] and 1.5 to 1.9,[16,19] respectively. Tupy and colleagues found a peritumoral white matter K^{trans} threshold of greater than 1.2 to differentiate glioblastoma from BM had 78% sensitivity and 79% specificity.[20]

Perfusion imaging can also differentiate HGG from PCNSL. In general, HGGs have higher rCBV[25–28] and rCBF[26,29] but lower K^{trans}[26,28–30] compared with PCNSL. This may be due to the extensive neovascularization seen in HGGs compared with PCNSLs.[27] PCNSLs also have greater disruption of the BBB, resulting in increased permeability of blood vessels compared with HGG.[31] As PCNSLs have heterogeneous hemodynamic properties, using one type of perfusion parameter may not suffice to adequately diagnose PCNSLs. In addition, the reported rCBV threshold to differentiate HGG from PCNSL ranges from greater than 2.67 to 4.76.[25,28] The optimal cutoff value of rCBF and K^{trans} ranges from greater than 1.202[29] and less than 0.187 to 0.429,[29,30] respectively.

Nonneoplastic lesions such as nonbacterial abscesses can mimic gliomas. For example, a nonbacterial cerebral abscess can have a contrast-enhancing rim around a central necrotic core and could be mistaken for a glioma.[26] HGG has higher rCBV[26,32,33] and rCBF[32] but lower K^{trans}[32] compared with nonbacterial abscesses.

Gliomas are classified based on their genotypes and distinguished with multiparametric perfusion imaging. Isocitrate dehydrogenase (IDH) wild-type (wt) gliomas have higher rCBV,[34–37] rCBF,[38,39] and K^{trans}[34,38,40] than IDH mutant gliomas. Commonly reported cutoff rCBV to differentiate between IDH wt from IDH mutant gliomas range from greater than 1.45 to 3.42,[36,37] and the optimal rCBF and K^{trans} cutoff values are greater than 2.71[39] and 0.035,[40] respectively. Gliomas with telomerase reverse transcriptase (TERT)

Table 1
Multiparametric MR perfusion imaging: gliomas

	DSC: CBV	ASL: CBF	DCE: K^{trans}
HGG vs BM	HGG > BM	HGG > BM	HGG > BM
HGG vs PCNSL	HGG > PCNSL	HGG > PCNSL	HGG < PCNSL
HGG vs cerebral abscess	HGG > cerebral abscess	HGG > cerebral abscess	HGG < cerebral abscess
IDH^{wt} vs IDH^{mut}	$IDH^{wt} > IDH^{mut}$	$IDH^{wt} > IDH^{mut}$	$IDH^{wt} > IDH^{mut}$
$TERT_p^{wt}$ vs $TERT_p^{mut}$	$TERT_p^{mut} > TERT_p^{wt}$	$TERT_p^{mut} > TERT_p^{wt}$	$TERT_p^{mut} < TERT_p^{wt}$
$EGFRvIII^{wt}$ vs $EGFRvIII^{mut}$	$EGFRvIII^{mut} > EGFRvIII^{wt}$	N/A	$EGFRvIII^{mut} > EGFRvIII^{wt}$
$MGMT_p^{unmeth}$ vs $MGMT_p^{met}$	$MGMT_p^{unmeth} > MGMT_p^{met}$	$MGMT_p^{unmeth} > MGMT_p^{met}$	$MGMT_p^{unmeth} > MGMT_p^{met}$
Oligo vs Astro (IDH-mut) of equal grade	Oligo > Astro	Oligo > Astro	Oligo > Astro
HGG vs LGG	HGG > LGG	HGG > LGG	HGG > LGG

Abbreviations: ASL, arterial spin labeling; Astro, astrocytoma; BM, brain metastases; CBF, cerebral blood flow; CBV, cerebral blood volume; DCE, dynamic contrast enhanced; DSC, dynamic susceptibility contrast; EGFRvIII, epidermal growth factor receptor variant III; HGG, high grade glioma; IDH, isocitrate dehydrogenase; Ktrans, volume transfer constant; LGG, lower grade glioma; met, methylated; unmeth, unmethylated; mut, mutant; MGMT, methylguanine-DNA methyltransferase; N/A, not available due to insufficient literary evidence; oligo, oligodendroglioma; p, promoter; PCNSL, primary central nervous system lymphoma; TERT, telomerase reverse transcriptase; wt, wild type.

promoter mutation have higher nCBV[41] and nCBF[41] but lower K^{trans}[42] than those without the mutation. rCBV[43] and K^{trans}[44] are higher in gliomas with epidermal growth factor receptor (EGFR) vIII mutation status than those without expression of the mutation. Although the perfusion parameters are conflicting for gliomas with methylguanine-DNA methyltransferase (MGMT) promoter methylation, in general, the rCBV,[34,45] rCBF,[46] and K^{trans}[8,34,45] are higher in gliomas without MGMT promoter methylation.

Multiparametric imaging can also help in differentiating IDH mutant glioma with 1p/19q codeletion (oligodendroglioma) from its 1p/19q non-codeleted counterpart (astrocytoma). Oligodendrogliomas (**Fig. 1**) have been reported to display higher nCBV,[47] rCBF,[48] and K^{trans}[49] than astrocytomas of the same grade.

Glioma Grading

Multiparametric imaging can facilitate histologic grading of gliomas. Gliomas of histologic grade III and IV will be referred to as high grade and those of grade I and II will be referred to as low grade. The rCBV,[6,50–52] rCBF,[39,53,54] and K^{trans}[50,55,56] are all higher for HGGs (**Fig. 2**) compared with low-grade gliomas (LGGs). The rCBV threshold for HGGs grading that is commonly reported in the literature is greater than 1.8 to 2.9.[51,52] Commonly reported rCBF and K^{trans} values for

HGGs range from greater than 2.08 to 2.52[39,54] and 0.079 to 0.42,[55,56] respectively. Computing rCBF with rCBV for glioma grading increased the area under the receiver operating characteristic curve to 0.92 compared with 0.78 when using rCBV alone.[9] HGGs are more aggressive and exist in a hypoxic microenvironment with more leaky, immature vessels, and they have higher rates of neoangiogenesis than LGGs.[26,57] These factors would account for HGGs having higher perfusion parameters than LGGs.

ASSESSING THERAPEUTIC RESPONSE

In the following section, we will provide perfusion parameters that facilitate monitoring treatment response after radiation, chemotherapy, and/or immunotherapy (**Table 2**).

Radiation Necrosis

Radiation necrosis is a severe brain tissue reaction to radiotherapy for brain tumors that can occur as soon as 3 months and several years but typically occurs 6 months to 2 years postirradiation.[58,59] The reported incidence of radiation necrosis after radiotherapy ranges from 5% to 25%.[59] Radiation necrosis commonly affects the periventricular white matter.[60] Conventional imaging features of recurrent glioma are similar to radiation necrosis.[61]

Compared with glioma recurrence, enhancing lesions from radiation necrosis (**Fig. 3**) have lower

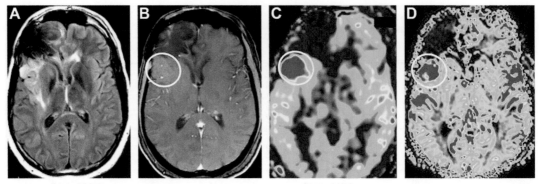

Fig. 1. High-grade oligodendroglioma. A 31 year old man with a history of a right frontal anaplastic oligodendroglioma. (*A*) Axial FLAIR and (*B*) axial T1-weighted contrast-enhanced MR images demonstrate gyral thickening with vague enhancement (*circle*) posterior to the prior resection site. (*C*) ASL and (*D*) DSC-MR perfusion images show significant elevation of CBF and rCBV (*circles*), respectively, in the area of FLAIR abnormality and disproportionate to the degree of enhancement consistent with residual high-grade oligodendroglioma.

rCBV,[18,62,63] rCBF,[62,64–66] and K[trans].[11,18,67,68] In contrast to neoangiogenesis and increased permeability of abnormally formed vessels in tumor recurrences, vascular damage from radiation necrosis results in decreased perfusion parameters.[18]

DSC, DCE, and ASL each showed moderately high sensitivity and specificity in differentiating radiation necrosis from tumor recurrence.[69] Each one had unique benefits that could contribute to accurately determining radiation necrosis. Specifically, contrast-free 3D pseudo-continuous ASL imaging has shown to be a promising alternative to DSC to distinguish radiation necrosis from tumor recurrence for long-term follow-up of patients with gliomas.[64] Another study demonstrated that DCE is helpful in the diagnosis of radiation necrosis with 98% sensitivity and 97% specificity, performing better than DSC.[70] Nael and colleagues demonstrated that multiparametric imaging improved the diagnostic accuracy of differentiating radiation

necrosis from glioblastoma recurrence with an accuracy of 92.8% compared with 85.8% and 75.5% when using DSC or DCE alone, respectively.[11] Although the threshold values to differentiate radiation necrosis tumor recurrence from radiation necrosis vary depending on the imaging parameters, commonly reported rCBV threshold values ranged from greater than 1.75 to 2.2,[11,63] rCBF greater than 1.1 to 1.41 [62,66] and K[trans] greater than 0.1 to 0.19,[11,68] respectively. At our institution, the primary indication for multiparametric perfusion imaging is distinguishing radiation necrosis from glioma recurrence.

Pseudoprogression

Pseudoprogression is an imaging diagnosis defined as an enlarging contrast-enhancing lesion. This typically occurs after chemoradiotherapy but can occur from radiotherapy alone.[71] These

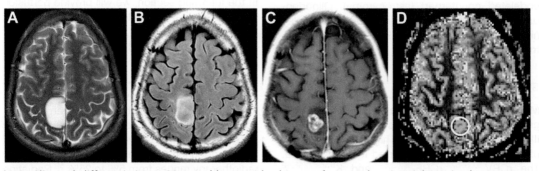

Fig. 2. Glioma dedifferentiation. A 28 year old man with a history of a nonenhancing right parietal astrocytoma, IDH-mutant, WHO grade 2. (*A*) Axial T2-weighted and (*B*) axial FLAIR images display a classic T2-FLAIR mismatch sign. (*C*) Axial T1-weighted contrast-enhanced MR image 6 years after chemoradiation therapy shows new heterogenous enhancement in the glioma. (*D*) DSC-MR perfusion image demonstrates elevation of rCBV (*circle*) in the area of enhancement favoring dedifferentiation to a higher-grade glioma rather than treatment changes. At the subsequent resection; pathology confirmed an astrocytoma, IDH mutant, *WHO grade 4.*

Table 2
Multiparametric MR perfusion imaging: monitor glioma treatment response

	DSC: CBV	ASL: CBF	DCE: K^{trans}
RN vs TR	RN < TR	RN < TR	RN < TR
PsP vs TR	PsP < TR	PsP < TR	PsP < TR
PR vs ThR	PR > ThR	PR > ThR	N/A

Abbreviations: ASL, arterial spin labeling; CBF, cerebral blood flow; CBV, cerebral blood volume; DCE, dynamic contrast enhanced; DSC, dynamic susceptibility contrast; K^{trans}, volume transfer constant; N/A, not available due to insufficient literary evidence; PR, pseudoresponse; PsP, pseudoprogression; RN, radiation necrosis; ThR, therapeutic response; TR, tumor recurrence.

contrast-enhancing lesions have been reported to occur in 20% of patients with radiotherapy-temozolomide therapy and can occur within 2 to 6 months, with a median of 3 months, after treatment.[61] Greater than 90% of gliomas with MGMT methylated promoter status progress to pseudoprogression.[72] It is theorized that pseudoprogression is a result of exaggerated local inflammatory tissue reaction and an increase in vascular permeability in response to effective treatment-induced cellular hypoxia.[61] However, this enhancement spontaneously stabilizes or decreases without a change in therapy.[73] Failing to differentiate between pseudoprogression and tumor progression could result in erroneously halting or changing effective therapy.

The Response Assessment in Neuro-Oncology (RANO) working group suggests that pseudoprogression cannot be differentiated from tumor progression in the first 12 weeks post-chemoradiotherapy and therefore, advocates for serial imaging after the first 3 to 6 months.[73] Advanced perfusion studies have higher diagnostic accuracy, exceeding 90%, in detecting pseudoprogression (**Fig. 4**) versus glioma recurrence or progression (**Fig. 5**) than conventional MR imaging.[73] Relative to tumor recurrence, a lesion with pseudoprogression has lower rCBV,[74–76] CBF,[77,78] and K^{trans}.[79–81] Overall, the rCBV threshold to distinguish pseudoprogression versus HGG is lower than 1.35 to 1.75,[74,75] CBF less than 0.995 to 1.02,[78] and K^{trans} less than 0.1302 to 0.347.[80,81] Combining rCBV from DSC with DCE enables a more accurate diagnosis of pseudoprogression than with DCE alone.[12] Choi and colleagues showed that adjunctive ASL can improve the diagnostic accuracy of DSC in differentiating pseudoprogression from tumor progression by 12.9%[13] compared with when DSC was used alone.

For patients with recurrent glioma, immune checkpoint inhibitors, such as nivolumab or pembrolizumab, can be used for treatment.[82] Immunotherapy-related treatment response could take up to 6 months to be accurately identified.[82]

There is a paucity of data on monitoring treatment response following immunotherapy. Song and colleagues demonstrated that out of the 19 patients with recurrent HGG who were treated with immune checkpoint inhibitors, 5 patients showed lesions with pseudoprogression.[82] Although these lesions showed a significant increase in contrast enhancement, initially; at the 6 month follow-up post-treatment, most patients demonstrated interval decrease in rCBV and

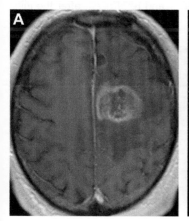
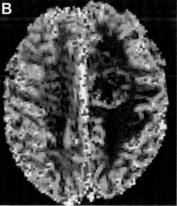
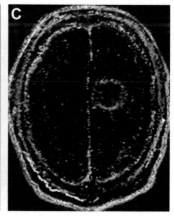

Fig. 3. Radiation necrosis. A 39 year old man with a history of a left frontal astrocytoma, IDH mutant, Grade 2 status postchemoradiation therapy. (*A*) Axial T1-weighted contrast-enhanced MR image shows rim enhancement at the prior resection site. (*B*) DSC and (*C*) DCE-MR perfusion images reveal no elevation of rCBV or K^{trans} in the area of the rim enhancement which favored radiation necrosis and was subsequently confirmed on pathology following re-resection.

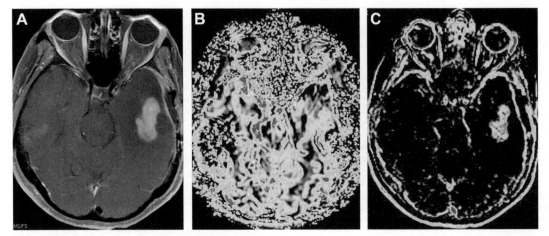

Fig. 4. Pseudoprogression. A 53 year old woman with a history of a left temporal glioblastoma on pembrolizumab. (*A*) Axial T1-weighted contrast-enhanced MR image shows enhancement at the prior resection site. (*B*) DSC and (*C*) DCE-MR perfusion images demonstrate no significant elevation of rCBV or Ktrans in the area of enhancement favoring pseudoprogression. This was confirmed following redo resection with pathology revealing only granulation tissue and reactive changes.

K^{trans}. For the patients whose tumors had progressed, there was an increase in these perfusion parameters.[82] Therefore, these findings emphasize the importance of adhering to the RANO working group guidelines recommending follow-up imaging of enhancing lesions after 3 to 6 months of treatment, including immunotherapy, to differentiate between pseudoprogression and tumor progression.[73]

Pseudoresponse

Pseudoresponse is a decrease in contrast enhancement, T2 or FLAIR signal, vasogenic edema, and mass effect due to vascular normalization of the BBB resulting from treatment with antiangiogenic agents such as bevacizumab and

cediranib.[61] Patients temporarily improve their symptoms as well.[61] Despite this initial favorable response to treatment, there is no true reduction in tumor size and no improvement in overall survival.[14,61] Norden and colleagues demonstrate that although combination therapy with bevacizumab and chemotherapy improved the 6 month progression-free survival, more people than expected showed diffuse and distant infiltrating disease with no significant change in the long-term outcome in patients with recurrent HGG.[83]

Advanced perfusion imaging parameters can help to differentiate true responders from nonresponders quantitatively. Post-antiangiogenic treatment demonstrates an early decrease in rCBV,[14,84] rCBF,[85] and $K^{trans5,84,86}$ after the initial

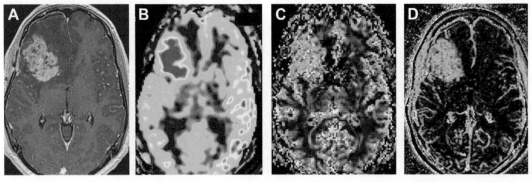

Fig. 5. Recurrent glioblastoma. A 31 year old man with a history of a right frontal glioblastoma on pembrolizumab. (*A*) Axial T1-weighted contrast-enhanced MR image shows heterogenous enhancement at the prior resection site. (*B*) ASL, (*C*) DSC, and (*D*) DCE-MR perfusion images demonstrate marked elevation of CBF, rCBV, and Ktrans, respectively, in the area of enhancement favoring glioblastoma recurrence which was confirmed on pathology following a redo resection.

dose of antiangiogenic therapy. However, for lesions with pseudoresponse, these reversed to abnormal values at longer follow-up or for those on a drug holiday.[5,14,85] Batchelor and colleagues demonstrated that the cerebral blood volume values initially decreased but increased to abnormal values at day 56 after treatment with ACD2171, an antiangiogenic agent, in patients with HGG.[14] Greater early decrease in K^{trans} correlated with increased progression-free survival post-antiangiogenic treatment.[61,86] Beppu and colleagues detected a reduction in rCBF up to 4 weeks after initiating bevacizumab followed by a rapid increase between 4 and 8 weeks which corresponded with an increase in tumor volume.[85] Therefore, the RANO working group recommended that the reduced enhancement should persist for at least 4 weeks before considering it a true antiangiogenic response.[87]

SUMMARY

MR perfusion imaging is useful to make clinical decisions in the diagnosis, management, and follow up of patients with gliomas. In our experience, multiparametric MR perfusion imaging improves on the proper identification of glioma recurrence or progression from treatment-related changes as compared with using a single MR perfusion technique.

DISCLOSURE

The authors have nothing to disclose.

REFERENCES

1. Miller KD, Ostrom QT, Kruchko C, et al. Brain and other central nervous system tumor statistics, 2021. CA Cancer J Clin 2021;71(5):381–406 [published Online First: 20210824].
2. Brown NF, Ottaviani D, Tazare J, et al. Survival Outcomes and Prognostic Factors in Glioblastoma. Cancers 2022;14(13). https://doi.org/10.3390/cancers14133161 [published Online First: 20220628].
3. Tan AC, Ashley DM, López GY, et al. Management of glioblastoma: State of the art and future directions. CA A Cancer J Clin 2020;70(4):299–312.
4. von Baumgarten L, Illerhaus G, Korfel A, et al. The Diagnosis and Treatment of Primary CNS Lymphoma. Dtsch Arztebl Int 2018;115(25):419–26.
5. van Dijken BRJ, van Laar PJ, Smits M, et al. Perfusion MRI in treatment evaluation of glioblastomas: Clinical relevance of current and future techniques. J Magn Reson Imaging 2019;49(1):11–22.
6. Gaudino S, Benenati M, Martucci M, et al. Investigating dynamic susceptibility contrast-enhanced perfusion-weighted magnetic resonance imaging in posterior fossa tumors: differences and similarities with supratentorial tumors. Radiol Med 2020;125(4):416–22 [published Online First: 20200108].
7. Kimura M, da Cruz LCH Jr. Multiparametric MR Imaging in the Assessment of Brain Tumors. Magn Reson Imaging Clin N Am 2016;24(1):87–122.
8. Ahn SH, Ahn SS, Park YW, et al. Association of dynamic susceptibility contrast- and dynamic contrast-enhanced magnetic resonance imaging parameters with molecular marker status in lower-grade gliomas: A retrospective study. NeuroRadiol J 2023;36(1):49–58 [published Online First: 20220509].
9. Bell LC, Stokes AM, Quarles CC. Analysis of postprocessing steps for residue function dependent dynamic susceptibility contrast (DSC)-MRI biomarkers and their clinical impact on glioma grading for both 1.5 and 3T. J Magn Reson Imaging 2020;51(2):547–53 [published Online First: 20190617].
10. Hirschler L, Sollmann N, Schmitz-Abecassis B, et al. Advanced MR Techniques for Preoperative Glioma Characterization: Part 1. J Magn Reson Imaging 2023;57(6):1655–75 [published Online First: 20230303].
11. Nael K, Bauer AH, Hormigo A, et al. Multiparametric MRI for Differentiation of Radiation Necrosis From Recurrent Tumor in Patients With Treated Glioblastoma. AJR Am J Roentgenol 2018;210(1):18–23 [published Online First: 20170927].
12. Bonm AV, Ritterbusch R, Throckmorton P, et al. Clinical Imaging for Diagnostic Challenges in the Management of Gliomas: A Review. J Neuroimaging 2020;30(2):139–45 [published Online First: 2020 0110].
13. Choi YJ, Kim HS, Jahng GH, et al. Pseudoprogression in patients with glioblastoma: added value of arterial spin labeling to dynamic susceptibility contrast perfusion MR imaging. Acta Radiol 2013;54(4):448–54 [published Online First: 20130430].
14. Batchelor TT, Sorensen AG, di Tomaso E, et al. AZD2171, a pan-VEGF receptor tyrosine kinase inhibitor, normalizes tumor vasculature and alleviates edema in glioblastoma patients. Cancer Cell 2007;11(1):83–95.
15. Ly KI, Gerstner ER. The Role of Advanced Brain Tumor Imaging in the Care of Patients with Central Nervous System Malignancies. Curr Treat Options Oncol 2018;19(8):40 [published Online First: 20180621].
16. Suh CH, Kim HS, Jung SC, et al. Perfusion MRI as a diagnostic biomarker for differentiating glioma from brain metastasis: a systematic review and meta-analysis. Eur Radiol 2018;28(9):3819–31.
17. Blasel S, Jurcoane A, Franz K, et al. Elevated peritumoural rCBV values as a mean to differentiate metastases from high-grade gliomas. Acta Neurochir 2010;152(11):1893–9.

18. Tong E, McCullagh KL, Iv M. Advanced Imaging of Brain Metastases: From Augmenting Visualization and Improving Diagnosis to Evaluating Treatment Response. Front Neurol 2020;11:270 [published Online First: 20200415].

19. Lin L, Xue Y, Duan Q, et al. The role of cerebral blood flow gradient in peritumoral edema for differentiation of glioblastomas from solitary metastatic lesions. Oncotarget 2016;7(42):69051–9.

20. Tupy R, Mirka H, Mracek J, et al. Tumor-related Perfusion Changes in White Matter Adjacent to Brain Tumors: Pharmacodynamic Analysis of Dynamic 3T Magnetic Resonance Imaging. Anticancer Res 2018;38(7):4149–52.

21. Bauer AH, Erly W, Moser FG, et al. Differentiation of solitary brain metastasis from glioblastoma multiforme: a predictive multiparametric approach using combined MR diffusion and perfusion. Neuroradiology 2015;57(7):697–703.

22. Artzi M, Liberman G, Blumenthal DT, et al. Differentiation between vasogenic edema and infiltrative tumor in patients with high-grade gliomas using texture patch-based analysis. J Magn Reson Imaging 2018. https://doi.org/10.1002/jmri.25939 [published Online First: 20180103].

23. Heynold E, Zimmermann M, Hore N, et al. Physiological MRI Biomarkers in the Differentiation Between Glioblastomas and Solitary Brain Metastases. Mol Imaging Biol 2021;23(5):787–95 [published Online First: 20210423].

24. Arsiwala TA, Sprowls SA, Blethen KE, et al. Ultrasound-mediated disruption of the blood tumor barrier for improved therapeutic delivery. Neoplasia 2021;23(7):676–91.

25. Chaganti J, Taylor M, Woodford H, et al. Differentiation of Primary Central Nervous System Lymphoma and High-Grade Glioma with Dynamic Susceptibility Contrast-Derived Metrics: Pilot Study. World Neurosurg 2021;151:e979–87 [published Online First: 20210518].

26. Guida L, Stumpo V, Bellomo J, et al. Hemodynamic Imaging in Cerebral Diffuse Glioma-Part A: Concept, Differential Diagnosis and Tumor Grading. Cancers 2022;14(6). https://doi.org/10.3390/cancers14061432 [published Online First: 20220310].

27. Makino K, Hirai T, Nakamura H, et al. Differentiating Between Primary Central Nervous System Lymphomas and Glioblastomas: Combined Use of Perfusion-Weighted and Diffusion-Weighted Magnetic Resonance Imaging. World Neurosurg 2018;112:e1–6 [published Online First: 20180213].

28. Kang KM, Choi SH, Chul-Kee P, et al. Differentiation between glioblastoma and primary CNS lymphoma: application of DCE-MRI parameters based on arterial input function obtained from DSC-MRI. Eur Radiol 2021;31(12):9098–109 [published Online First: 20210518].

29. Xi YB, Kang XW, Wang N, et al. Differentiation of primary central nervous system lymphoma from high-grade glioma and brain metastasis using arterial spin labeling and dynamic contrast-enhanced magnetic resonance imaging. Eur J Radiol 2019;112:59–64 [published Online First: 20190108].

30. Lu S, Wang S, Gao Q, et al. Quantitative Evaluation of Diffusion and Dynamic Contrast-Enhanced Magnetic Resonance Imaging for Differentiation Between Primary Central Nervous System Lymphoma and Glioblastoma. J Comput Assist Tomogr 2017;41(6):898–903.

31. Suh CH, Kim HS, Jung SC, et al. MRI as a diagnostic biomarker for differentiating primary central nervous system lymphoma from glioblastoma: A systematic review and meta-analysis. J Magn Reson Imaging 2019;50(2):560–72 [published Online First: 20190114].

32. Haris M, Gupta RK, Singh A, et al. Differentiation of infective from neoplastic brain lesions by dynamic contrast-enhanced MRI. Neuroradiology 2008;50(6):531–40.

33. Hakyemez B, Erdogan C, Bolca N, et al. Evaluation of different cerebral mass lesions by perfusion-weighted MR imaging. J Magn Reson Imaging 2006;24(4):817–24.

34. Zhang HW, Lyu GW, He WJ, et al. DSC and DCE Histogram Analyses of Glioma Biomarkers, Including IDH, MGMT, and TERT, on Differentiation and Survival. Acad Radiol 2020;27(12):e263–71 [published Online First: 20200123].

35. Wu H, Tong H, Du X, et al. Vascular habitat analysis based on dynamic susceptibility contrast perfusion MRI predicts IDH mutation status and prognosis in high-grade gliomas. Eur Radiol 2020;30(6):3254–65 [published Online First: 20200220].

36. Kilincer A, Cebeci H, Seher N, et al. Can Dynamic Susceptibility Contrast Perfusion Imaging be Utilized to Detect Isocitrate Dehydrogenase Gene Mutation in Gliomas? Turk Neurosurg 2022;32(5):826–33.

37. Hempel J-M, Schittenhelm J, Klose U, et al. In Vivo Molecular Profiling of Human Glioma. Clin Neuroradiol 2019;29(3):479–91.

38. Brendle C, Hempel JM, Schittenhelm J, et al. Glioma Grading and Determination of IDH Mutation Status and ATRX loss by DCE and ASL Perfusion. Clin Neuroradiol 2018;28(3):421–8 [published Online First: 20170509].

39. Hou H, Chen W, Diao Y, et al. 3D Amide Proton Transfer-Weighted Imaging for Grading Glioma and Correlating IDH Mutation Status: Added Value to 3D Pseudocontinuous Arterial Spin Labelling Perfusion. Mol Imaging Biol 2023;25(2):343–52 [published Online First: 20220812].

40. Hu Y, Chen Y, Wang J, et al. Non-Invasive Estimation of Glioma IDH1 Mutation and VEGF Expression by Histogram Analysis of Dynamic Contrast-Enhanced

MRI. Front Oncol 2020;10:593102 [published Online First: 20201208].

41. Park YW, Ahn SS, Park CJ, et al. Diffusion and perfusion MRI may predict EGFR amplification and the TERT promoter mutation status of IDH-wildtype lower-grade gliomas. Eur Radiol 2020;30(12):6475–84 [published Online First: 20200812].

42. Ivanidze J, Lum M, Pisapia D, et al. MRI Features Associated with TERT Promoter Mutation Status in Glioblastoma. J Neuroimaging 2019;29(3):357–63.

43. Akbari H, Bakas S, Pisapia JM, et al. In vivo evaluation of EGFRvIII mutation in primary glioblastoma patients via complex multiparametric MRI signature. Neuro Oncol 2018;20(8):1068–79.

44. Arevalo-Perez J, Thomas AA, Kaley T, et al. T1-Weighted Dynamic Contrast-Enhanced MRI as a Noninvasive Biomarker of Epidermal Growth Factor Receptor vIII Status. AJNR Am J Neuroradiol 2015;36(12):2256–61 [published Online First: 20150903].

45. Stumpo V, Guida L, Bellomo J, et al. Hemodynamic Imaging in Cerebral Diffuse Glioma-Part B: Molecular Correlates, Treatment Effect Monitoring, Prognosis, and Future Directions. Cancers 2022;14(5). https://doi.org/10.3390/cancers14051342 [published Online First: 20220305].

46. Han Y, Yan LF, Wang XB, et al. Structural and advanced imaging in predicting MGMT promoter methylation of primary glioblastoma: a region of interest based analysis. BMC Cancer 2018;18(1):215 [published Online First: 20180221].

47. Lee MK, Park JE, Jo Y, et al. Advanced imaging parameters improve the prediction of diffuse lower-grade gliomas subtype, IDH mutant with no 1p19q codeletion: added value to the T2/FLAIR mismatch sign. Eur Radiol 2020;30(2):844–54.

48. Wang N, Xie S-y, Liu H-m, et al. Arterial Spin Labeling for Glioma Grade Discrimination: Correlations with IDI I1 Genotype and 1p/19q Status. Translational Oncology 2019;12(5):749–56.

49. Lee JY, Ahn KJ, Lee YS, et al. Differentiation of grade II and III oligodendrogliomas from grade II and III astrocytomas: a histogram analysis of perfusion parameters derived from dynamic contrast-enhanced (DCE) and dynamic susceptibility contrast (DSC) MRI. Acta Radiol 2018;59(6):723–31 [published Online First: 20170901].

50. Liang J, Liu D, Gao P, et al. Diagnostic Values of DCE-MRI and DSC-MRI for Differentiation Between High-grade and Low-grade Gliomas: A Comprehensive Meta-analysis. Acad Radiol 2018;25(3):338–48 [published Online First: 20171206].

51. Soliman RK, Gamal SA, Essa AA, et al. Preoperative Grading of Glioma Using Dynamic Susceptibility Contrast MRI: Relative Cerebral Blood Volume Analysis of Intra-tumoural and Peri-tumoural Tissue. Clin Neurol Neurosurg 2018;167:86–92 [published Online First: 20180108].

52. Daboudi M, Papadaki E, Vakis A, et al. Brain SPECT and perfusion MRI: do they provide complementary information about the tumour lesion and its grading? Clin Radiol 2019;74(8):652.e1.

53. Ma H, Wang Z, Xu K, et al. Three-dimensional arterial spin labeling imaging and dynamic susceptibility contrast perfusion-weighted imaging value in diagnosing glioma grade prior to surgery. Exp Ther Med 2017;13(6):2691–8 [published Online First: 20170420].

54. ElBeheiry AA, Emara DM, Abdel-Latif AA-B, et al. Arterial spin labeling in the grading of brain gliomas: could it help? Egyptian Journal of Radiology and Nuclear Medicine 2020;51(1):235.

55. Jiang JS, Hua Y, Zhou XJ, et al. Quantitative Assessment of Tumor Cell Proliferation in Brain Gliomas with Dynamic Contrast-Enhanced MRI. Acad Radiol 2019;26(9):1215–21 [published Online First: 20181108].

56. Zhao M, Guo LL, Huang N, et al. Quantitative analysis of permeability for glioma grading using dynamic contrast-enhanced magnetic resonance imaging. Oncol Lett 2017;14(5):5418–26 [published Online First: 20170906].

57. Kim R, Choi SH, Yun TJ, et al. Prognosis prediction of non-enhancing T2 high signal intensity lesions in glioblastoma patients after standard treatment: application of dynamic contrast-enhanced MR imaging. Eur Radiol 2017;27(3):1176–85 [published Online First: 20160629].

58. Na A, Haghigi N, Drummond KJ. Cerebral radiation necrosis. Asia Pac J Clin Oncol 2014;10(1):11–21 [published Online First: 20131031].

59. Donovan EK, Parpia S, Greenspoon JN. Incidence of radionecrosis in single-fraction radiosurgery compared with fractionated radiotherapy in the treatment of brain metastasis. Curr Oncol 2019;26(3):e328–33 [published Online First: 20190601].

60. Mamlouk MD, Handwerker J, Ospina J, et al. Neuroimaging findings of the post-treatment effects of radiation and chemotherapy of malignant primary glial neoplasms. NeuroRadiol J 2013;26(4):396–412 [published Online First: 20130827].

61. Fatterpekar GM, Galheigo D, Narayana A, et al. Treatment-related change versus tumor recurrence in high-grade gliomas: a diagnostic conundrum–use of dynamic susceptibility contrast-enhanced (DSC) perfusion MRI. AJR Am J Roentgenol 2012;198(1):19–26.

62. Xu Q, Liu Q, Ge H, et al. Tumor recurrence versus treatment effects in glioma: A comparative study of three dimensional pseudo-continuous arterial spin labeling and dynamic susceptibility contrast imaging. Medicine (Baltim) 2017;96(50):e9332.

63. Kuo F, Ng NN, Nagpal S, et al. DSC Perfusion MRI-Derived Fractional Tumor Burden and Relative CBV Differentiate Tumor Progression and Radiation

Necrosis in Brain Metastases Treated with Stereo-tactic Radiosurgery. AJNR Am J Neuroradiol 2022; 43(5):689–95 [published Online First: 20220428].

64. Wang YL, Chen S, Xiao HF, et al. Differentiation be-tween radiation-induced brain injury and glioma recurrence using 3D pCASL and dynamic suscepti-bility contrast-enhanced perfusion-weighted imag-ing. Radiother Oncol 2018;129(1):68–74 [published Online First: 20180202].

65. Liu J, Li C, Chen Y, et al. Diagnostic performance of multiparametric MRI in the evaluation of treatment response in glioma patients at 3T. J Magn Reson Im-aging 2020;51(4):1154–61 [published Online First: 20190820].

66. Hou H, Diao Y, Yu J, et al. Differentiation of true pro-gression from treatment response in high-grade gli-oma treated with chemoradiation: a comparison study of 3D-APTW and 3D-PcASL imaging and DWI. NMR Biomed 2023;36(1):e4821 [published Online First: 20220917].

67. Park JE, Kim JY, Kim HS, et al. Comparison of Dy-namic Contrast-Enhancement Parameters between Gadobutrol and Gadoterate Meglumine in Posttreat-ment Glioma: A Prospective Intraindividual Study. AJNR Am J Neuroradiol 2020;41(11):2041–8 [pub-lished Online First: 20201015].

68. Bisdas S, Naegele T, Ritz R, et al. Distinguishing recurrent high-grade gliomas from radiation injury: a pilot study using dynamic contrast-enhanced MR imaging. Acad Radiol 2011;18(5):575–83 [published Online First: 20110321].

69. Wang L, Wei L, Wang J, et al. Evaluation of perfusion MRI value for tumor progression assessment after glioma radiotherapy: A systematic review and meta-analysis. Medicine (Baltim) 2020;99(52): e23766.

70. Morabito R, Alafaci C, Pergolizzi S, et al. DCE and DSC perfusion MRI diagnostic accuracy in the follow-up of primary and metastatic intra-axial brain tumors treated by radiosurgery with cyberknife. Ra-diat Oncol 2019;14(1):65 [published Online First: 20190415].

71. Brandsma D, Stalpers L, Taal W, et al. Clinical fea-tures, mechanisms, and management of pseudo-progression in malignant gliomas. Lancet Oncol 2008;9(5):453–61.

72. Brandes AA, Franceschi E, Tosoni A, et al. MGMT promoter methylation status can predict the inci-dence and outcome of pseudoprogression after concomitant radiochemotherapy in newly diag-nosed glioblastoma patients. J Clin Oncol 2008; 26(13):2192–7.

73. Thust SC, van den Bent MJ, Smits M. Pseudoprogres-sion of brain tumors. J Magn Reson Imaging 2018; 48(3):571–89 [published Online First: 20180507].

74. Shi W, Qu C, Wang X, et al. Diffusion kurtosis imaging combined with dynamic susceptibility contrast-enhanced MRI in differentiating high-grade glioma recurrence from pseudoprogression. Eur J Radiol 2021;144:109941 [published Online First: 20210831].

75. Gahramanov S, Muldoon LL, Varallyay CG, et al. Pseudoprogression of glioblastoma after chemo- and radiation therapy: diagnosis by using dynamic susceptibility-weighted contrast-enhanced perfu-sion MR imaging with ferumoxytol versus gadoteri-dol and correlation with survival. Radiology 2013; 266(3):842–52 [published Online First: 20121130].

76. Kim M, Park JE, Emblem K, et al. Vessel Type Deter-mined by Vessel Architectural Imaging Improves Dif-ferentiation between Early Tumor Progression and Pseudoprogression in Glioblastoma. AJNR Am J Neuroradiol 2021;42(4):663–70 [published Online First: 20210204].

77. Le Fevre C, Constans JM, Chambrelant I, et al. Pseudoprogression versus true progression in glio-blastoma patients: A multiapproach literature review. Part 2 - Radiological features and metric markers. Crit Rev Oncol Hematol 2021;159:103230 [pub-lished Online First: 20210127].

78. Jovanovic M, Radenkovic S, Stosic-Opincal T, et al. Differentiation between progression and pseudo-progresion by arterial spin labeling MRI in patients with glioblastoma multiforme. J buon 2017;22(4): 1061–7.

79. Thomas AA, Arevalo-Perez J, Kaley T, et al. Dynamic contrast enhanced T1 MRI perfusion differentiates pseudoprogression from recurrent glioblastoma. J Neuro Oncol 2015;125(1):183–90.

80. Jing H, Yan X, Li J, et al. The Value of Dynamic Contrast-Enhanced Magnetic Resonance Imaging (DCE-MRI) in the Differentiation of Pseudoprogres-sion and Recurrence of Intracranial Gliomas. Contrast Media Mol Imaging 2022;2022:5680522 [published Online First: 20220722].

81. Yun TJ, Park CK, Kim TM, et al. Glioblastoma treated with concurrent radiation therapy and temozolomide chemotherapy: differentiation of true progression from pseudoprogression with quantitative dynamic contrast-enhanced MR imaging. Radiology 2015; 274(3):830–40 [published Online First: 20141021].

82. Song J, Kadaba P, Kravitz A, et al. Multiparametric MRI for early identification of therapeutic response in recurrent glioblastoma treated with immune check-point inhibitors. Neuro Oncol 2020;22(11):1658–66.

83. Norden AD, Young GS, Setayesh K, et al. Bevacizu-mab for recurrent malignant gliomas: efficacy, toxicity, and patterns of recurrence. Neurology 2008;70(10):779–87.

84. Choi SH, Jung SC, Kim KW, et al. Perfusion MRI as the predictive/prognostic and pharmacodynamic biomarkers in recurrent malignant glioma treated with bevacizumab: a systematic review and a time-to-event meta-analysis. J Neuro Oncol 2016; 128(2):185–94 [published Online First: 20160423].

85. Beppu T, Sato Y, Sasaki T, et al. Comparisons Between PET With 11C-Methyl-l-Methionine and Arterial Spin Labeling Perfusion Imaging in Recurrent Glioblastomas Treated With Bevacizumab. Clin Nucl Med 2019;44(3):186–93.

86. Sorensen AG, Batchelor TT, Zhang WT, et al. A "vascular normalization index" as potential mechanistic biomarker to predict survival after a single dose of cediranib in recurrent glioblastoma patients. Cancer Res 2009;69(13):5296–300 [published Online First: 20090623].

87. Wen PY, Chang SM, Van den Bent MJ, et al. Response Assessment in Neuro-Oncology Clinical Trials. J Clin Oncol 2017;35(21):2439–49 [published Online First: 20170622].

Clinical Interpretation of Intravoxel Incoherent Motion Perfusion Imaging in the Brain

Christian Federau, MD, MSc[a,b,*]

KEYWORDS

- Intravoxel incoherent motion • IVIM • Perfusion • Imaging • MR imaging

KEY POINTS

- Intravoxel incoherent motion, IVIM, perfusion imaging extracts information of blood motion in biological tissue from diffusion-weighted MR images.
- IVIM measures local perfusion in a quantitative manner and does not require the injection of an intravenous contras agent.
- Currently, the clinical interpretation of IVIM perfusion maps should be predominantly done on the IVIM perfusion fraction maps.
- Improvements in image quality of the IVIM pseudo-diffusion maps, using advanced postprocessing tools involving artificial intelligence, could provide additional local perfusion information in the clinical setting, not otherwise available with other perfusion techniques.
- D* maps should be interpreted with caution in tissue with low perfusion, because D* would be the pseudo-diffusion coefficient of an "empty compartment," and is therefore not properly defined.
- Partial volume effects between brain parenchyma and the cerebrospinal fluid compartment and turbulence within the cerebrospinal fluid compartment might lead to "artefactually increased perfusion fraction."

INTRODUCTION

Magnetic resonance diffusion-weighted signal measures the relative loss of signal in the tissue due to the incoherent motion of water molecules.[1] At high b-values, those incoherent motions occur are mostly occurring due to by thermal diffusion, but at low b-value below 200 s/mm^2, a measurable portion occurs due to blood motion inside the vascular bed, mainly in the smaller vessels and the capillaries.[2] Intravoxel incoherent motion (IVIM) is a mathematical method that uses, in its original and most applied form, a bi-exponential signal equation model to distinguish the microcirculatory effects from the thermal diffusion effects. The various IVIM perfusion parameters are obtained by fitting the signal equation model to the measured signal at various b-values, wherein usually half of them is obtained at values below 200 s/mm^2. Although the standard approach to process the IVIM signal involves a two-step segmented approach, several algorithms have been proposed to improve the IVIM parameter estimation quality, including Bayesian inference algorithms[3,4] and deep learning strategies.[5,6] Simplified methods[7,8] and models combining IVIM and diffusion tensor imaging have been proposed.[9,10]

In the last decade, a large body of evidence has been published, which demonstrates the feasibility of IVIM perfusion imaging. This includes theoretic calculations, phantoms studies, ex vivo studies, correlation with histology, correlation with physiologically and pharmaceutically induced perfusion state changes, correlation with standard perfusion

a AI Medical AG, Goldhaldenstr 22a, Zollikon 8702, Switzerland; b University of Zürich, Zürich, Switzerland
* AI Medical AG, Zollikon, Switzerland.
E-mail address: christian@ai-medical.ch

Magn Reson Imaging Clin N Am 32 (2024) 85–92
https://doi.org/10.1016/j.mric.2023.07.002
1064-9689/24/© 2023 Elsevier Inc. All rights reserved.

parameters, and demonstration of clinical applicability.[11] The main domain of clinical application of IVIM is oncology,[12] where IVIM can provide useful information on tumor microvascular structural and functional abnormality. In neurology, IVIM can be used to study cerebral perfusion changes at the microvascular level in various neurologic disorders, such as in diabetes,[13] small vessel disease,[14] stroke,[15] or for predicting cerebral hyperperfusion after carotid endarterectomy[16] IVIM found application in clinical setting where perfusion imaging is relevant, but contrast injection contraindicated, such as in placenta imaging,[17] for example, for discriminating intrauterine growth restriction,[18] and in kidney diseases, for example, to determine delayed graft functions in following kidney transplantation.[19] Overall, IVIM is a promising technique that has the potential to provide valuable insights into tissue microstructure and perfusion in various clinical settings. In this article, the author describes the IVIM parameters and their clinical meaning and reviews several known interpretation pitfalls.

UNDERSTANDING THE INTRAVOXEL INCOHERENT MOTION PERFUSION PARAMETERS IN NORMAL TISSUE

The IVIM parameters consist of the diffusion coefficient D and the IVIM perfusion parameters, which are the perfusion fraction f, the pseudo-diffusion coefficient D*, and the blood flow-related parameter fD*. It is important to understand that diffusion coefficient D is not equal to the thermal diffusion coefficient, but should rather be understood as the "perfusion-free apparent diffusion coefficient." The perfusion coefficient f can be interpreted as the portion of volume (more precisely of signal generating volume) of blood flowing incoherently in a given voxel. The pseudo-diffusion coefficient D* provides information on the speed of blood flow in the tissue, in a similar way that the diffusion coefficient D provides information on the speed of water molecules in the tissue. Note that D* also includes thermal motion of the blood constituents, but those can be considered negligible in most situations. Note that the information contained in D and D* should be differentiated for the ballistic speed but should rater be understood as the "mixing" speed of the particles under consideration. The blood flow-related parameter fD* as been shown, as its name indicates, to be related to blood flow. Of all three IVIM perfusion parameters, by far the most used in the clinical setting is the perfusion fraction f. The pseudo-diffusion coefficient D* maps are often very noisy, and the fD* maps do in our experience, seldomly provide additional information compared with the f maps, but its use has been relatively limited in the literature.[20]

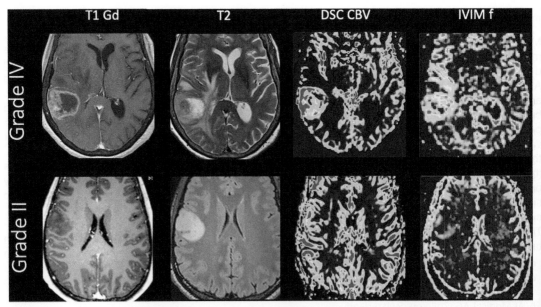

Fig. 1. Hyperperfusion due to neoangiogenesis is a well-known landmark of high-grade tumors compared with low grade. In this example, a hyperperfused ring can be easily seen on both DSC and IVIM in the high-grade tumor, whereas the low-grade tumor does not show any sign of hyperperfusion.

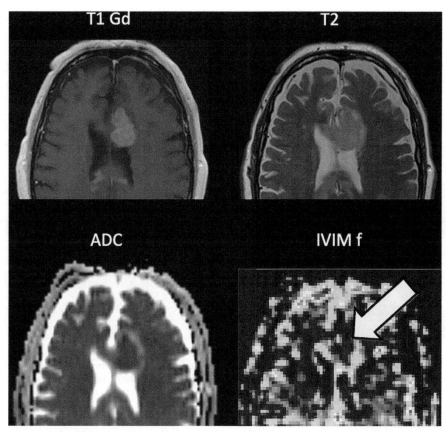

Fig. 2. Some cases of cerebral lymphoma might be difficult to differentiate from high-grade glioma. Perfusion imaging can be helpful to differential those two entities, as lymphoma is constituted of densely packed white blood cells, without any hyperperfusion due to neoangiogenesis as in high-grade glioma. In this case, the imaging findings of homogeneous contrast uptake, decreased apparent diffusion coefficient (ADC), and reduced IVIM perfusion fraction (*arrow*) were suggestive of lymphoma, which was confirmed on the biopsy.

UNDERSTANDING THE INTRAVOXEL INCOHERENT MOTION PERFUSION PARAMETERS IN PATHOLOGIC TISSUE
Oncology

Changes in blood flow characteristics are an important landmark of many tumors. Blood flow measurements can be used, for example, for tumor diagnosis, tumor grading, therapy monitoring, and prognosis assessment. Several antiangiogenic drugs were developed to control tumor growth by restricting the formation of new vessels. IVIM has been shown to provide relevant clinical perfusion information for grading brain glioma (**Fig. 1**),[21,22] differentiating high-grade glioma from lymphoma (**Fig. 2**),[23] monitoring treatment response,[24] and predicting survival and clinical outcome.[25–27]

Further, a particular and unique property of the IVIM perfusion method can be exploited and can shine in the context of oncology: its direct dependence on the underlying microvascular network architecture.[2] Therefore, it can be hypothesized that relevant perfusion information, not visible with other perfusion methods, could be revealed by IVIM, for example, early tumor recurrence (**Fig. 3**, see also **Fig. 6** in ref[23]), but insufficient knowledge on this topic is currently available and should be further investigated.

Stroke

The application of IVIM to stroke is more challenging compared with oncology, because the quality of the IVIM fit depends on the perfusion fraction.[28] D and f have been shown to be more robust in the context of low perfusion, compared with D*[29] In low-perfused tissue, D* maps should be interpreted with caution, because D* becomes the pseudo-diffusion coefficient of an "empty compartment," and is therefore not properly defined.

Consistent with the known pathophysiology of strokes, the perfusion fraction has been shown

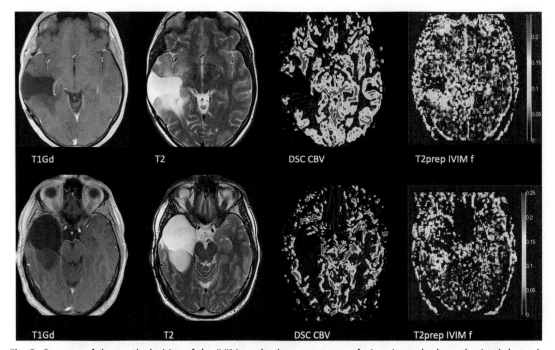

Fig. 3. Because of the particularities of the IVIM method to measure perfusion, it can be hypothesized that relevant perfusion information, not visible with other perfusion methods, could be revealed by IVIM. In those two cases, hyperperfusion suggestive of tumor recurrence was observed with IVIM but not DSC, in the posterior part of resection cavity of those high-grade glioma, suggestive of tumor recurrence.

to be reduced in the stroke core (**Fig. 4**).[30] Further, the fact that IVIM measures perfusion locally, that is, independently of speed and path of the blood flow to the tissue, is a particularly appealing property in the context of stroke. Indeed, this property could be of high value in assessing regions of presumed low collateral flow within the penumbra in hyperacute stroke.[31] In a preliminary study, within the penumbra of hyperacute stroke, regions with "visually evident penumbra perfusion lesions" were observed, which all converted to infarcted regions on follow-up imaging, regardless of thrombectomy treatment.[15] Therefore, IVIM has the

potential to refine the boundaries of the viability of penumbral tissue and improve selection criteria for successful revascularization treatment.[31] Finally, IVIM could be of clinical interest to confirm cerebral death, as it can demonstrate in such cases lack of cerebral perfusion with retained perfusion in the territory of the external carotid artery,[32] therefore excluding a technical deficiency in the intracerebral measurement.

Pearls and Pitfalls

When interpreting IVIM perfusion maps, it is important to keep in mind that there can be multiple

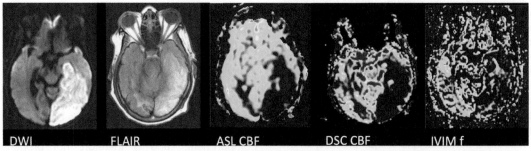

Fig. 4. Example of a large extensive stroke of the left-sided posterior cerebral artery. The hypoperfusion in the infarct core is clearly visible on the arterial spin labeling (ASL) CBF, dynamic susceptibility contrast (DSC) CBF, and IVIM f.

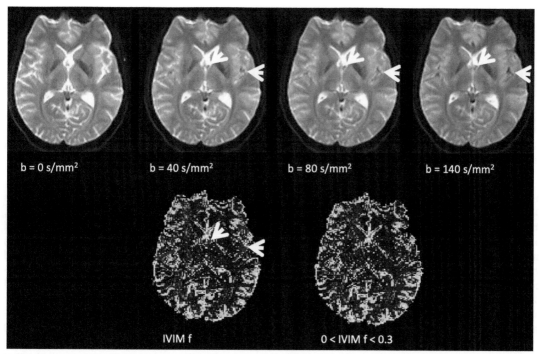

b = 0 s/mm²   b = 40 s/mm²   b = 80 s/mm²   b = 140 s/mm²

IVIM f   0 < IVIM f < 0.3

Fig. 5. Turbulence can lead to strong incoherent motions in the CSF, already visible at low values (*arrow* pointing at the Foramen of Monro and the Sylvian cistern). Those turbulences lead to artifactually very high "perfusion fraction" in the subarachnoidal and ventricular spaces, which can be removed by cropping the IVIM f maps between 0 and 0.3.

sources of incoherent motion in biological tissue. IVIM is sensitive to blood motion in all vessels within a voxel, not just capillaries. Various artifacts may also occur, such as partial volume effects and differences in relaxation times in different organs. In the brain, the cerebrospinal fluid is a particular source of artifacts on the IVIM perfusion maps.

First, turbulence in the CSF can lead to strong incoherent motions (**Fig. 5**), but of course those occur in the subarachnoidal and ventricular space and are therefore easily identifiable. Because those turbulence results in a very high f, much larger than any observed physiologic f in the brain parenchyma, the image can be made more

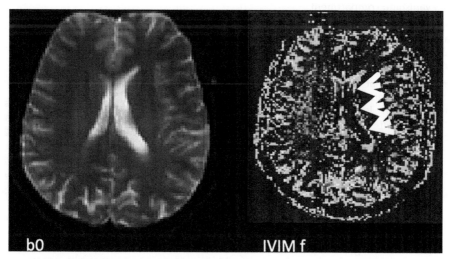

b0   IVIM f

Fig. 6. Partial volume effects at the border of the CSF compartment and the brain parenchyma (*arrows*) results in artifactually high perfusion fraction and should not be misinterpreted.

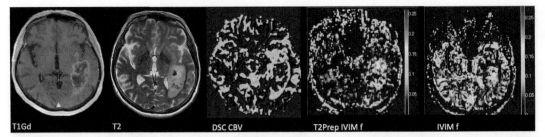

Fig. 7. CSF effects on the IVIM signal can be decreased using CSF attenuation pulses such as T2 prep IVIM, which can significantly increase the contrast of pathologies on the IVIM perfusion maps.

appealing by adding a cutoff for f, usually above 0.3 (see **Fig. 5**). Second, partial volume effects at the border of the CSF compartment and the brain parenchyma can result in artifactually high perfusion fraction, because of the contrast between the free diffusing water molecules of the CSF compartment and the restricted diffusion in the brain parenchyma (**Fig. 6**). Because of those cerebro-spinal fluid (CSF) effects on IVIM signal, the use of MR imaging sequences including CSF attenuation pulses has been suggested, to increase the contrast of the IVIM perfusion maps (**Fig. 7**). In particular, a T2 preparation (T2prep) pulse can be used to suppress the CSF signal while preserving a maximum the blood signal.[33] On the other side, IVIM can also be used for visualizing slow cerebrospinal fluid motion[34] and the glymphatic system.[35]

> **Pearls and pitfalls of clinical intravoxel incoherent motion perfusion imaging**
>
> In stroke, cerebral death or other low-perfused disease, one should avoid to interpret the D* maps, because D* is the pseudo-diffusion coefficient of a vanishing compartment.
>
> Partial volume effects between brain parenchyma and the cerebrospinal fluid compartment can lead to artifactually increased perfusion fraction.
>
> Turbulent cerebrospinal flow, in particular at the foramina of Monroe and in the depth of different sulci, can lead to "artefactually increased perfusion fraction," but can be easily interpreted through their anatomic localization.

DISCUSSION AND SUMMARY

The IVIM method is of interest to provide perfusion information in the clinical context of various pathologies. In general, the higher the perfusion fraction, the better the quality of the images. For this reason, the IVIM method is particularly adequate

for the evaluation of hyperperfused lesions, such as high-grade brain tumor, but as seen above, clinical application of IVIM in disease with reduced perfusion such as stroke and cerebral death is possible. Different properties of the IVIM method can be of higher relevance depending on the pathologies, such as the dependence of the IVIM signal on the structure of the microvascular network for high-grade brain tumor and the independence of the incoming flow for stroke. Several pitfalls should be remembered when reading cases with IVIM perfusion maps, in particular that partial volume with the CSF compartment can lead to artifactually high perfusion fraction and that in hypoperfused region, D* is not properly defined anymore and therefore should be interpreted with caution.

CONFLICTS OF INTEREST/COMPETING INTERESTS

C. Federau: Founder and CEO of AI Medical AG.

REFERENCES

1. Bihan DL, Iima M, Federau C, et al. Intravoxel Incoherent Motion (IVIM) MRI : Principles and Applications (online). Jenny Stanford Publishing; 2018. Accessed at: https://www.taylorfrancis.com/books/e/9780429427275. Accessed December 8, 2020.
2. Van VP, Schmid F, Spinner G, Kozerke S, Federau C. Simulation of intravoxel incoherent perfusion signal using a realistic capillary network of a mouse brain. NMR in Biomedicine (online serial). 2021;34. Accessed at: https://onlinelibrary.wiley.com/doi/10.1002/nbm.4528. Accessed March 24, 2023.
3. Spinner GR, Federau C, Kozerke S. Bayesian inference using hierarchical and spatial priors for intravoxel incoherent motion MR imaging in the brain: Analysis of cancer and acute stroke. Med Image Anal 2021;73:102144.
4. While PT. A comparative simulation study of Bayesian fitting approaches to intravoxel incoherent motion modeling in diffusion-weighted MRI:

Bayesian Fitting Approaches to IVIM Modeling in DWI. Magn Reson Med 2017;78:2373–87.

5. Kaandorp MPT, Zijlstra F, Federau C, While PT. Deep learning intravoxel incoherent motion modeling: Exploring the impact of training features and learning strategies. Magn Reson Med 2023;90(1):312–28.

6. Huang H-M. An unsupervised convolutional neural network method for estimation of intravoxel incoherent motion parameters. Phys Med Biol 2022;67: 215018.

7. Conklin J, Heyn C, Roux M, et al. A Simplified Model for Intravoxel Incoherent Motion Perfusion Imaging of the Brain. AJNR Am J Neuroradiol 2016;37: 2251–7.

8. Wang X, Cao M, Chen H, Ge J, Suo S, Zhou Y. Simplified Perfusion Fraction from Diffusion-Weighted Imaging in Preoperative Prediction of IDH1 Mutation in WHO Grade II–III Gliomas: Comparison with Dynamic Contrast-Enhanced and Intravoxel Incoherent Motion MRI. Radiology and Oncology (online serial). Sciendo; 2020;1. Accessed at: https://content.sciendo.com/view/journals/raon/ahead-of-print/article-10.2478-raon-2020-0037/article-10.2478-raon-2020-0037.xml. Accessed July 24, 2020.

9. Rauh SS, Maier O, Gurney-Champion OJ, et al. Model-based reconstructions for intravoxel incoherent motion and diffusion-tensor imaging parameter map estimations. NMR in Biomedicine (online serial). Epub 2023 Mar 18. Accessed at: https://onlinelibrary.wiley.com/doi/10.1002/nbm.4927. Accessed April 10, 2023.

10. Dietrich O, Cai M, Tuladhar AM, et al. Integrated intravoxel incoherent motion tensor and diffusion tensor brain MRI in a single fast acquisition. NMR in Biomedicine (online serial). Epub 2023 Feb 6. Accessed at: https://onlinelibrary.wiley.com/doi/10.1002/nbm.4905. Accessed April 10, 2023.

11. Federau C. Intravoxel incoherent motion MRI as a means to measure in vivo perfusion: A review of the evidence. NMR Biomed 2017;30.

12. Iima M. Perfusion-driven Intravoxel Incoherent Motion (IVIM) MRI in Oncology: Applications, Challenges, and Future Trends. MRMS 2021;20: 125–38.

13. van Bussel FC, Backes WH, Hofman PA, et al. On the interplay of microvasculature, parenchyma, and memory in type 2 diabetes. Diabetes Care 2015;38:876–82.

14. Wong SM, Zhang CE, van Bussel FCG, et al. Simultaneous investigation of microvasculature and parenchyma in cerebral small vessel disease using intravoxel incoherent motion imaging. Neuroimage 2017;14:216–21.

15. Federau C, Wintermark M, Christensen S, et al. Collateral blood flow measurement with intravoxel incoherent motion perfusion imaging in hyperacute brain stroke. Neurology 2019;92:e2462–71.

16. Takahashi T, Uwano I, Akamatsu Y, et al. Prediction of cerebral hyperperfusion following carotid endarterectomy using intravoxel incoherent motion magnetic resonance imaging. J Stroke Cerebrovasc Dis 2023;32:106909.

17. Jiang L, Sun T, Liao Y, et al. Probing the ballistic microcirculation in placenta using flow-compensated and non-compensated intravoxel incoherent motion imaging. Magn Reson Med 2021;85: 404–12.

18. Antonelli A, Capuani S, Ercolani G, et al. Human placental microperfusion and microstructural assessment by intra-voxel incoherent motion MRI for discriminating intrauterine growth restriction: a pilot study. J Matern Fetal Neonatal Med 2022;35: 9667–74.

19. Hashim E, Yuen DA, Kirpalani A. Reduced Flow in Delayed Graft Function as Assessed by IVIM Is Associated With Time to Recovery Following Kidney Transplantation. J Magn Reson Imag 2021;53: 108–17.

20. Federau C, O'Brien K, Birbaumer A, et al. Functional mapping of the human visual cortex with intravoxel incoherent motion MRI. PLoS One 2015;10: e0117706.

21. Federau C, Meuli R, O'Brien K, et al. Perfusion measurement in brain gliomas with intravoxel incoherent motion MRI. AJNR Am J Neuroradiol 2014;35: 256–62.

22. Togao O, Hiwatashi A, Yamashita K, et al. Differentiation of high-grade and low-grade diffuse gliomas by intravoxel incoherent motion MR imaging. Neuro Oncol 2016;18:132–41.

23. Federau C. Measuring Perfusion. Magn Reson Imag Clin N Am 2021;29:233–42.

24. Guo Y, Dai G, Xiong X, et al. Intravoxel incoherent motion radiomics nomogram for predicting tumor treatment responses in nasopharyngeal carcinoma. Translational Oncology 2023;31:101648.

25. Xia X, Wen L, Zhou F, et al. Predictive value of DCE-MRI and IVIM-DWI in osteosarcoma patients with neoadjuvant chemotherapy. Front Oncol 2022;12: 967450.

26. Puig J, Sánchez-González J, Blasco G, et al. Intravoxel Incoherent Motion Metrics as Potential Biomarkers for Survival in Glioblastoma. PLoS One 2016;11:e0158887.

27. Federau C, Cerny M, Roux M, et al. IVIM perfusion fraction is prognostic for survival in brain glioma. Clin Neuroradiol 2017;27:485–92.

28. Merisaari H, Federau C. Signal to noise and b-value analysis for optimal intra-voxel incoherent motion imaging in the brain. In: Vegh V, editor. PLoS One 2021;16:e0257545.

29. Meeus EM, Novak J, Withey SB, et al. Evaluation of intravoxel incoherent motion fitting methods in low-perfused tissue. J Magn Reson Imag 2017;45: 1325–34.

30. Federau C, Sumer S, Becce F, et al. Intravoxel incoherent motion perfusion imaging in acute stroke: initial clinical experience. Neuroradiology 2014;56: 629–35.

31. McKinley R, Marshall R. Advanced MRI in acute stroke: Is the whole penumbra salvageable? Neurology 2019;92:983–4.

32. Federau C, Nguyen A, Christensen S, et al. Cerebral perfusion measurement in brain death with intravoxel incoherent motion imaging. Neurovasc Imaging 2016;2:9.

33. Federau C, O'Brien K. Increased brain perfusion contrast with T_2-prepared intravoxel incoherent motion (T2prep IVIM) MRI. NMR Biomed 2015;28: 9–16.

34. Yamada S, Hiratsuka S, Otani T, et al. Usefulness of intravoxel incoherent motion MRI for visualizing slow cerebrospinal fluid motion. Fluids Barriers CNS 2023;20:16.

35. Gomolka RS, Hablitz LM, Mestre H, et al. Loss of aquaporin-4 results in glymphatic system dysfunction via brain-wide interstitial fluid stagnation. Elife 2023;12:e82232.

Cerebrovascular Reserve Imaging
Problems and Solutions

David J. Mikulis, MD, FRCP(C)

KEYWORDS

- Cerebrovascular disease • Cerebrovascular reactivity • Cerebral blood flow • MR perfusion imaging
- CT perfusion imaging

KEY POINTS

- A major function of the cerebral vasculature is to increase blood flow in support of the increased energy demand associated with neuronal signaling.
- Cerebrovascular reactivity (CVR) can measure blood flow augmentation, a valuable predictor of effective collateral blood and stroke risk in patients with steno-occlusive disease (SOD).
- Resting perfusion methods, commonly applied in patients with (SOD), have a limited ability to distinguish effective from ineffective collateral blood flow.
- Despite the high clinical potential for assessing cerebrovascular diseases, CVR is not a current standard of practice primarily due to a lack of standardization.
- A solution for standardizing CVR for clinical use is presented.

INTRODUCTION

The human brain with an estimated 80 to 100 billion neurons and approximately 1000 synaptic connections per neuron represents the pinnacle of biological complexity. If the neuronal networks were not complex enough, there are supporting glial and vascular networks that somehow must weave through the spatial confines of the neural net to provide the metabolic needs of the entire cellular assembly. Indeed, there are complex interactions between neuronal and nonneuronal elements that contribute to management of the tissue environment enabling optimal brain performance while managing valuable energy resources. From a blood flow perspective, the most relevant interactions are between the neurons, glial cells, and vascular cells with the latter including endothelial, smooth muscle, and contractile pericytes. These cells form the neuro-glio-vascular unit (NGVU). The NGVU became a crucial element in conserving cardiac output due to its ability to spatially regulate blood flow, a capability shared only by the skin. NGVU modulation of blood flow is tightly linked to the metabolic demand tuned to the spatial distribution of neural network activity. This avoids the need to increase blood flow to the entire brain when only aspecific neural networks become more active. The importance of local flow modulation may seem insignificant until the magnitude of brain blood flow changes in neural networks is considered. Because signaling within neural networks is associated with a threefold increase in energy demand,[1,2] the vasculature responds with increases in blood flow on the order of 50% over a resting baseline.[3,4] Somewhat surprisingly this flow increase is three times greater than the increase in oxygen consumption associated the increase in signaling.[3] As a result, there is a somewhat paradoxic increase in venous oxygen despite the increase in metabolic activity. This circulatory response will become important

The Krembil Brain Institute, Institute of Medcial Science, Department of Medical Imaging, The University of Toronto, The University Health Network, The Toronto Western Hospital, 399 Bathurst Street, Room 3MC-431, Toronto, ON M5T 2S8, Canada
E-mail address: David.Mikulis@uhn.ca

Magn Reson Imaging Clin N Am 32 (2024) 93–109
https://doi.org/10.1016/j.mric.2023.09.002
1064-9689/24/© 2023 Elsevier Inc. All rights reserved.

later in the discussion of MR imaging mapping of blood flow changes following vasodilatory stimuli.

A common theme in the evolution of a species is conservation of energy. Along these lines, humans are a striking example of the "energy premium" associated with the evolution of an energy hungry brain. Energy requirements drove significant changes in the body and brain during the transition from apex primates to sapiens concerning cardiac output, blood flow, skeletal muscle mass, and brain size. The higher energy demands of the larger human brain meant more work for the heart via increased cardiac output directed to the brain away from the rest of the body. Although the brain represents only 2% of body weight, it consumes up to 20% of the cardiac output.[5] It has been hypothesized therefore that a diversion of the cardiac output was necessary to support the enlarging brain requiring a compromise between skeletal muscle mass and brain size. Skeletal muscle decreased as brain size increased. We became smarter but weaker.

Another adaptation made by the growing brain, possibly to conserve space in a dense cellular network, was to sacrifice intracellular energy storage. Although glycogen is abundant in skeletal muscle, decreasing amounts are seen in the heart and brain. Although glycogen occupies approximately 2% of the cell volume in adult human cardiomyocytes,[6] its cerebral concentrations are so low that it is unlikely to act as a conventional energy reserve.[7] Although skeletal muscle can survive ischemic conditions up to 2 hours or more, the absence of cerebral energy stores severely limits brain survivability during ischemia. The often quoted "time is brain" concept concerns cerebral survivability during ischemic conditions underscoring the fact that the brain needs a constant source of glucose and oxygen provided by a healthy cervico-cerebral vascular system. "Brain is energy" is actually the central foundation of the homeostatic equation. Because there are limited energy stores in the brain, constant delivery of energy substrates by the vasculature is critical. An efficient distribution system that matches the metabolic needs within spatially distinct neural networks, which have highly variable energy requirements over time, is a necessity. A system such as this is exactly what has evolved, thereby conserving cardiac work. The system has contractile properties that manage vascular resistance and therefore blood flow along the entire course of the vascular tree from the level of the aortic arch (that contracts after closure of the aortic valve acting as a propulsive "second heart"), to the pericytes along capillaries.

Because there are numerous diseases that can impair the ability of the vasculature to provide an adequate source of cerebral blood flow (CBF) in the setting of acute and chronic disease conditions, assessing the ability of the vascular system to carry out this primary role in regulating blood flow would seem desirable. At issue is whether resting perfusion metrics, including blood flow, cerebral blood volume (CBV), mean transit time (MTT), time between the site of the measured arterial input function (AIF) and the peak tissue signal collaterals (Tmax), time from the tissue arrival of the bolus to the peak of the bolus signal time to peak (TTP), and blood arrival time, are adequate for this purpose. Or is a test of the ability of the vasculature to increase blood flow to a vasodilatory stimulus a more accurate measure? Somewhat surprisingly, the two different medical services, cardiology and neurology responsible for assessing circulations controlling blood flow in the most highly energetic human organs, are seemingly at odds with each other. Cardiology considers a vasodilatory stressor (cardiovascular reactivity known as "the cardiac stress test") essential for assessing disease within the coronary circulation. Neurology applies resting perfusion measurements instead of using a vasodilatory stressor for measuring cerebrovascular reactivity (CVR). Subsequently, widespread clinical application of the cardiac stress test has been adopted, but there has not been adoption of a "brain stress test." Part of the reason for this may be that cardiac research has benefited from a large number of clinical trials typically recruiting thousands of patients. From the neurology perspective, there are far fewer clinical trials recruiting fewer subjects. In fact, two of the most important and influential, but also controversial studies, one examining CVR,[8,9] and the other using oxygen extraction fraction,[10] disagreed on the clinical value of vascular dynamics. Although CVR research is increasing, it has not kept pace with research related to the cardiac stress test. A 2023 PubMed search revealed that there has been a slower rise in CVR publications compared with the cardiac stress test or even to that of already well-established CT scanning of the abdomen used as a control (**Fig. 1**).

The major theme of this article therefore examines resting cerebral perfusion metrics and CVR primarily for assessing the efficacy of collateral blood flow. A case will be made that application of resting perfusion metrics is effective for determining the presence of collateral blood flow but struggles to determine the *efficacy* of these collateral pathways especially as the degree and extent of steno-occlusive disease (SOD) increases. The concept of "effective collaterals" is based on the fundamental role of the vasculature to increase

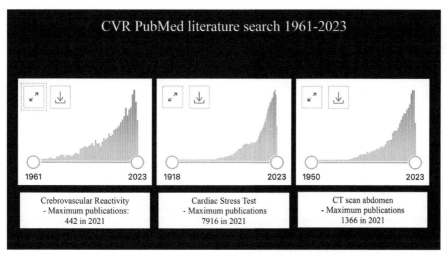

Fig. 1. PubMed literature search using search terms "Crebrovascular Reactivity," "Cardiac Stress Test," and "CT Acan Abdomen."

blood flow in response to increases in metabolic demand made possible by the ability of the cerebral vessels to dilate. CVR therefore is the critical element in the circulatory response for meeting increased metabolic demand.

CVR directly tests the ability of the vasculature to dilate but in doing so assumes that the average metabolic demand of the brain over time is relatively constant. Both CVR and resting perfusion metrics make this assumption. Issues concerning the major components of CVR testing including application of vasodilatory stimuli and mapping of associated blood flow changes will be thoroughly discussed. Ideally, the vasodilatory stimulus should only invoke action on the primary effector of the flow control system, which is vascular smooth muscle component of the NGVU, without influencing the other components. Finally, the potential value of CVR for assessing diseases other than stenoses of the major cerebral supply vessels will be discussed.

Regulation of Cerebral Blood Flow

CBF is regulated by altering the tone of vascular smooth muscle enabling control of vessel diameter and thereby flow resistance. There are, however, several incompletely understood mechanisms influencing arterial smooth muscle tone. The dominant mechanisms are blood pressure (BP), endogenous nitric oxide, glial cell modulators, and carbon dioxide (CO_2). Autoregulation relates to "reflex" changes in smooth muscle tone induced by mechanical stretching of smooth muscle as BP increases and modulates voltage-dependent Ca2+ channels.[11] Smooth muscle tone is also influenced by endothelial cells and neurons via release

endothelial nitric oxide synthase (eNOS) and neuronal nitric oxide synthase (nNOS) vasodilators. Glial cells release arachidonic acid (vasoconstrictor) and prostaglandins (vasodilators) depending on tissue levels of neurotransmitters, oxygen, pH, and metabolites.[12] CO_2 influences smooth muscle tone through its effect on regulation of intracellular hydrogen ion concentration.[13]

Cerebrovascular Reactivity

CVR can be quantified as the ratio between the changes in blood flow per unit change in an applied vasodilatory stimulus. The relationship follows a sigmoidal curve (**Fig. 2**).[13] Cerebrovascular reserve is defined as the amount of vasodilatory capacity or increase in vessel diameter that remains for a given level of blood flow. The first CVR report in humans was published by Kety and Schmidt in 1948 using a nitrous oxide method for measuring total CBF and carbon dioxide as the stimulus.[14] Since that time, there has been an exponential growth in publications reaching an annual high of 442 in 2021. The main driver of this increase may be the perception in the ischemic stroke community that for a given stenosis of a large supply artery, patients with hemodynamic impairment, that is, reduced CVR, have a higher risk of ischemic stroke. This has been well documented in the older CVR literature in **Table 1**.[15–18] Why then has CVR testing not entered the mainstream of clinical practice? There are three main reasons. The first is the relative simplicity of obtaining resting cerebral perfusion metrics using dynamic susceptibility contrast-enhanced MR imaging or dynamic contrast-enhanced CT. Both require a bolus of contrast

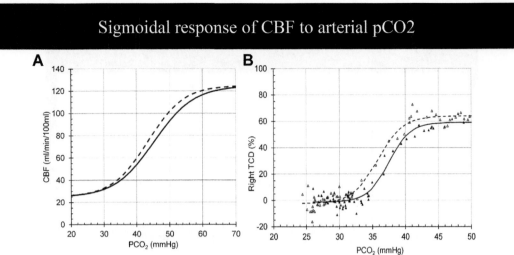

Fig. 2. CBF responses to P_{CO_2} to at P_{O_2} = 150 mm Hg (*solid line*) and P_{O_2} = 50 parentheses (*dashed line*). (*A*) Model response. (*B*) Example transcranial Doppler measurements of middle cerebral artery blood flow velocities.

with whole brain imaging with study durations of 90 seconds or less. The second reason is the lack of standardization of CVR testing. There are numerous ways to apply vasodilatory stimuli, and there are numerous ways to map blood flow changes. Unfortunately, the multiplicity of tools has resulted in inconsistency in CVR results. One of the more important inconsistencies is the fact that tissue blood flow responses in the setting of SOD will vary depending on the strength and/or duration of the stimulus yielding significant differences in the appearances of CVR maps (**Fig. 3**). The third reason is that CVR testing is more time-consuming compared with the time required to setup and then image a bolus of injected contrast. Finally, there is insufficient prospective clinical evidence supporting the added value of CVR over resting perfusion methods.

Cerebrovascular Reactivity Versus Resting Perfusion

Cerebral autoregulation can be global or local. The response to a drop in BP in a healthy individual is generalized relaxation of smooth muscle tone in all of the cerebral arteries that maintains resting

Table 1
The consequences of steal physiology

Author (journal)	CVR method	Subjects	Follow-up	Ischemic risk	Comment
Silvestrini (Jama 2000)	TCD breath-hold	94 prospective	28.5 mo	Annual risk TIA or stroke 3.4 higher	Asymptomatic carotid stenosis (≥70%)
Markus (Brain 2001)	TCD carbogen	107 prospective	21 mo	14.4 odds ratio TIA or stroke	Asymptomatic occlusion (3 mo) or ≥70% stenosis (2 y)
Blaser (Stroke 2002)	TCD carbogen	143 propsective	19 d	5.2 times higher risk of disabling stroke per month	Recent (0–92 d, median 10 d) ischemic event and 80–95% stenosis
Schoof (J of T&C Surgery 2007)	TCD carbogen	2797 prospective	Stroke post-cardiac surgery	28.3 odds ratio for stroke	If high grade stenosis ≥80%) or occlusion and decreased CVR present

See Reference section for complete documentation of listed studies

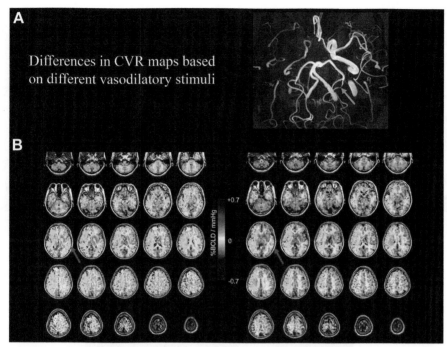

Fig. 3. CVR study with rapid (*left map*) and slow (*right*) map increases in CO2 each to 10 mmHg above resting baseline in 77 yo woman with atherosclerotic occlusion of the distal RICA and high-grade stenosis of left P2 branch (*blue arrow*). Yellow-red indicate increases in blood flow whereas blue indicates decrease in blood flow ("steal physiology"). Note differences in the left hemisphere (*red arrows*) depending on the nature of the stimulus.

perfusion. In an individual with SOD, there is a pressure drop across the lesion that invokes smooth muscle relaxation in the distal vasculature thus maintaining resting blood flow at normal or near normal levels. However, consumption of vasodilatory reserve has acute and chronic consequences. The acute consequence is that for a given stenosis, symptomatic patients with a significant loss of vascular reserve have a higher risk of permanent ischemic injury than those patients with a similar degree of stenosis who have retained vascular reserve—more commonly termed "hemodynamic" reserve (see **Table 1**). The chronic consequence is that normal augmentation of blood flow responses during neuronal activation are diminished to varying degrees depending on the degree to which vascular reserve has been consumed to maintain resting CBF. Under these circumstances, the blood flow increase in response to neural activity is reduced. The consequence of the reduced flow response in the absence of ictal events is the development cortical atrophy.[19,20] The adaptation of the cerebral circulation to SOD is variable. There is the ability to recruit collateral blood flow resources by amplification of existing collaterals or developing new vessels (angiogenesis). There is a substantial literature on collateral circulation; however, the major points relevant to this discussion are (1) the

compensatory status of preexisting collateral pathways and (2) and the time frame over which SOD disease develops. The presence of an effective preexisting circle of Willis network and/or preexisting connections between vascular territories over the pial surface can fully compensate even for an acute vascular occlusion. Acute balloon occlusion of large cerebral supply arteries has been used in settings where sacrifice of the supply artery is a treatment necessity, for example, in patients with traumatic carotid cavernous fistulae. Slowly progressive stenosis eventually leading to occlusion of a large supply artery can provide the time needed for development of new collateral vessels (angiogenesis) or development of increased capacity in existing. **Fig. 4** is an example of a patient who developed transient ischemic attacks (TIAs) from a sudden thrombotic internal carotid occlusion secondary to a stenosing atherosclerotic plaque. TIAs were thought to be hemodynamic in nature based on increased mean transit time (MTT) on CT perfusion. However, the TIAs were subsequently proved to be embolic based on the following points (1) the CVR map showed near normal hemodynamics, (2) the symptoms were alleviated via medical management alone (anticoagulation), and (3) MR imaging showed tiny embolic infarcts. The CVR changed patient management

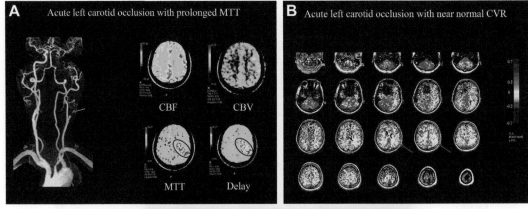

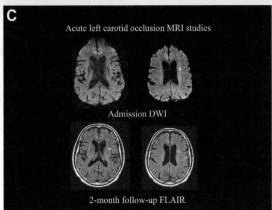

Fig. 4. (A) 76 yo patient seen in emergency room (ER) with regular episodes of right-sided facial droop, slurred speech, right sided arm and leg weakness, CTA indicated a left carotid occlusion (*red arrow*) with no string sign. CT perfusion map showed red areas involving left primary motor cortex indicating MTT > 4 sec compared to the remainder of the brain. Heparinization failed to control the TIAs and by-pass surgery was planned. (B) An urgent CVR study revealed near normal hemodynamic reserve (*red arrows*) indicating effective collaterals. The patient was managed conservatively. Symptoms persisted for 10 days and then stopped. The patient was subsequently discharged and continued asymptomatic at 2 month follow-up. Note the consistently higher CVR always seen in the cerebellum and brainstem. (C) MRI indicated only small areas of acute ischemic injury in the left hemisphere on admission with minimal progression on follow-up at 2 months.

(see **Fig. 4**). Importantly, MTT was not able to discern that the slow filling collaterals were actually effective.

Given sufficient time collateral circulation including neoangiogenesis can develop, however, the effectiveness of this collateralization can vary considerably. Resting perfusion imaging using boluses of intravenously administered contrast agents are the current standard of practice in symptomatic patients for testing the efficacy of collaterals in acute and chronic SOD.[21] However, an accurate measurement of blood flow metrics requires selection of an appropriate AIF for deconvolution with the tissue signal during bolus administration of a contrast agent. A significant problem with bolus perfusion methods is locating and measuring the AIF. Often the vessel with SOD is so narrowed or occluded that a reliable AIF cannot

be generated on this vessel, thus requiring selection of a healthy vessel elsewhere. Selection of a vessel that is not directly involved in perfusing the tissue of interest violates the model on which the deconvolution is based. Nevertheless, resting perfusion methods have dominated assessment of collaterals despite the fact that the three primary blood flow metrics, CBF, CBV, and MTT, have shown limited utility. However, a shift toward measurement of *timing* metrics such as TTP and Tmax has evolved.[21] Unfortunately, studies have shown mixed results when comparing one resting blood flow method against another such as CT perfusion against multiphase computed tomographic angiography (CTA) (**Figs. 5** and **6**).[22–24] Furthermore, the gold standard digital subtraction angiography (DSA) grading scale, adopted for use in clinical trials, also uses timing metrics based on the

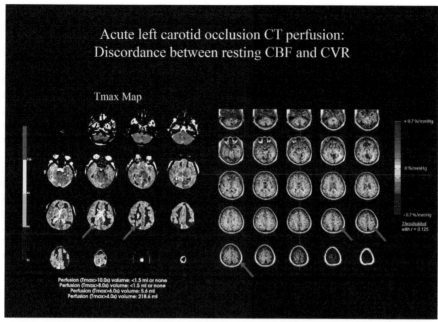

Fig. 5. Despite steal physiology in most of the left middle cerebral artery (MCA) territory (*red arrows right panel*), the longest Tmax values are in the right hemisphere (*red arrows left panel*).

subjective assessment of how quickly the cerebral vessels fill during direct arterial injection of contrast. A recent study assessing the performance of this scale was conducted using 30 pretreatment AP and lateral video loops chosen

from the THRACE randomized controlled trial study in patients with proximal cerebral artery occlusion.[25] These video loops were sent to 19 readers for assessment of collateral efficacy. The conclusion from the study was that "Concordance

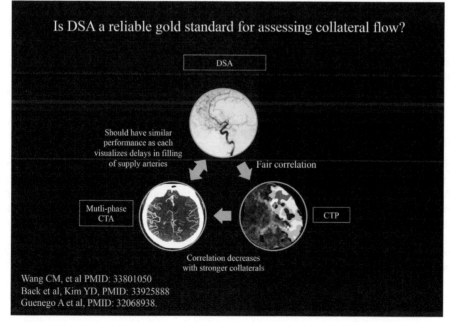

Fig. 6. DSA and CTA are subjective assessments prone to variance based on rater differences. CTP is objective and quantitative but has become dependent on timing metrics. By comparison, the fundamental flow metrics that compose the "Central Volume Principle" CBV = CBF × MTT have surprisingly shown limited clinical utility.

rates were poor among trained and experienced readers, and not improved by pre-test training or dichotomized grading." This research study revealed *"important limitations"* for collateral flow assessment within the definition of the American Society of Interventional and Therapeutic Radiology/Society of Interventional Radiology (ASITN/SIR) scale. In summary, it would seem that there are significant limitations in the use of timing metrics for the evaluation of collateral efficacy. It is sensible therefore, to consider that a better solution to this dilemma, is to show the ability of blood flow to increase when challenged by a vasodilatory stimulus as this is the normal vascular response to the metabolic requirement of highly energetic tissue. Increases in blood flow approaching 50% over baseline have been documented during activation of the cerebral cortex indicating the importance of flow augmentation in active neural networks.[3,4] From a metabolic perspective, it is interesting to note that not all of the blood flow increase is necessarily accounted for by increased oxygen utilization, which only increases by approximately 15% over baseline during neuronal activation.[3] Theories for this considerable increase in flow therefore include additional factors such as an increase in the surface area for oxygen transfer along the length of the microvasculature and removal of metabolic waste. Because blood flow increases are necessary for maintaining the health of cerebral tissue, it would seem that the most effective test of the circulatory system is not to assess the system at rest, but to challenge its capacity to increase flow through application of CVR methodology. However, the challenge of implementing CVR testing needs to overcome the existing disparity in available methods for administering the vasodilatory stimulus and for mapping tissue blood flow responses while doing so.

Cerebrovascular Reactivity Optimization and Standardization

Before beginning the discussion of CVR methodologies, an important aspect of the interpretation of CVR maps must be understood. The issue arises from the fact that interconnections exist throughout the vascular network brain that can result in a reverse "Robin Hood" phenomenon where vascular beds that have normal levels of vascular reserve can steal flow from those beds with reduced vascular reserve. This occurs because vascular beds distal to a stenosis consume vascular reserve through vasodilation to maintain resting blood flow at normal levels. As a result, these beds are unable to lower resistance to the same degree as healthy beds. When a global vasodilatory stimulus is applied, a steal phenomenon ensues where blood flow follows the path of least resistance. Flow is diverted away from beds with a limited ability to vasodilate. This has been termed vascular "steal." Some vascular beds are maximally vasodilated at rest and are therefore vulnerable to decreases in BP resulting in hemodynamic TIAs. Providing a global vascular stimulus can reveal and map the extent of these steal regions. However, the extent of steal physiology depends on the magnitude of the stimulus provided because a mild stimulus may not be sufficient to reveal the full extent of marginalized vascular beds. Two important issues are raised by this phenomenon. The first is what magnitude of vascular stimulus should be applied, and the second is how can the reproducibility within and across subjects be ensured for accurate clinical decision-making?

Control of the vasodilatory stimulus: The ideal CVR method would be to use the neuronal component of the NGVU to induce vasodilation. It is the most desirable but least achievable method. There is no conceivable way to activate each neuronal network within a vascular territory of interest because innumerable neuronal networks exist within a given vascular territory and no single task paradigm would be effective in activating these networks. Interestingly, recent work has shown that for a given vasodilatory stimulus that induces steal physiology in the primary motor cortex, different fMR imaging task responses can be observed from visible to no observable activation.[26,27] It is expected that further increases in arterial CO_2 with greater steal could eventually extinguish the ability of active neurons to increase CBF, but this would require further testing for confirmation.

With this background, the following is an example of our research effort over the last 20 years to optimize and standardize CVR methodology to meet the challenges of translating CVR from a research tool to full clinical standard of practice.[28] It is an example only and other investigators may find more optimal strategies, but is does highlight problems requiring a solution. The following details the current status of the approach addressing the two primary challenges derived from the definition of CVR itself, that is, the need to deliver a known stimulus and the ability to map whole brain blood flow changes.

There are numerous ways to provide a vasodilatory challenge. These include BP manipulation, pharmacologic challenges, and carbon dioxide inhalation. All of the methods can suffer from difficulty reproducing the stimulus and achieving a repeatable and quantifiable stimulus. CVR can be obtained using manipulation of BP but reproducibly controlling BP to targeted levels is difficult and is associated with safety concerns. Pharmacologic manipulation for controlling blood flow is problematic as well. Acetazolamide is typically used for this purpose. However, it has unpredictable time courses and is considered to be a supramaximal stimulus that would induce vasodilation beyond the range of normal increases in CBF seen with neuronal activation.[3,4] A vasodilatory stimulus can be achieved using breath-holding techniques but the levels to which arterial CO_2 accumulates are unknown within and between individuals. Methods using simple inhalation of increased levels of inspired CO_2 induce unknown changes in arterial P_{CO_2} due to unpredictable respiratory responses in the form of increasing minute ventilation. The ability to control arterial CO_2 levels would be ideal as CO_2 is benign and can be rapidly absorbed and removed from the blood via the lungs. Fortunately, accurate control of CO_2 was made possible by advances in respiratory physiology that enabled targeting of selected arterial values of CO_2. This led to the development of two approaches: end-tidal forcing[29] and sequential gas delivery (SGD).[30] Arterial CO_2 levels targeted using SGD has been validated against arterial blood sampling and is the only method available having had this validation.[30–32] Fig. 7 indicates the high degree of accuracy and reproducibility of the CO_2 stimulus achieved with SGD over time benefitting assessment of interval changes in CVR critical for informing optimal patient management. Note that an increase in the CO_2 stimulus of 10 mm Hg over resting values was chosen. The reasoning behind this is that 6% to 8% increases in CBF per mm Hg increase in arterial P_{CO_2}.[33] Therefore, a 10 mm Hg in arterial P_{CO_2} would increase CBF by 60% to 80% covering the 50% increase in CBF seen with neuronal activation. The ramp increase in P_{CO_2} briefly exceeds this step increase in CBF but also includes a hypocapnic component that enables calculation of relative vascular resistance that may eventually be used to replace conventional CVR maps.[34] Details are beyond the scope of this document and the reader is referred to the cited reference for further information. Finally, there is an additional consideration regarding the application of CO_2 for selectively influencing vascular smooth muscle tone independent of the remaining elements of the NGVU. There is controversy in the literature, as to whether or not elevated CO_2 levels affect neuronal activity directly.[35] Because no consensus has been

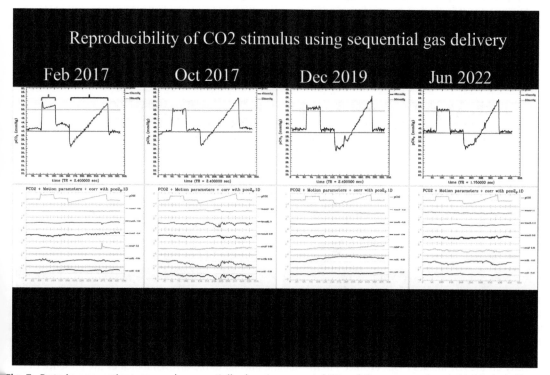

Fig. 7. Data in one patient scanned sequentially showing repeatability of the measured end-tidal (exhaled) CO_2 values to the preprogrammed end-tidal CO_2 targets used for each CVR session more than four different CVR sessions. Red bracket is the step stimulus and blue bracket is the ramp stimulus. Bottom graphs indicate head motion in six different axes during MR imaging data acquisition (in millimeters).

reached, it is assumed that the influence is insignificant for the purposes of measuring CVR. Nevertheless, continued monitoring of this issue in the research literature is warranted.

Mapping changes in CBF: The MR imaging pulse sequence used to map blood flow changes should be able to measure CBF accurately and quantitatively in the setting of advanced cerebrovascular disease with good signal to noise ratio (SNR), no signal drift, no required contrast administration, immunity to skull base susceptibility artifacts, and with very short scan times. Whole brain coverage is needed with good spatial resolution $\leq$ 3 mm isotropic voxels, and the sequence should be capable of mapping whole brain blood flow changes every 1.5 to 2 seconds in order to capture dynamic changes in the CO_2 vasodilatory protocol as seen in **Fig. 7**. As of this writing, there is no available MR imaging pulse sequence that fits all of these requirements. The only pulse sequence capable of meeting most of these needs is the blood oxygenation dependent (BOLD) sequence. It matches all the requirements except for: (1) its sensitivity to inhomogeneous magnetic fields at the skull base limiting assessment of cerebral tissues in this region, (2) nonlinearity of the signal with blood flow, and (3) signal drift. Fortunately, the extent of "invisible" brain secondary to susceptibility artifact is limited to small regions, and signal drift can be corrected using high bandpass filtering. The major issue is that the BOLD signal is nonlinear with blood flow and also

depends on blood volume. The main nonlinearity assuming constant tissue metabolism is that increasing blood flow washes out deoxyhemoglobin approaching an asymptote at 100% oxygen saturation. Therefore, greater increases in CBF are associated with smaller increases in the BOLD signal. There is also the effect of the nonlinear relationship between CBF and CBV described the Grubb constant where CBV = 0.80 CBF 0. 38. The relationship indicates a rapid initial increase in CBV followed by a long shallow increase. Despite these issues, from a physiologic perspective and within the boundaries of Stage 1 and 2 ischemia where Stage 3 indicates ischemic tissue injury, the BOLD signal always increases with CBF. Furthermore, we are not aware of any publication where CBF and CBV behave inversely to each thus violating the Grubb relationship. BOLD is therefore a reasonable surrogate for measuring changes in blood flow. Measuring CBF with MR imaging arterial spin labeling (ASL) is an interesting alternative to BOLD especially because there is a linear relationship between CBF and ASL. However, the acquisition is plagued by poor temporal resolution, and significant loss of magnetization in labeled blood water protons due to T1 relaxation effects to the point where signal to noise is compromised. This is especially so in the setting of longer collateral pathways that develop in increasingly severe SOD. An additional problem seen in advanced SOD occurs when the labeled water remains in supply arteries including the pial

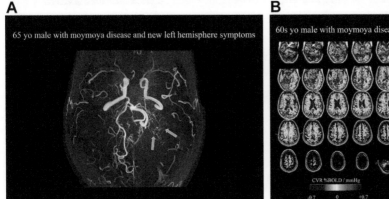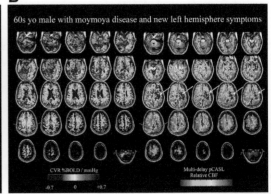

Fig. 8. (*A*) MRA shows bilateral ICA occlusions distal to the posterior communicating arteries and left PCA occlusion with moya collaterals (*arrows*). (*B*) CVR shows areas of steal physiology in both hemispheres. Compared with areas with CVR steal physiology, ASL in general shows somewhat larger regions with marked reduction in CBF. Note that the areas of concentrated spin label in the collateral moya vessels seen near the left PCA occlusion in (*A*) (*white arrows*). The tissue in the vicinity of this collateral site has mostly positive reactivity. The high signal intensity on the ASL images (ASL "artifact") in the midline (medial to *red arrows*) indicates the presence of collaterals with what seems to be a significant reduction in CBF in the adjacent frontal lobe gray matter bilaterally. The CVR map however indicates that most of the right anterior cerebral artery territory has positive CVR. The left ACA territory has steal physiology in the poster half of the left ACA territory. ICA, internal carotid artery; MRA, magnetic resonance angiography; PCA, posterior cerebral artery.

circulation. This labeled blood water may not reach the microcirculation. Because the spatial resolution of the scan cannot distinguish the small pial vessels on the brain surface from the micro-vasculature within the cerebral cortex, the cortex can appear to have a range of perfusion values from adequate to artifactually increased perfusion (**Fig. 8**) even when the most recent multi-delay ASL acquisitions are applied. In terms of ASL mapping, the true status of the vasodilatory capacity in the tissues is uncertain. The discordance between CVR and ASL in this case is concerning as surgical decisions can be influenced by the maps. In addition, ASL acquisitions do not have the less than 2 seconds whole brain temporal resolution for monitoring rapid changes in CBF that BOLD offers. We hope that continued ASL development would

eventually offer a solution enabling replacement of BOLD for CVR studies.

CVR metrics speed and magnitude of response: The CO_2 stimulation paradigm seen in **Fig. 7** was developed after considerable debate over many years. The protocol begins with a baseline CO_2 level that is the individual subjects' resting level. The paradigm lasts 13.5 minutes and consists of an STEP and RAMP stimulus. Note that the speed in the rise and fall of the CO_2 change occurs in one breath. The response of the BOLD signal is slower and exponential in nature.[36] In healthy patients, the duration of the plateau is long and all vascular beds reach a maximum value before the fall in CO_2. This is not the case in patients with SOD. Some vascular beds continue to rise without pla-teauing before the drop in CO_2. Therefore, in order

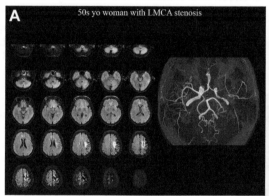
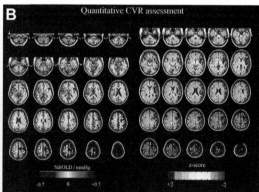

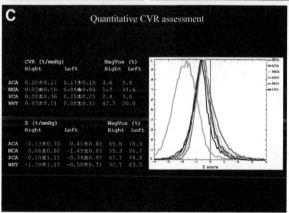

Fig. 9. (A) The FLAIR image indicates an old ischemic infarct in the left hemisphere. The MRA shows an occluded left MCA. (B) CVR indicates steal physiology persisting throughout the left MCA territory around the LMCA infarct. Z-score map indicates that the CVR in all other vascular territories is within normal limits (within two standard deviations) relative to a healthy control population. The left MCA territory is more than two standard deviations below the normal population as it should be since there is steal physiology in this territory. (C) Segmentation of patient gray matter into vascular territories from a standard vascular territory template enables quantification of CVR magnitude of response for each vascular territory. This provides a mean CVR magnitude and a total voxel count of negative responding voxels (steal) for each vascular territory. Rapid visualization of the distribution of the voxels is made possible by plotting the histograms of each vascular territory as shown in the graph. Note that the healthy territories have mean z-score distributions only minimally decreased (shifted to the left) compared with the healthy population.FLAIR, fluid attenuated inversion recovery; LMCA, left middle cerebral artery.

to accurately measure the magnitude of the flow response in patients, a longer slower RAMP increase in signal is required. Modeling the rise in the BOLD signal as a first order exponential enables measurement of the exponential constant representing the speed of response of a vascular bed.[36] The protocol therefore provides two CVR metrics representing biomarkers of vascular responses that have significant impact in measuring effectiveness of collateral circulations in patients with SOD, and the impact of non-SOD diseases on intraparenchymal vascular performance.[37,38]

CVR atlases: The design of functional neuroimaging studies that have examined disease states in patients depends on group data from healthy individuals. In conventional functional imaging studies, image data are typically merged from a group of healthy controls and compared against merged data from a patient population with a specific disease condition. This approach has proven effective in determining the effect of a disease condition on cerebral structure and function. The inherent problem with this approach is the inability to detect disease-related affects in patients. The reason for this is that signal-to-noise ratios in the acquired functional images of individual subjects are typically insufficient to detect disease-related effects. For example, fMR imaging techniques have been available for over 30 years, but no single diagnostic application of this tool has yet been developed. Although CVR uses the same BOLD image acquisitions used for fMR imaging studies on 3T systems (highly recommended field strength for CVR studies), the magnitude of the stimulus-induced signal changes is typically 50% to 100% stronger than those seen with fMR imaging activation of neural networks. Our approach to the diagnostic assessment of vascular disease in individual subjects takes advantage of the greater CVR signal changes and combines this advantage with the development of control atlases enabling voxelwise z-scoring of individual patient responses.[39] These responses can be viewed as z-score maps and histograms enabling quantitative assessment

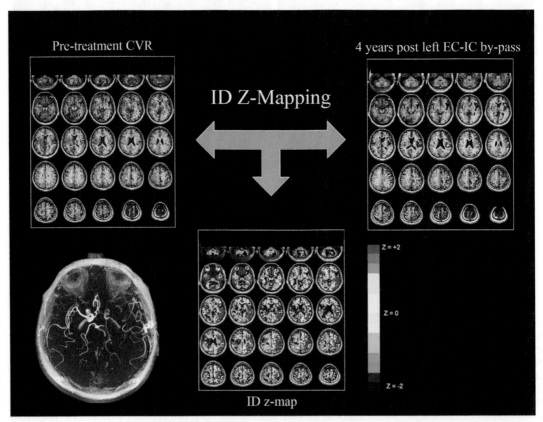

Fig. 10. Patient with distal left ICA occlusion treated with left EC-IC bypass. The "interval difference (ID) difference map" controls for differences in session-to-session variance caused by normal variations in physiology, magnet performance, and head positioning. The ID difference therefore grades the effects of management decisions in terms quantitative z-scores by comparing the patient's own ID difference map against a group ID difference atlas made from healthy controls. EC-IC, external carotid-internal carotid.

of the degree to which an individual patient differs from a healthy population (**Fig. 9**). The only drawback to this approach is that it requires building a healthy control atlas against which an individual patient can be assessed. In the ideal world, the atlases are generated on a single MR imaging platform used in scanning patients and controls. However, we have shown that the results are highly comparable on platforms from different vendors provided that the BOLD pulse sequence parameters are matched.[40] It has also been shown using a quantitative CO_2 stimulus that there is little age dependence on CVR between the third and seventh decades in disease-free controls. Areas of reduced CVR begin to develop after the seventh decade predominantly in the white matter of the frontal lobes.[41]

The control data collected for CVR atlas formation can be broken down into two separate atlases: one for the speed of response and one for the magnitude of response. From a clinical perspective, the assessment of large supply artery SOD has been the primary application of CVR testing. Under these circumstances, the relevant clinical information is primarily derived from the magnitude atlas. However, there are disease conditions where the disease itself has limited impact on large supply arteries but does have an impact on the brain parenchymal circulation. This is where

the speed of response metric has shown considerable promise (see below).

We have also developed interval difference (ID) atlases. An ID image can be made from a healthy control scanned on two different days. The ID images from a group of controls are then merged into a common brain space creating an ID atlas. Comparing the patient ID map against the ID atlas can account for changes in the disease condition and the effects of management over time while controlling for differences in physiology, head positioning, and magnet performance.[42] Voxelwise interval difference z-score maps are then available for quantitative assessment of the temporal differences (**Fig. 10**).

Finally, during the acquisition of CVR data, it is recommended that BP and head movement are monitored. The effect of elevated BP often seen with induction of the CO_2 stimulus is believed to improve CVR, but the degree to which it influences CVR maps has not been formally studied. We have assumed that increases in BP greater than 10 mm Hg could significantly alter the results of CVR studies and as a result, monitoring of BP as frequently as possible before, during, and after the CO_2 stimuli is recommended. In our experience, translation or rotational head motion in excess of 3 mm should also raise concerns.

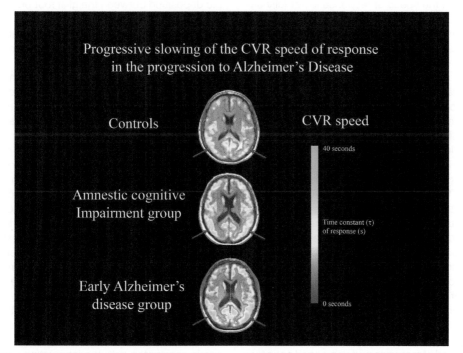

Fig. 11. Merged speed of response data from a healthy control group, amnestic cognitive impairment group, and early Alzheimer's disease group. Arrows indicate progressive slowing of the speed of response in temporoparietal regions of the brain associated with worsening cognitive impairment.

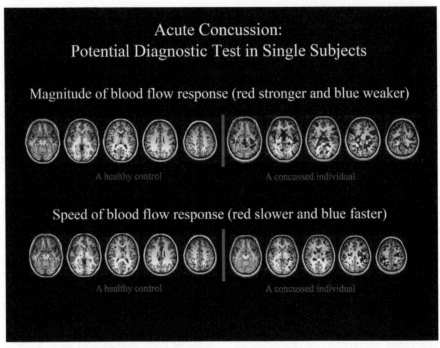

Fig. 12. Z-score maps thresholded at two standard deviations showing faster and stronger CVR responses in a patient scanned in the first week after concussion. There is a clear increase in the extent of abnormal CVR compared with the healthy control. Note that much of the change is in white matter the primary site of the concussive injury. The etiology of this "supernormal" CVR response remains unknown.

The speed of response CVR metric: The biological basis of the speed of response is not fully understood but multiple factors could be involved. If it can be assumed that the CO_2 stimulus used to increase blood flow only affects the vascular component of the NGVU, the speed of smooth muscle response may be the primary factor. Secondary factors may include vessel compliance, cerebral compliance, endothelial dysfunction, modulation of autonomic tone, mitochondrial disease, venous hypertension, trauma, migraine pathophysiology, drugs including ion channel blockers, sickle cell disease, infection (COVID), and subarachnoid hemorrhage to name a few. We have studied two diseases that have shown remarkable findings. The first is amnestic cognitive impairment (aMCI) the precursor of Alzheimer's disease (AD).[38] Compared with controls from a healthy control atlas, patients with aMCI demonstrated a significant slowing of the speed of response in temporoparietal cortex areas where amyloid deposition is prominent in AD. Furthermore, there was even greater slowing in the same regions in patients diagnosed with early AD (**Fig. 11**). A statistically significant correlation was also observed between a slower speed of response and decreased cognitive performance. Interestingly, a mouse model of AD showed concentric rings of amyloid deposition surrounding the microvasculature with much of the deposition between the glial foot processes of the NGVU. It would seem that encirclement of vessels by amyloid could decrease vascular compliance possibly made worse by glio-endothelial interference from amyloid deposition.[43] Because one of the earliest changes in the brain in patients who later develop AD is vascular in nature,[44] these studies justify further examination of CVR as a more available and potentially earliest marker for screening patients with amnestic MCI.

Another example of the value of the speed of response measurement is in concussed individuals. Concussion diagnosis has been elusive. CVR using quantitative stimuli has demonstrated high receiver operating characteristic (ROC) values between 0.90 and 0.95 based on both tails of the z-score distributions in the chronic stages of the injury when associated with persistence of symptoms. In the acute phase of the injury, the high z-scores were found in the tail of the distributions, indicating a faster speed and stronger magnitude of response specifically in the white matter (**Fig. 12**). This pattern of CVR metrics has not been reported in any other condition. Dysautonomia associated with the innervation of pial and parenchymal vessels has been suggested as a possible cause.

SUMMARY

The vasculature plays a vital role in meeting the metabolic demands of the tissues in any organ. Despite the similarity in high blood flow demand by the brain and heart, evaluation of the vasculature in these organs has taken very different paths. The difference is based on the established value of measuring cardiac blood flow augmentation. A cardiac stress test was developed for the heart, but resting perfusion metrics have become the mainstay in the brain. Because both organs depend on strong flow augmentation, it is somewhat perplexing that such a difference even exists. A simple reason may be that the heart feels pain when there is insufficient flow, but the brain does not. Perhaps a more significant reason is that there are myriad methods for measuring CVR, but standardization has never been achieved. This article has served to demonstrate advances that act as an example of how a "brain stress test" can be successfully standardized and implemented using a clinically tested method where most of the CVR studies were carried out in patients with the most severe SOD. The CVR protocol provides precise quantitative vasodilatory stimuli enabling acquisition of two CVR metrics: the speed and magnitude of the flow responses. They can be thought of biomarkers of vascular health and performance with acceptable image acquisition times at 13.5 minutes. These metrics have provided significant advantages in clinical and research settings.

With regard to patient research issues, current CVR methods apply nonquantifiable stimuli. CVR data generated from such stimuli will likely regress to the mean over a population thus providing reasonable hypothesis testing capability. However, an increased number of subjects needed to reach statistical significance are required. The consequences are increasing study costs and an increase in patient burden. Furthermore, the accuracy and reproducibility of studies using uncontrolled vasodilatory stimuli are uncertain.

Based on our clinical experience of more than 1200 patient CVR studies, we believe that the management of individual patients with cerebrovascular disease requires precisely controlled reproducible stimuli to optimize the diagnosis, appropriate treatment planning, and monitoring of treatment efficacy. Despite the fact that for a given stenosis, many studies have shown that the risk of permanent ischemic injury is up to five times higher in patients with hemodynamic impairment than without, there are no prospective outcome studies using a controlled vasodilatory stimulus. In a recent review of cerebral hemodynamics and oxygen extraction studies, it was stated that *"There is a great opportunity, and clinical need, to prove the therapeutic efficacy of hemodynamic assessment in patients with atherosclerotic asymptomatic extracranial carotid stenosis, and symptomatic internal carotid occlusion and intracranial stenosis. A better understanding of the long-term metabolic and physiologic impact of chronic regional hemodynamic impairment and the mechanism of hemodynamic stroke is needed."*[45] Moving forward, new approaches for assessing the ability of the vasculature to meet the metabolic needs of the brain including resting state BOLD techniques and artificial intelligence methods may eventually replace current CVR methods. This development would be most welcomed, but assessment of the need to move away from resting perfusion measures remains the same. The challenge for the future is therefore on the shoulders of the next generation of stroke neurology and vascular neuroradiology/neurosurgery to conduct the requisite clinical trials designed to compare CVR against resting perfusion metrics that are the current standard of practice. This represents an opportunity to improve patient care that is both compelling and long overdue.

CLINICS CARE POINTS

- The solution described for implementing cerebrovascular reactivity (CVR) was derived from testing in a clinical population based on more than 1200 patient examinations.
- The method has become a focal point in the clinical assessment of patients with advanced cerebrovascular disease who are now being seen in a newly formed "Revascualrization Clinic."
- Although standardized CVR methodology has shown defacto clinical utility, the need for randomized clinical trials comparing CVR metrics versus resting perfusion metrics is needed.

DISCLOSURE

D.J. Mikulis holds minor equity in Thornhill Medical Inc vendor of the Respiract enabling precise breath to breath control of arterial CO_2 for accurate delivery of vasoactive stimuli during CVR studies.

FUNDING

The Canadian Institutes of Health Research research grant #130459; Physicians' Services

Incorporated Foundation of Ontario research grant; American Society of Neuroradiology Foundation research grant; Center for Aging and Brain Health Innovation Ontario - research grant; General Electric – Investigator Sponsored Research.

REFERENCES

1. Attwell D, Laughlin SB. An energy budget for signaling in the grey matter of the brain. JCBFM 2001;21(10):1133–45.

2. Harris JJ, Jolivet R, Attwell D, et al. Synaptic energy use and supply. Neuron 2012;75:762–1145.

3. Davis TL, Kwong KK, Weisskoff RM, et al. Calibrated functional MRI: mapping the dynamics of oxidative metabolism. Proc Natl Acad Sci U S A 1998;95(4):1834–9.

4. Ito H, Ibaraki M, Kanno I, et al. Changes in cerebral blood flow and cerebral oxygen metabolism during neural activation measured by positron emission tomography: comparison with blood oxygenation level-dependent contrast measured by functional magnetic resonance imaging. J Cereb Blood Flow Metab 2005;25(3):371–7.

5. Data based on "body, Physics of." Macmillan Encyclopedia of Physics. New York: Macmillan; 1996.

6. Shelley HJ. Glycogen reserves and their changes at birth and in anoxia. Br Med Bull 1961;2:137–43.

7. Rich LR, Harris W, Brown AM. The Role of Brain Glycogen in Supporting Physiological Function. Front Neurosci 2019;13:1176.

8. Kuroda S, Kawabori M, Hirata K, et al. Clinical significance of STA-MCA double anastomosis for hemodynamic compromise in post-JET/COSS era. Acta Neurochir 2014;156:77–83.

9. Ogasawara K, Ogawa A. [JET study (Japanese EC-IC Bypass Trial)]. Nihon Rinsho 2006;64(suppl 7):524–7.

10. Powers WJ, Clarke WR, Grubb RL, et al. Extracranial-intracranial bypass surgery for stroke prevention in hemodynamic cerebral ischemia: the Carotid Occlusion Surgery Study randomized trial. JAMA 2011;306:1983–92.

11. Knot HJ, Nelson MT. Regulation of arterial diameter and wall [Ca2+] in cerebral arteries of rat by membrane potential and intravascular pressure. J Physiol 1998;508(Pt 1):199–209.

12. Attwell D, Buchan AM, Charpak S, et al. Glial and neuronal control of brain blood flow. Nature 2010;468(7321):232–43.

13. Duffin J, Mikulis DJ, Fisher JA. Control of Cerebral Blood Flow by Blood Gases. Front Physiol 2021;12:640075.

14. Kety SS, Schmidt CF. The effects of altered arterial tensions of carbon dioxide and oxygen on cerebral blood flow and cerebral oxygen consumption of normal young men. J Clin Invest 1948;27(4):484–92.

15. Silvestrini M, Vernieri F, Pasqualetti P, et al. Impaired cerebral vasoreactivity and risk of stroke in patients with asymptomatic carotid artery stenosis. JAMA 2000;283(16):2122–7.

16. Markus H, Cullinane M. Severely impaired cerebrovascular reactivity predicts stroke and TIA risk in patients with carotid artery stenosis and occlusion. Brain 2001;124(Pt 3):457–67.

17. Blaser T, Hofmann K, Buerger T, et al. Risk of stroke, transient ischemic attack, and vessel occlusion before endarterectomy in patients with symptomatic severe carotid stenosis. Stroke 2002;33(4):1057–62.

18. Schoof J, Lubahn W, Baeumer M, et al. Impaired cerebral autoregulation distal to carotid stenosis/occlusion is associated with increased risk of stroke at cardiac surgery with cardiopulmonary bypass. J Thorac Cardiovasc Surg 2007;134(3):690–6.

19. Fierstra J, Poublanc J, Han JS, et al. Steal physiology is spatially associated with cortical thinning. J Neurol Neurosurg Psychiatry 2010;81(3):290–3.

20. Lee JJ, Shimony JS, Jafri H, et al. Hemodynamic Impairment Measured by Positron-Emission Tomography Is Regionally Associated with Decreased Cortical Thickness in Moyamoya Phenomenon. AJNR Am J Neuroradiol 2018;39(11):2037–44.

21. Wouters A, Christensen S, Straka M, et al. A Comparison of Relative Time to Peak and Tmax for Mismatch-Based Patient Selection. Front Neurol 2017;8:539.

22. Wang CM, Chang YM, Sung PS, et al. Hypoperfusion Index Ratio as a Surrogate of Collateral Scoring on CT Angiogram in Large Vessel Stroke. J Clin Med 2021;10(6):1296.

23. Baek JH, Kim YD, Lee KJ, et al. Low Hypoperfusion Intensity Ratio Is Associated with a Favorable Outcome Even in Large Ischemic Core and Delayed Recanalization Time. J Clin Med 2021;10(9):1869.

24. Guenego A, Fahed R, Albers GW, et al. Hypoperfusion intensity ratio correlates with angiographic collaterals in acute ischaemic stroke with M1 occlusion. Eur J Neurol 2020;27(5):864–70.

25. Ben Hassen W, Malley C, Boulouis G, et al. Inter- and intraobserver reliability for angiographic leptomeningeal collateral flow assessment by the American Society of Interventional and Therapeutic Neuroradiology/Society of Interventional Radiology (ASITN/SIR) scale. J Neurointerv Surg 2019;11(4):338–41.

26. van Niftrik CHB, Hiller A, Sebök M, et al. Heterogeneous motor BOLD-fMRI responses in brain areas exhibiting negative BOLD cerebrovascular reactivity indicate that steal phenomenon does not always result from exhausted cerebrovascular reserve capacity. Magn Reson Imaging 2023;103:124–30.

27. Para AE, Sam K, Poublanc J, et al. Invalidation of fMRI experiments secondary to neurovascular uncoupling in patients with cerebrovascular disease. J Magn Reson Imaging 2017;46(5):1448–55.

28. Sobczyk O, Fierstra J, Venkatraghavan L, et al. Measuring Cerebrovascular Reactivity: Sixteen Avoidable Pitfalls. Front Physiol 2021;12:665049.

29. Robbins PA, Swanson GD, Micco AJ, et al. A fast gas-mixing system for breath-to-breath respiratory control studies. J Appl Physiol 1982;52:1358–62.

30. Ito S, Mardimae A, Han J, et al. Non-invasive prospective targeting of arterial PCO2 in subjects at rest. J Physiol 2008;586:3675–82.

31. Slessarev M, Han J, Mardimae A, et al. Prospective targeting and control of end-tidal CO2 and O2 concentrations. J Physiol 2007;581:1207–19.

32. Fisher JA, Iscoe S, Duffin J. Sequential gas delivery provides precise control of alveolar gas exchange. Respir Physiol Neurobiol 2016;225:60–9.

33. Kety SS, Schmidt CF. The effects of altered arterial tension of carbon dioxide and oxygen on cerebral blood flow and cerebral oxygen consumption of normal men. J Clin Investig 1948;27:484–92.

34. Duffin J, Sobczyk O, Crawley A, et al. The role of vascular resistance in BOLD responses to progressive hypercapnia. Hum Brain Mapp 2017;38(11):5590–602.

35. Xu F, Uh J, Brier MR, et al. The influence of carbon dioxide on brain activity and metabolism in conscious humans. J Cereb Blood Flow Metab 2011;31(1):58–67.

36. Poublanc J, Crawley AP, Sobczyk O, et al. Measuring cerebrovascular reactivity: the dynamic response to a step hypercapnic stimulus. J Cereb Blood Flow Metab 2015;35(11):1746–56.

37. Shafi R, Poublanc J, Venkatraghavan L, et al. A Promising Subject-Level Classification Model for Acute Concussion Based on Cerebrovascular Reactivity Metrics. J Neurotrauma 2021;38(8):1036–47.

38. Holmes KR, Tang-Wai D, Sam K, et al. Slowed Temporal and Parietal Cerebrovascular Response in Patients with Alzheimer's Disease. Can J Neurol Sci 2020;47(3):366–73.

39. Sobczyk O, Battisti-Charbonney A, Poublanc J, et al. Assessing cerebrovascular reactivity abnormality by comparison to a reference atlas. J Cereb Blood Flow Metab 2015;35:213–20.

40. Sobczyk O, Sayin ES, Sam K, et al. The Reproducibility of Cerebrovascular Reactivity Across MRI Scanners. Front Physiol 2021;12:668662.

41. McKetton L, Cohn M, Tang-Wai DF, et al. Cerebrovascular Resistance in Healthy Aging and Mild Cognitive Impairment. Front Aging Neurosci 2019;11:79.

42. Sobczyk O, Crawley AP, Poublanc J, et al. Identifying Significant Changes in Cerebrovascular Reactivity to Carbon Dioxide. AJNR Am J Neuroradiol 2016;37(5):818–24.

43. Kimbrough IF, Robel S, Roberson ED, et al. Vascular amyloidosis impairs the gliovascular unit in a mouse model of Alzheimer's disease. Brain 2015;138(Pt 12):3716–33.

44. Iturria-Medina Y, Sotero RC, Toussaint PJ, et al, Alzheimer's Disease Neuroimaging Initiative. Early role of vascular dysregulation on late-onset Alzheimer's disease based on multifactorial data-driven analysis. Nat Commun 2016;7:11934.

45. Derdeyn CP. Hemodynamics and oxygen extraction in chronic large artery steno-occlusive disease: Clinical applications for predicting stroke risk. J Cereb Blood Flow Metab 2018;38(9):1584–97.

MR Perfusion Imaging of the Lung

Fernando U. Kay, MD, PhD[a],*, Ananth J. Madhuranthakam, PhD[a,b]

KEYWORDS

- Lung perfusion • Magnetic resonance imaging (MRI) • Arterial spin labeling (ASL)
- Fourier decomposition (FD) • Hyperpolarized 129-Xenon (129-xe) MRI
- Contrast-enhanced (CE) MRI

KEY POINTS

- Lung perfusion is an important quantitative biomarker in various pulmonary diseases.
- Several contrast-enhanced and non–contrast-enhanced methods have been developed to assess lung perfusion on MRI.
- Lung perfusion imaging using MRI presents multiple benefits, notably avoiding ionizing radiation and concerns associated with iodinated contrast.
- Non–contrast-enhanced MRI lung perfusion is an ideal modality for patients with renal dysfunction and for those who are pregnant.
- The broader clinical adoption of MRI lung perfusion hinges on the integration of advanced technology into clinical scanners, collaborative research efforts, and rigorous validation.

INTRODUCTION

Lung perfusion and ventilation are fundamental biological functions that hold potential as quantitative biomarkers for advancing our comprehension and management of lung diseases.[1] Lung perfusion is regulated by a web of intricate biological and physiologic mechanisms, which can be severely disrupted by common respiratory ailments such as chronic obstructive pulmonary disease (COPD), pulmonary embolism (PE), and pulmonary hypertension (PH), leading to secondary impairment of lung perfusion.[2–4] Consequently, lung perfusion presents an intuitive target for quantitative imaging, enabling clinicians to gain detailed insights into the underlying disease processes and explore potential therapeutic interventions.

In response to the pressing need for non-invasive, accurate, and precise techniques to investigate lung perfusion in vivo, there has been an upswing in the development of various imaging modalities.[5] These modalities come with distinct features such as spatial resolution, type of tracer, the presence or absence of ionizing radiation, and field of view coverage, all designed with the goal to enhance the standard of lung perfusion imaging while addressing the shortcomings of preceding techniques.

MRI offers a unique avenue for probing lung perfusion without exposing patients to ionizing radiation. Despite challenges such as low signal intensity due to air-filled sacs, the alveoli, diminished proton density in the lung, increased magnetic field inhomogeneities due to air-tissue interfaces, and susceptibility to respiratory motion and cardiovascular pulsations, MRI brings numerous advantages to the table. Its capacity for high-resolution angiography combined with perfusion imaging facilitates in-depth examination of thoracic vascular abnormalities and their functional consequences.[6] A noteworthy feature of MRI is the ability to assess lung perfusion without intravenous contrast agents,[7] making it particularly beneficial for patients with kidney disease, allergies, or those who are pregnant. Additionally,

[a] Department of Radiology, University of Texas Southwestern Medical Center, 5323 Harry Hines Boulevard, Dallas, TX 75390, USA; [b] Advanced Imaging Research Center, University of Texas Southwestern Medical Center, North Campus 2201 Inwood Road, Dallas, TX 75390-8568, USA
* Corresponding author.
E-mail address: Fernando.Kay@UTSouthwestern.edu

Magn Reson Imaging Clin N Am 32 (2024) 111–123
https://doi.org/10.1016/j.mric.2023.09.006
1064-9689/24/© 2023 Elsevier Inc. All rights reserved.

the quantitative imaging capabilities of MRI enable accurate measurement of perfusion parameters, which can be used for longitudinal assessment to monitor disease progression or response to therapy.

The aim of this review is to delve into the prevalent MRI techniques employed for evaluating lung perfusion, highlighting their specific features, the challenges they entail, and the strides made toward incorporating them into routine clinical practice.

LUNG PERFUSION: PHYSIOLOGIC PERSPECTIVE

Pioneering physiologic studies upended the initial belief that lungs were functionally homogeneous, revealing instead a distinct functional heterogeneity that persists regardless of anatomic segmentation.[8–12] Alongside this, an abundance of research has shed light on how posture and gravity markedly influence lung function. Imaging methods have depicted that both ventilation and perfusion are inclined toward gravity-dependent regions of the lung.

The gravitational model is built upon the balance between the perfusion pressure in pulmonary circulation and the regional resistances, which are governed by local gradients in tissue and alveolar pressures.[13,14] The conventional model[15] suggests that alveolar pressures outweigh arterial and venous pressures in non-dependent regions. In contrast, in dependent regions, arterial and venous pressures prevail over alveolar pressures, resulting in a more pronounced perfusion gradient in dependent regions compared to non-dependent areas.

The previously unchallenged view that gravity is the sole determinant of the vertical distribution of pulmonary perfusion has been recently questioned by research utilizing high-resolution imaging in animal models and humans. This research emphasizes the considerable influence of the lungs' inherent microarchitectural features on the heterogeneity of lung perfusion.[16–22] A comprehensive understanding of the determinants of regional lung perfusion is pivotal for grasping disease mechanisms and devising focused therapeutic strategies. For example, insights from studies demonstrating more uniform pulmonary perfusion in the prone position[23,24] have been instrumental in creating novel ventilation strategies for patients with acute alveolar injury.[25] These strategies aim to alleviate the adverse effects of increased intra-alveolar positive end-expiratory pressures, which can reduce lung perfusion,[26] while concurrently ameliorating the ventilation-perfusion mismatch common in the collapsed dorsal regions of the lung when in the supine position.[27]

MRI, akin to other noninvasive imaging techniques, has proven invaluable in unraveling the complex and dynamic nature of lung perfusion physiology. For instance, MRI has suggested the presence of differences in lung perfusion between inspiration and expiration.[28] However, evaluating in vivo perfusion necessitates a nuanced approach, as lung density distributions can significantly influence the measurements, leading to deviations when compared to data from excised lungs adjusted for lung density.[29]

Assessing regional pulmonary perfusion presents distinct methodological challenges, chiefly due to the specialized microarchitecture of the lungs. Unlike the densities of solid organs such as the liver or brain, which hover around 1 g/cm^3, the average lung density is substantially lower, at approximately 0.26 g/cm^3 as estimated by computed tomography (CT).[30] This underscores the critical need for a standardized methodology to quantify lung perfusion biomarkers for clinical use, ensuring a fair evaluation of the spatial and temporal heterogeneity in perfusion.

MRI TECHNIQUES FOR LUNG PERFUSION IMAGING
Contrast-enhanced Methods

Contrast-enhanced (CE) MRI perfusion utilizes the T1 shortening effects that occur upon administration of gadolinium-based contrast agents (GBCA), thereby facilitating lung perfusion assessment via the tracer dilution technique.[31] This approach is especially advantageous for dynamically imaging anatomic structures such as the heart and lungs. In 1994, Wilke and colleagues[32] and Eichenberger and colleagues[33] independently demonstrated the efficacy of gadolinium-enhanced ultrafast MRI in assessing ischemic heart disease.[32,33]

In a landmark study in 1996, Hatabu and colleagues extended the application of GBCA to pulmonary perfusion imaging (**Fig. 1**). They successfully employed CE inversion recovery turbo fast low-angle shot (FLASH) technique with high temporal resolution and an ultra-short echo time (TE) of 1.4 millisecond for noninvasive MR imaging of pulmonary perfusion in humans and a porcine model simulating PE.[34] This technique, which was among the first to perform 2-dimensional (2D) qualitative analyses of lung perfusion, overcame the challenges posed by magnetic inhomogeneities often seen due to the lung's complex arrangement of air and soft tissue within the alveoli. Around the same time, Amundsen and colleagues (1997)[35] and Berthezène and colleagues (1999)[36] adopted similar techniques to identify regional perfusion impairments from PE, finding a

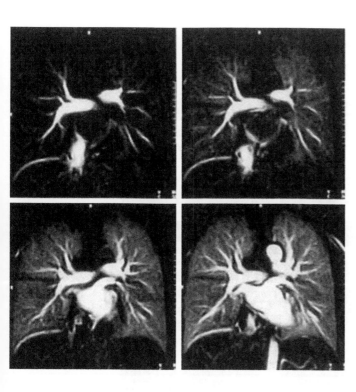

Fig. 1. Dynamic contrast-enhanced MR imaging process was used to examine the pulmonary perfusion in a healthy volunteer. The imaging was performed using an ultra-short CE inversion recovery turbo fast low-angle shot sequence. Images were obtained over a period of 20 seconds during the injection of gadolinium-based contrast agent and subtracted from the pre-contrast image. The process captured 45 dynamic images every 1.7 seconds in the same coronal plane that included the pulmonary hila (area where blood vessels and airways enter the lung). The contrast agent arrival resulted in increased signal intensity in the perfused lung areas, seen by subtracting pre-contrast images from the post-contrast ones. (Reprinted with permissions from reference[34].)

strong agreement between qualitative CE MRI perfusion and lung scintigraphy perfusion.[37] Additionally, Amundsen and colleagues (2000) utilized perfusion MR imaging to explore first-pass characteristics in patients with pneumonia or COPD, uncovering distinct contrast enhancement patterns and signal intensity curves that distinguished these conditions from normal lung and PE.[38]

Subsequently, the practicality of using dynamic CE MRI for quantitative assessment of pulmonary perfusion was confirmed. In a study by Hatabu and colleagues (1999), a pig model with induced PE was used to evaluate the use of the indicator dilution principle in extracting quantitative parameters of regional lung perfusion. The results were benchmarked against absolute pulmonary perfusion measurements obtained using colored microspheres, and a correlation was observed with absolute lung perfusion.[39] Initial quantitative experiments employing this methodology in humans lent support to the gravitational model of lung perfusion distribution.[40]

Recognizing the limitations of 2D MRI sequences in clinical practice, particularly their constrained spatial resolution and insufficient anatomic coverage for comprehensive imaging of the lungs, there has been a paradigm shift toward 3D MRI. Fink and colleagues (2003) and Ohno and colleagues (2004) spearheaded this development by introducing a CE 3D MRI sequence optimized for lung perfusion assessment.[41,42] This innovative technique employed a spoiled gradient echo (GRE) method with an ultra-short echo time (TE) of 0.6 to 0.8 millisecond, full lung coverage, and high temporal resolution (**Fig. 2**). Ohno and colleagues (2004) leveraged the high-resolution imaging afforded by 3D acquisition to provide quantitative pixel-by-pixel perfusion analysis employing an algebraic application of the tracer-dilution theory, enabling the detection of multiple segmental perfusion defects in a patient with chronic thromboembolic PH (CTEPH) in their feasibility study, which paralleled results from lung perfusion scintigraphy.

Ohno and colleagues (2007) and Ley and colleagues (2007) also implemented quantitative CE 3D MRI perfusion imaging to explore hemodynamic parameter differences in patients with different classes of PH (I, II, and III) as compared to healthy individuals.[43,44] A significant increase in mean transit time across all PH classes was discovered, corresponding to increases in invasive measurements of pulmonary vascular resistance. This phenomenon was attributed to pathologic changes in peripheral pulmonary arteries, which led to increased pulmonary arterial pressure.

In conclusion, studies have suggested an optimal gadolinium (Gd) dose of 0.05 to 0.1 mmol/kg of body weight to maximize the signal-to-noise ratio without saturation effects that may distort the arterial input function.[45,46] High-concentration GBCAs do not seem to provide benefits over lower concentration agents for

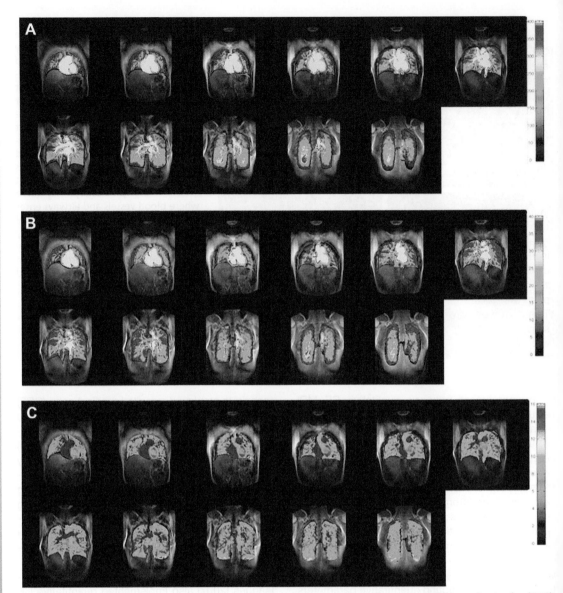

Fig. 2. Dynamic contrast-enhanced perfusion imaging performed with a 3-dimensional (3D) gradient echo (GRE) sequence. Color-coded regional quantitative parameters of lung perfusion were calculated for a volunteer using the deconvolution method: (*A*) pulmonary blood flow; (*B*) pulmonary blood volume; (*C*) mean transit time (Reprinted with permissions from reference[42]).

lung perfusion assessment.[46] Injection rates of 3 mL/s or more are recommended for optimal separation of pulmonary and systemic components of lung parenchyma perfusion.[47]

Non-contrast Enhanced Methods

The use of GBCAs in CE MRI perfusion techniques brings several constraints. The first is the additional cost associated with GBCAs. Secondly, there is a potential for allergic reactions and concerns regarding gadolinium accumulation in the body, which has previously been associated with

nephrogenic systemic fibrosis (NSF),[48] and deposition in structures such as the basal ganglia.[49] Thirdly, supply chain uncertainties, which have been exacerbated in the post-coronavirus disease 2019COVID era, could impact the availability of GBCAs.[50] Lastly, the use of GBCAs imposes limitations on the frequency and repetition of imaging sequences due to safety considerations.

Arterial Spin Labeling

In contrast to CE MRI, arterial spin labeling (ASL) has gained prominence as a non-CE MRI technique for measuring lung perfusion. ASL utilizes a unique strategy where water protons in the blood are magnetically labeled to serve as endogenous tracers, eliminating the need for external contrast agents.[51] There are 2 main methodologies within ASL, namely pulsed ASL and continuous ASL.

Pulsed ASL has been more widely used and was first introduced for lung perfusion imaging by Mai and colleagues in 1999.[52] In this approach, 2 images are acquired. First, a control image, where a spatially selective 180-degree radiofrequency pulse inverts the longitudinal magnetization in an imaging slice but without affecting the magnetization of blood water protons outside the slice. Next, a label image is obtained using a non-selective inversion pulse that inverts the magnetization of blood water protons. Subsequently, perfusion-weighted images are produced by calculating pixel-wise differences between the 2 images. This method integrated *half-Fourier* acquisition single-shot *turbo spin-echo*(HASTE) imaging, which reduced susceptibility to magnetic field inhomogeneities in the lungs and allowed for shorter image acquisition times suitable for breath-holding.[53] The signal measurements in this method were initially validated in an animal model with artificial pulmonary artery occlusion[54] and later in a PE case.[55] Various pulsed ASL variants have been developed, with a focus on evaluating the reliability of quantitative measurements acquired from pulmonary blood flow[56–62] (**Fig. 3**).

Continuous ASL, though potentially capable of producing larger signal changes in lung tissue, has faced challenges due to its use of long, off-resonance inversion pulses that result in prominent magnetization transfer effects between water and macromolecular protons.[63] This can cause signal losses and biases in lung perfusion measurements. Additionally, hardware constraints and concerns about specific absorption ratios limit the application of continuous ASL. However, Roberts and colleagues (1999) conducted human lung perfusion studies using a respiratory-triggered continuous ASL sequence and validated signal intensity changes in an animal study with balloon occlusion of the pulmonary artery.[64,65]

To address some of the challenges associated with continuous ASL, pseudo-continuous ASL has been introduced. This technique reduces magnetization transfer effects, decreases subtraction errors, improves labeling efficiency, and is more compatible with existing radiofrequency amplifiers.[66] Seith and colleagues (2020) developed an electrocardiogram (ECG)-triggered pseudo-continuous ASL sequence with a balanced steady-state free-precession (SSFP) readout for quantitative assessment and visualization of pulmonary blood flow under free-breathing conditions.[67] They found that the course of labeled blood through the lung was highly dependent on the individual's cardiac cycle duration. Furthermore, a subsequent prospective study involving patients with suspected acute PE showed that free-breathing pseudo-continuous ASL MRI had high sensitivity and specificity compared to computed tomography pulmonary angiography (CTPA) for the detection of PE[68] (**Fig. 4**).

Fourier Decomposition

Fourier decomposition (FD) is a non-CE method that has been developed to enable simultaneous measurements of lung perfusion (Q) and ventilation (V), facilitating the acquisition of V/Q maps.[69] Bauman and colleagues (2009) introduced this method, which uses an optimized 2D SSFP sequence to acquire high-temporal-resolution images without the need for respiratory or electrocardiographic (ECG) gating. To account for respiratory motion and align lung structures over time, a non-rigid image registration algorithm was employed.[70] Fourier analysis was then applied to the aligned images to separate the signal contributions from ventilation and perfusion. This enabled the examination of specific regions within the pulmonary parenchyma based on the variation of signal intensity over time. The method was validated qualitatively against single-photon emission computed tomography (SPECT)/CT and CE MRI perfusion.[71,72]

Following the introduction of the FD method, several variations have been developed. One such variation is the SElf-gated Non-Contrast-Enhanced FUnctional Lung imaging (SENCEFUL) method, which uses a quasi-random FLASH sequence.[73] Another variation, known as "phase-resolved functional lung imaging (PREFUL)," was introduced by Voskrebenzev and colleagues in 2018.[74] PREFUL utilizes a standard spoiled GRE sequence with a temporal resolution ranging from 288 to 324 milliseconds, akin to the original FD method. However, PREFUL incorporates an image-sorting algorithm that effectively increases the temporal resolution down to 33 millisecond. This enhancement allows for the calculation of time to peak, ventilation-perfusion maps, and fractional ventilation flow-volume loops, thereby providing a more comprehensive and quantitative understanding of regional lung function.[74,75] Furthermore, perfusion maps derived from PREFUL were validated against SPECT and CE MRI perfusion, exhibiting a reasonable correlation with these quantitative references in subjects with COPD, cystic fibrosis (CF), and CTEPH.[76] PREFUL's ability

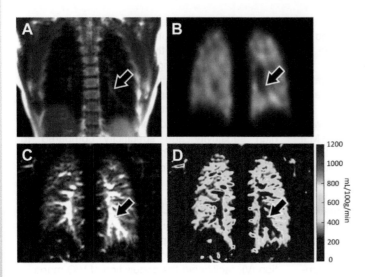

Fig. 3. Coronal proton density-weighted MR image (*A*), single photon emission computed tomography (SPECT) perfusion image using technetium-99 m-macroaggregated albumin (^{99m}Tc-MAA) (*B*), MR perfusion-weighted image acquired using non-contrast pulsed ASL called "flow alternating inversion recovery (FAIR)" (*C*), and the quantitative perfusion map derived from FAIR perfusion (*D*) in a 33-year old healthy female volunteer. The non-contrast perfusion measured using FAIR demonstrates similar qualitative assessment as measured by SPECT. Arrows indicate signals from major vessels that are visible on FAIR perfusion images (*C*, *D*), and seen as regions of photopenia on SPECT images (*B*). (Reprinted with permission from Ref.[62])

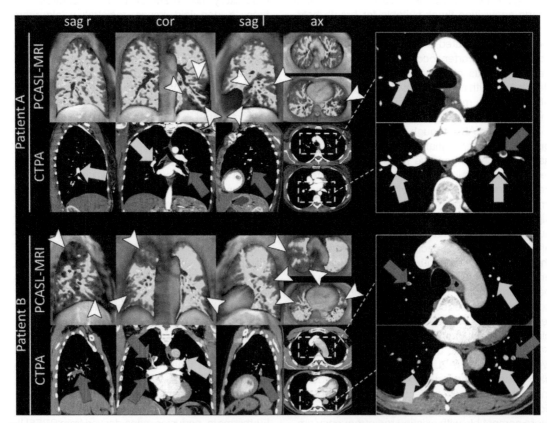

Fig. 4. State-of-the art non-CE perfusion imaging of the lung using free-breathing pseudo-continuous ASL (PCASL-MRI) in 2 patients with pulmonary embolism. Perfusion deficits shown by arrowheads on the colored perfusion map overlays are matched by filling defects in the branches of the pulmonary artery (*red arrows*) on computed tomography pulmonary angiography (CTPA). Patent branches are shown by green arrows for comparison (Reprinted with permissions from Ref[68]).

to produce quantitative lung ventilation, perfusion, and V/Q maps in a single study, without the need for gas inhalation or intravenous contrast, has captured significant attention in ongoing research, enhancing the potential of lung MRI for routine monitoring of conditions, such as post-lung transplant complications[77] (**Fig. 5**).

Hyperpolarized 129-Xe MRI

Hyperpolarized 129-Xe has recently gained approval for clinical evaluation of lung ventilation in both adults and pediatric patients aged 12 years and above. Beyond its utility in assessing ventilation, 129-Xe offers additional promise in its capacity to provide biomarkers for regional gas exchange within the lungs, achieved through the measurement of Xe uptake by tissue and blood.[78] Moreover, there has been significant evidence

suggesting that a decline in the relative regional distribution ratio between Xe dissolved in red blood cells and that in the lung parenchyma tissue can serve as an indicator of compromised alveolar-capillary diffusion or a decrease in pulmonary perfusion.[79,80] With these findings, there emerges a compelling case for the use of 129-Xe MR in assessing lung perfusion, thereby offering a comprehensive examination of lung physiology,[81] which requires further validation.

READINESS FOR CLINICAL TRANSLATION

Despite the array of imaging approaches for measuring lung perfusion using MRI, clinical translation has been slow. This can be partially attributed to competition with other functional methods, such as scintigraphy, SPECT/CT, and multi-energy CT. However, a recent consensus

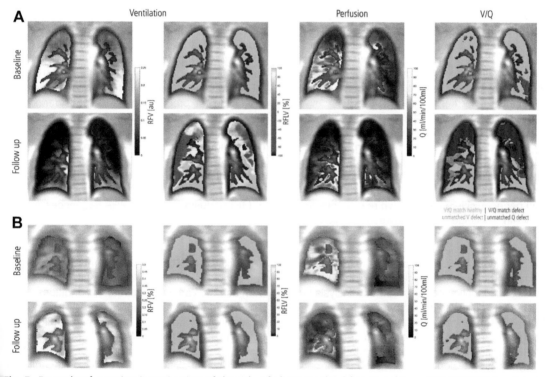

Fig. 5. Example of ongoing investigation of the role of phase-resolved functional lung MRI (PREFUL) for detecting complications of lung transplant. Panel (*A*) shows ventilation, perfusion, and ventilation-perfusion (V/Q maps) in a patient who developed progressive bronchiolitis obliterans syndrome as a complication of lung transplant. Over the course of 38 months, the forced expiratory volume in the first second of expiration (FEV1) declined from 95% of the predicted value at baseline to 47%. The regional fractional ventilation (RFV) declined from 0.20 to 0.08 (a decrease of 39%), the regional flow volume loop (RFVL) declined from 0.99 to 0.70 (a decrease of 71%), and perfusion (Q) declined from 54 mL/min/100 mL to 25 mL/min/100 mL (a decrease of 46%). The ventilation-perfusion (V/Q)–matched defect increased from less than 1% to 35%. Panel (*B*) displays images of another patient after transplant with uneventful course. Over 36 months, her FEV1 decreased from 95% to 47% (similar to Panel A). However, her RFV increased from 0.18 to 0.33 (an increase of 176%), and her RFVL remained constant at 0.99. Perfusion values remained stable at 39 mL/min/100 mL and 37 mL/min/100 mL, respectively (95% of baseline values). The V/Q-matched defect was 0% in both examinations. (Reproduced with permission from reference[77].)

document from the Fleischner Society has acknowledged the clinical readiness of chest MRI, including perfusion methods, for applications in CF, lung cancer, and CTEPH.[6]

In CF, CT is typically the reference modality for diagnosis[82] and for monitoring longitudinal response to therapy.[83,84] Concerns regarding the cumulative effects of ionizing radiation exposure in young patients have prompted the search for alternatives.[85] Lung perfusion abnormalities, which result from disrupted pulmonary function due to airway obstruction, have been suggested as surrogates for disease severity.[86] Various MRI-based lung perfusion measurement techniques have been proposed for evaluating CF, with preliminary evidence indicating comparable performance between CE and non-CE methods.[87–90]

MRI has also become significant in the evaluation of PH, offering a comprehensive assessment of cardiac morphology and function, which can be used for prognosis, monitoring, and determination of etiology, especially in classes II and IV.[91] CE MRI perfusion is highly sensitive for diagnosing CTEPH,[92,93] and emerging evidence suggests that MRI perfusion may also serve as a noninvasive method for evaluating pulmonary vascular resistance, a marker of disease severity.[43,94,95]

For characterizing lung lesions such as nodules and masses, perfusion MRI is well-accepted. By using variations of CE MRI perfusion techniques, studies have analyzed dynamic changes in lung lesion signals, with varied diagnostic performance.[96] Protocols with high temporal resolution (about 1 second per acquisition) have shown reasonable accuracy in distinguishing between benign and malignant lung nodules, comparable to dynamic perfusion CT and *fluorodeoxyglucose* FDG PET/CT but without ionizing radiation exposure.[97–99] Combining diffusion-weighted imaging (DWI) enhances diagnostic accuracy. A meta-analysis suggests that DWI MRI is comparable or superior to FDG PET/CT for characterizing solitary pulmonary nodules.[100] This supports the potential of combining DWI MRI with CE MRI perfusion as a robust methodology for lung lesion characterization, warranting further validation. Additionally, studies by Ohno and colleagues in 2004 and 2007 highlighted the potential of CE 3D MRI for predicting postoperative lung function in lung cancer patients by precisely delineating tumor extent and its relation to adjacent lung tissue.[101,102]

In COPD, MRI perfusion has been extensively studied as a promising method for assessing physiologic responses without ionizing radiation. Studies have offered insights into differential lung perfusion responses to tobacco smoke and electronic nicotine delivery systems, potentially aiding in understanding lung injury patterns from these products.[103] Additionally, Tsuchiya and colleagues (2016) showed that phase-contrast MRI can detect decreases in pulmonary blood flow associated with reductions in lung volume and increases in lung fibrosis area in interstitial lung disease.[104] Hueper and colleagues (2013) investigated measures of regional pulmonary microvascular perfusion using MRI and their relationships to global lung perfusion and diffusing capacity.[105] Recent studies have also explored the validation and repeatability of phase-resolved functional lung (PREFUL) MRI in COPD patients compared to other methods like CE perfusion MRI.[106–108] However, due to the complexity of COPD and the need for further validation and standardization of techniques, MRI perfusion has not yet been integrated into routine clinical practice for COPD.

While MRI has been successfully integrated into clinical programs for diagnosing PE,[109] chest magnetic resonance angiography (MRA) and MRI perfusion are still under development. They show promise but require additional validation and regulatory approval before broad adoption in standard clinical practice.[6] Notably, non-contrast MRA and MRI perfusion techniques for PE are especially promising for pregnant patients, considering the unresolved concerns about the safety of GBCA for fetal health.[110] Feasibility studies have shown good alignment of MRI perfusion with conventional methods in evaluating segmental perfusion abnormalities in PE.[111] However, more recent studies question the additional diagnostic value of MRI perfusion over CE MRA sequences.[112]

CONCLUSION AND FUTURE DIRECTIONS

In conclusion, MRI perfusion is emerging as a versatile tool for assessing lung perfusion and function across various respiratory conditions. The lack of ionizing radiation makes it particularly appealing for longitudinal studies and applications in younger populations. While progress has been made, particularly in CF, lung cancer, and CTEPH, the clinical translation of MRI perfusion techniques has been limited by the need for further validation, standardization, and comparison with established imaging modalities. Future directions in the field should focus on rigorous validation studies, optimization of protocols, and exploring novel applications. Additionally, as the technology evolves, reducing scan times and improving resolution may render MRI perfusion more feasible for routine clinical use. Collaborative efforts between clinicians, researchers, and regulatory bodies are essential to establish MRI perfusion as a reliable and standard tool in respiratory medicine.

CLINICS CARE POINTS

- For conditions like CF and lung cancer, MRI perfusion techniques have shown significant potential, especially given the concerns regarding the cumulative effects of ionizing radiation exposure in young patients.

- MRI, especially non-contrast MRA and MRI perfusion techniques, is promising for the evaluation of PE in specific populations, such as pregnant patients, due to concerns about the safety of GBCA for fetal health.

- Being relatively new techniques, MRI lung perfusion sequences demand advanced technical know-how, as well as hardware and software capabilities. While there is emerging evidence about the utility of MRI lung perfusion in clinical practice, further validation and standardization is necessary before wide implementation.

DISCLOSURES

No disclosures.

REFERENCES

1. West JB. State of the art: ventilation-perfusion relationships. Am Rev Respir Dis 1977;116(5):919–43.
2. Collaborators GBDCRD. Prevalence and attributable health burden of chronic respiratory diseases, 1990-2017: a systematic analysis for the Global Burden of Disease Study 2017. Lancet Respir Med 2020;8(6):585–96.
3. Smith SB, Geske JB, Kathurla P, et al. Analysis of National Trends in Admissions for pulmonary embolism. Chest 2016;150(1):35–45.
4. Hoeper MM, Humbert M, Souza R, et al. A global view of pulmonary hypertension. Lancet Respir Med 2016;4(4):306–22.
5. Hopkins SR, Wielputz MO, Kauczor HU. Imaging lung perfusion. J Appl Physiol (1985) 2012; 113(2):328–39.
6. Hatabu H, Ohno Y, Gefter WB, et al. Expanding applications of pulmonary MRI in the clinical evaluation of lung disorders: fleischner society position paper. Radiology 2020;297(2):286–301.
7. Ley S, Ley-Zaporozhan J. Pulmonary perfusion imaging using MRI: clinical application. Insights Imaging 2012;3(1):61–71.
8. West JB, Dollery CT. Distribution of blood flow and ventilation-perfusion ratio in the lung, measured with radioactive carbon dioxide. J Appl Physiol 1960;15:405–10.
9. West JB, Dollery CT, Hugh-Jones P. The use of radioactive carbon dioxide to measure regional blood flow in the lungs of patients with pulmonary disease. J Clin Invest 1961;40(1):1–12.
10. Martin CJ, Cline F Jr, Marshall H. Lobar alveolar gas concentrations; effect of body position. J Clin Invest 1953;32(7):617–21.
11. Rahn H, Sadoul P, Farhi LE, et al. Distribution of ventalation and perfusion in the lobes of the dog's lung in the supine and erect position. J Appl Physiol 1956;8(4):417–26.
12. Anthonisen NR, Milic-Emili J. Distribution of pulmonary perfusion in erect man. J Appl Physiol 1966; 21(3):760–6.
13. Hughes JM, Glazier JB, Maloney JE, et al. Effect of lung volume on the distribution of pulmonary blood flow in man. Respir Physiol 1968;4(1):58–72.
14. Banister J, Torrance RW. The effects of the tracheal pressure upon flow: pressure relations in the vascular bed of isolated lungs. Q J Exp Physiol Cogn Med Sci 1960;45:352–67.
15. West JB. Regional differences in the lung. Chest 1978;74(4):426–37.
16. Reed JH Jr, Wood EH. Effect of body position on vertical distribution of pulmonary blood flow. J Appl Physiol 1970;28(3):303–11.
17. Greenleaf JF, Ritman EL, Sass DJ, et al. Spatial distribution of pulmonary blood flow in dogs in left decubitus position. Am J Physiol 1974;227(1): 230–44.
18. Beck KC, Rehder K. Differences in regional vascular conductances in isolated dog lungs. J Appl Physiol (1985) 1986;61(2):530–8.
19. Hakim TS, Lisbona R, Dean GW. Gravity-independent inequality in pulmonary blood flow in humans. J Appl Physiol (1985) 1987;63(3):1114–21.
20. Lisbona R, Dean GW, Hakim TS. Observations with SPECT on the normal regional distribution of pulmonary blood flow in gravity independent planes. J Nucl Med 1987;28(11):1758–62.
21. Hakim TS, Dean GW, Lisbona R. Effect of body posture on spatial distribution of pulmonary blood flow. J Appl Physiol (1985) 1988;64(3):1160–70.
22. Hakim TS, Dean GW, Lisbona R. Quantification of spatial blood flow distribution in isolated canine lung. Invest Radiol 1988;23(7):498–504.
23. Suzuki H, Sato Y, Shindo M, et al. Prone positioning improves distribution of pulmonary perfusion: noninvasive magnetic resonance imaging study in healthy humans. Eur Radiol 2008;18(3):522–8.
24. Nyren S, Mure M, Jacobsson H, et al. Pulmonary perfusion is more uniform in the prone than in the supine position: scintigraphy in healthy humans. J Appl Physiol (1985) 1999;86(4):1135–41.
25. Guerin C, Reignier J, Richard JC, et al. Prone positioning in severe acute respiratory distress syndrome. N Engl J Med 2013;368(23):2159–68.

26. Nieman GF, Paskanik AM, Bredenberg CE. Effect of positive end-expiratory pressure on alveolar capillary perfusion. J Thorac Cardiovasc Surg 1988;95(4):712–6.

27. Puybasset L, Gusman P, Muller JC, et al. Regional distribution of gas and tissue in acute respiratory distress syndrome. III. Consequences for the effects of positive end-expiratory pressure. CT Scan ARDS Study Group. Adult Respiratory Distress Syndrome. Intensive Care Med 2000; 26(9):1215–27.

28. Cao JJ, Wang Y, Schapiro W, et al. Effects of respiratory cycle and body position on quantitative pulmonary perfusion by MRI. J Magn Reson Imaging 2011;34(1):225–30.

29. Hopkins SR, Henderson AC, Levin DL, et al. Vertical gradients in regional lung density and perfusion in the supine human lung: the Slinky effect. J Appl Physiol (1985) 2007;103(1):240–8.

30. Rosenblum LJ, Mauceri RA, Wellenstein DE, et al. Density patterns in the normal lung as determined by computed tomography. Radiology 1980;137(2): 409–16.

31. Meier P, Zierler KL. On the theory of the indicator-dilution method for measurement of blood flow and volume. J Appl Physiol 1954;6(12):731–44.

32. Wilke N, Jerosch-Herold M, Stillman AE, et al. Concepts of myocardial perfusion imaging in magnetic resonance imaging. Magn Reson Q 1994;10(4): 249–86.

33. Eichenberger AC, Schuiki E, Kochli VD, et al. Ischemic heart disease: assessment with gadolinium-enhanced ultrafast MR imaging and dipyridamole stress. J Magn Reson Imaging 1994;4(3):425–31.

34. Hatabu H, Gaa J, Kim D, et al. Pulmonary perfusion: qualitative assessment with dynamic contrast-enhanced MRI using ultra-short TE and inversion recovery turbo FLASH. Magn Reson Med 1996;36(4):503–8.

35. Amundsen T, Kvaerness J, Jones RA, et al. Pulmonary embolism: detection with MR perfusion imaging of lung–a feasibility study. Radiology 1997; 203(1):181–5.

36. Berthezene Y, Croisille P, Wiart M, et al. Prospective comparison of MR lung perfusion and lung scintigraphy. J Magn Reson Imaging 1999;9(1):61–8.

37. Amundsen T, Torheim G, Kvistad KA, et al. Perfusion abnormalities in pulmonary embolism studied with perfusion MRI and ventilation-perfusion scintigraphy: an intra-modality and inter-modality agreement study. J Magn Reson Imaging 2002; 15(4):386–94.

38. Amundsen T, Torheim G, Waage A, et al. Perfusion magnetic resonance imaging of the lung: characterization of pneumonia and chronic obstructive pulmonary disease. A feasibility study. J Magn Reson Imaging 2000;12(2):224–31.

39. Hatabu H, Tadamura E, Levin DL, et al. Quantitative assessment of pulmonary perfusion with dynamic contrast-enhanced MRI. Magn Reson Med 1999; 42(6):1033–8.

40. Levin DL, Chen Q, Zhang M, et al. Evaluation of regional pulmonary perfusion using ultrafast magnetic resonance imaging. Magn Reson Med 2001; 46(1):166–71.

41. Fink C, Bock M, Puderbach M, et al. Partially parallel three-dimensional magnetic resonance imaging for the assessment of lung perfusion–initial results. Invest Radiol 2003;38(8):482–8.

42. Ohno Y, Hatabu H, Murase K, et al. Quantitative assessment of regional pulmonary perfusion in the entire lung using three-dimensional ultrafast dynamic contrast-enhanced magnetic resonance imaging: Preliminary experience in 40 subjects. J Magn Reson Imaging 2004;20(3):353–65.

43. Ohno Y, Hatabu H, Murase K, et al. Primary pulmonary hypertension: 3D dynamic perfusion MRI for quantitative analysis of regional pulmonary perfusion. AJR Am J Roentgenol 2007;188(1):48–56.

44. Ley S, Mereles D, Risse F, et al. Quantitative 3D pulmonary MR-perfusion in patients with pulmonary arterial hypertension: correlation with invasive pressure measurements. Eur J Radiol 2007;61(2): 251–5.

45. Nikolaou K, Schoenberg SO, Brix G, et al. Quantification of pulmonary blood flow and volume in healthy volunteers by dynamic contrast-enhanced magnetic resonance imaging using a parallel imaging technique. Invest Radiol 2004;39(9):537–45.

46. Fink C, Puderbach M, Ley S, et al. Contrast-enhanced three-dimensional pulmonary perfusion magnetic resonance imaging: intraindividual comparison of 1.0 M gadobutrol and 0.5 M Gd-DTPA at three dose levels. Invest Radiol 2004;39(3): 143–8.

47. Matsuoka S, Uchiyama K, Shima H, et al. Effect of the rate of gadolinium injection on magnetic resonance pulmonary perfusion imaging. J Magn Reson Imaging 2002;15(1):108–13.

48. Attari H, Cao Y, Elmholdt TR, et al. A systematic review of 639 Patients with Biopsy-confirmed Nephrogenic Systemic Fibrosis. Radiology 2019; 292(2):376–86.

49. Frenzel T, Apte C, Jost G, et al. Quantification and assessment of the chemical form of residual gadolinium in the brain after repeated administration of gadolinium-based contrast agents: comparative study in rats. Invest Radiol 2017;52(7):396–404.

50. Cavallo JJ, Pahade JK. Practice Management Strategies for Imaging Facilities Facing an Acute Iodinated Contrast Media Shortage. AJR Am J Roentgenol 2022;219(4):666–70.

51. Williams DS, Detre JA, Leigh JS, et al. Magnetic resonance imaging of perfusion using spin

inversion of arterial water. Proc Natl Acad Sci U S A 1992;89(1):212–6.

52. Mai VM, Hagspiel KD, Christopher JM, et al. Perfusion imaging of the human lung using flow-sensitive alternating inversion recovery with an extra radiofrequency pulse (FAIRER). Magn Reson Imaging 1999;17(3):355–61.

53. Mai VM, Berr SS. MR perfusion imaging of pulmonary parenchyma using pulsed arterial spin labeling techniques: FAIRER and FAIR. J Magn Reson Imaging 1999;9(3):483–7.

54. Mai VM, Hagspiel KD, Altes T, et al. Detection of regional pulmonary perfusion deficit of the occluded lung using arterial spin labeling in magnetic resonance imaging. J Magn Reson Imaging 2000;11(2):97–102.

55. Mai VM, Chen Q, Bankier AA, et al. Effect of lung inflation on arterial spin labeling signal in MR perfusion imaging of human lung. J Magn Reson Imaging 2001;13(6):954–9.

56. Buxton RB, Frank LR, Wong EC, et al. A general kinetic model for quantitative perfusion imaging with arterial spin labeling. Magn Reson Med 1998;40(3):383–96.

57. Hatabu H, Tadamura E, Prasad PV, et al. Noninvasive pulmonary perfusion imaging by STAR-HASTE sequence. Magn Reson Med 2000;44(5):808–12.

58. Wang T, Schultz G, Hebestreit H, et al. Quantitative perfusion mapping of the human lung using 1H spin labeling. J Magn Reson Imaging 2003;18(2):260–5.

59. Bolar DS, Levin DL, Hopkins SR, et al. Quantification of regional pulmonary blood flow using ASL-FAIRER. Magn Reson Med 2006;55(6):1308–17.

60. Martirosian P, Boss A, Fenchel M, et al. Quantitative lung perfusion mapping at 0.2 T using FAIR True-FISP MRI. Magn Reson Med 2006;55(5):1065–74.

61. Henderson AC, Prisk GK, Levin DL, et al. Characterizing pulmonary blood flow distribution measured using arterial spin labeling. NMR Biomed 2009;22(10):1025–35.

62. Greer JS, Maroules CD, Oz OK, et al. Non-contrast quantitative pulmonary perfusion using flow alternating inversion recovery at 3T: A preliminary study. Magn Reson Imaging 2018;46:106–13.

63. Detre JA, Leigh JS, Williams DS, et al. Perfusion imaging. Magn Reson Med 1992;23(1):37–45.

64. Roberts DA, Gefter WB, Hirsch JA, et al. Pulmonary perfusion: respiratory-triggered three-dimensional MR imaging with arterial spin tagging–preliminary results in healthy volunteers. Radiology 1999;212(3):890–5.

65. Roberts DA, Rizi RR, Lipson DA, et al. Dynamic observation of pulmonary perfusion using continuous arterial spin-labeling in a pig model. J Magn Reson Imaging 2001;14(2):175–80.

66. Alsop DC, Detre JA, Golay X, et al. Recommended implementation of arterial spin-labeled perfusion MRI for clinical applications: A consensus of the ISMRM perfusion study group and the European consortium for ASL in dementia. Magn Reson Med 2015;73(1):102–16.

67. Seith F, Pohmann R, Schwartz M, et al. Imaging pulmonary blood flow using pseudocontinuous arterial spin labeling (PCASL) with balanced steady-state free-precession (bSSFP) readout at 1.5T. J Magn Reson Imaging 2020;52(6):1767–82.

68. Othman AE, Liang C, Komma Y, et al. Free-breathing Arterial Spin Labeling MRI for the detection of pulmonary embolism. Radiology 2023;307(3):e221998.

69. Bauman G, Puderbach M, Deimling M, et al. Non-contrast-enhanced perfusion and ventilation assessment of the human lung by means of fourier decomposition in proton MRI. Magn Reson Med 2009;62(3):656–64.

70. Zapke M, Topf HG, Zenker M, et al. Magnetic resonance lung function–a breakthrough for lung imaging and functional assessment? A phantom study and clinical trial. Respir Res 2006;7(1):106.

71. Bauman G, Lutzen U, Ullrich M, et al. Pulmonary functional imaging: qualitative comparison of Fourier decomposition MR imaging with SPECT/CT in porcine lung. Radiology 2011;260(2):551–9.

72. Bauman G, Scholz A, Rivoire J, et al. Lung ventilation- and perfusion-weighted Fourier decomposition magnetic resonance imaging: in vivo validation with hyperpolarized 3He and dynamic contrast-enhanced MRI. Magn Reson Med 2013;69(1):229–37.

73. Fischer A, Weick S, Ritter CO, et al. SElf-gated Non-Contrast-Enhanced FUnctional Lung imaging (SENCEFUL) using a quasi-random fast low-angle shot (FLASH) sequence and proton MRI. NMR Biomed 2014;27(8):907–17.

74. Voskrebenzev A, Gutberlet M, Klimes F, et al. Feasibility of quantitative regional ventilation and perfusion mapping with phase-resolved functional lung (PREFUL) MRI in healthy volunteers and COPD, CTEPH, and CF patients. Magn Reson Med 2018;79(4):2306–14.

75. Voskrebenzev A, Kaireit TF, Klimes F, et al. PREFUL MRI depicts dual bronchodilator changes in COPD: a retrospective analysis of a randomized controlled trial. Radiol Cardiothorac Imaging 2022;4(2):e210147.

76. Behrendt L, Voskrebenzev A, Klimes F, et al. Validation of automated perfusion-weighted phase-resolved functional lung (PREFUL)-MRI in patients with pulmonary diseases. J Magn Reson Imaging 2020;52(1):103–14.

77. Vogel-Claussen J, Kaireit TF, Voskrebenzev A, et al. Phase-resolved Functional Lung (PREFUL) MRI-derived Ventilation and Perfusion Parameters

Predict Future Lung Transplant Loss. Radiology 2023;307(4):e221958.

78. Qing K, Ruppert K, Jiang Y, et al. Regional mapping of gas uptake by blood and tissue in the human lung using hyperpolarized xenon-129 MRI. J Magn Reson Imaging 2014;39(2):346–59.

79. Mansson S, Wolber J, Driehuys B, et al. Characterization of diffusing capacity and perfusion of the rat lung in a lipopolysaccharide disease model using hyperpolarized 129Xe. Magn Reson Med 2003; 50(6):1170–9.

80. Driehuys B, Cofer GP, Pollaro J, et al. Imaging alveolar-capillary gas transfer using hyperpolarized 129Xe MRI. Proc Natl Acad Sci U S A 2006; 103(48):18278–83.

81. Eddy RL, Parraga G. Pulmonary xenon-129 MRI: new opportunities to unravel enigmas in respiratory medicine. Eur Respir J 2020;55(2).

82. Sly PD, Brennan S, Gangell C, et al. Lung disease at diagnosis in infants with cystic fibrosis detected by newborn screening. Am J Respir Crit Care Med 2009;180(2):146–52.

83. Davis SD, Fordham LA, Brody AS, et al. Computed tomography reflects lower airway inflammation and tracks changes in early cystic fibrosis. Am J Respir Crit Care Med 2007;175(9):943–50.

84. Davis SD, Brody AS, Emond MJ, et al. Endpoints for clinical trials in young children with cystic fibrosis. Proc Am Thorac Soc 2007;4(4):418–30.

85. de Jong PA, Mayo JR, Golmohammadi K, et al. Estimation of cancer mortality associated with repetitive computed tomography scanning. Am J Respir Crit Care Med 2006;173(2):199–203.

86. Eichinger M, Optazaite DE, Kopp-Schneider A, et al. Morphologic and functional scoring of cystic fibrosis lung disease using MRI. Eur J Radiol 2012;81(6):1321–9.

87. Wielputz MO, Puderbach M, Kopp-Schneider A, et al. Magnetic resonance imaging detects changes in structure and perfusion, and response to therapy in early cystic fibrosis lung disease. Am J Respir Crit Care Med 2014;189(8):956–65.

88. Schraml C, Schwenzer NF, Martirosian P, et al. Noninvasive pulmonary perfusion assessment in young patients with cystic fibrosis using an arterial spin labeling MR technique at 1.5 T. Magma 2012;25(2): 155–62.

89. Bauman G, Puderbach M, Heimann T, et al. Validation of Fourier decomposition MRI with dynamic contrast-enhanced MRI using visual and automated scoring of pulmonary perfusion in young cystic fibrosis patients. Eur J Radiol 2013;82(12):2371–7.

90. Kunz AS, Weng AM, Wech T, et al. Non-contrast pulmonary perfusion MRI in patients with cystic fibrosis. Eur J Radiol 2021;139:109653.

91. Kiely DG, Levin D, Hassoun P, et al. EXPRESS: Statement on imaging and pulmonary hypertension from the Pulmonary Vascular Research Institute (PVRI). Pulm Circ 2019;9(3). 2045894019841990.

92. Rajaram S, Swift AJ, Telfer A, et al. 3D contrast-enhanced lung perfusion MRI is an effective screening tool for chronic thromboembolic pulmonary hypertension: results from the ASPIRE Registry. Thorax 2013;68(7):677–8.

93. Johns CS, Swift AJ, Rajaram S, et al. Lung perfusion: MRI vs. SPECT for screening in suspected chronic thromboembolic pulmonary hypertension. J Magn Reson Imaging 2017;46(6):1693–7.

94. Ohno Y, Koyama H, Nogami M, et al. Dynamic perfusion MRI: capability for evaluation of disease severity and progression of pulmonary arterial hypertension in patients with connective tissue disease. J Magn Reson Imaging 2008;28(4):887–99.

95. Ohno Y, Koyama H, Yoshikawa T, et al. Contrast-enhanced multidetector-row computed tomography vs. Time-resolved magnetic resonance angiography vs. contrast-enhanced perfusion MRI: assessment of treatment response by patients with inoperable chronic thromboembolic pulmonary hypertension. J Magn Reson Imaging 2012;36(3):612–23.

96. Ohno Y, Kauczor HU, Hatabu H, et al. International Workshop for Pulmonary Functional I. MRI for solitary pulmonary nodule and mass assessment: Current state of the art. J Magn Reson Imaging 2018; 47(6):1437–58.

97. Ohno Y, Hatabu H, Takenaka D, et al. Solitary pulmonary nodules: potential role of dynamic MR imaging in management initial experience. Radiology 2002;224(2):503–11.

98. Ohno Y, Koyama H, Takenaka D, et al. Dynamic MRI, dynamic multidetector-row computed tomography (MDCT), and coregistered 2-[fluorine-18]-fluoro-2-deoxy-D-glucose-positron emission tomography (FDG-PET)/CT: comparative study of capability for management of pulmonary nodules. J Magn Reson Imaging 2008;27(6):1284–95.

99. Ohno Y, Nishio M, Koyama H, et al. Solitary pulmonary nodules: Comparison of dynamic first-pass contrast-enhanced perfusion area-detector CT, dynamic first-pass contrast-enhanced MR imaging, and FDG PET/CT. Radiology 2015;274(2): 563–75.

100. Basso Dias A, Zanon M, Altmayer S, et al. Fluorine 18-FDG PET/CT and diffusion-weighted MRI for malignant versus benign pulmonary lesions: a meta-analysis. Radiology 2019;290(2):525–34.

101. Ohno Y, Hatabu H, Higashino T, et al. Dynamic perfusion MRI versus perfusion scintigraphy: prediction of postoperative lung function in patients with lung cancer. AJR Am J Roentgenol 2004; 182(1):73–8.

102. Ohno Y, Koyama H, Nogami M, et al. Postoperative lung function in lung cancer patients: comparative

analysis of predictive capability of MRI, CT, and SPECT. AJR Am J Roentgenol 2007;189(2):400–8.

103. Nyilas S, Bauman G, Korten I, et al. MRI shows lung perfusion changes after vaping and smoking. Radiology 2022;304(1):195–204.

104. Tsuchiya N, Yamashiro T, Murayama S. Decrease of pulmonary blood flow detected by phase contrast MRI is correlated with a decrease in lung volume and increase of lung fibrosis area determined by computed tomography in interstitial lung disease. Eur J Radiol 2016;85(9):1581–5.

105. Hueper K, Parikh MA, Prince MR, et al. Quantitative and semiquantitative measures of regional pulmonary microvascular perfusion by magnetic resonance imaging and their relationships to global lung perfusion and lung diffusing capacity: the multiethnic study of atherosclerosis chronic obstructive pulmonary disease study. Invest Radiol 2013;48(4):223–30.

106. Kaireit TF, Voskrebenzev A, Gutberlet M, et al. Comparison of quantitative regional perfusion-weighted phase resolved functional lung (PREFUL) MRI with dynamic gadolinium-enhanced regional pulmonary perfusion MRI in COPD patients. J Magn Reson Imaging 2019;49(4):1122–32.

107. Pohler GH, Loffler F, Klimes F, et al. Validation of phase-resolved functional lung (PREFUL) magnetic resonance imaging pulse wave transit time

108. Pohler GH, Klimes F, Behrendt L, et al. Repeatability of phase-resolved functional lung (PREFUL)-MRI ventilation and perfusion parameters in healthy subjects and COPD Patients. J Magn Reson Imaging 2021;53(3):915–27.

109. Nagle SK, Schiebler ML, Repplinger MD, et al. Contrast enhanced pulmonary magnetic resonance angiography for pulmonary embolism: Building a successful program. Eur J Radiol 2016;85(3):553–63.

110. Pahade JK, Litmanovich D, Pedrosa I, et al. Quality initiatives: imaging pregnant patients with suspected pulmonary embolism: what the radiologist needs to know. Radiographics 2009;29(3):639–54.

111. Kluge A, Gerriets T, Stolz E, et al. Pulmonary perfusion in acute pulmonary embolism: agreement of MRI and SPECT for lobar, segmental and subsegmental perfusion defects. Acta Radiol 2006;47(9):933–40.

112. Revel MP, Sanchez O, Lefort C, et al. Diagnostic accuracy of unenhanced, contrast-enhanced perfusion and angiographic MRI sequences for pulmonary embolism diagnosis: results of independent sequence readings. Eur Radiol 2013;23(9):2374–82.

compared to echocardiography in chronic obstructive pulmonary disease. J Magn Reson Imaging 2022;56(2):605–15.

Perfusion Imaging for the Heart

Amit R. Patel, MD[a,b,*], Christopher M. Kramer, MD[a,b]

KEYWORDS

- Myocardial perfusion imaging • Stress cardiac MR imaging • Coronary artery disease
- Diagnostic accuracy • Revascularization • Myocardial ischemic burden
- Coronary microvasculature

KEY POINTS

- Myocardial perfusion imaging in stress cardiac MR imaging is recommended by US and European Guidelines.
- Cardiac magnetic resonance (CMR) has high diagnostic accuracy for detecting hemodynamically significant coronary artery disease.
- Stress perfusion CMR is a noninvasive, cost-effective alternative to guide coronary revascularization.
- Quantifying blood flow and perfusion reserve enhances ischemic burden assessment.
- CMR enables evaluation of coronary microvasculature, a key factor in angina.

BACKGROUND

Perfusion imaging of the myocardium and other cardiac structures allows one to differentiate tissues not only based on the extent and integrity of the vascular bed within any given tissue of the heart but also based on the differential supply of blood flow into the tissue itself. This can be achieved most commonly through the use of exogenous contrast agents such as gadolinium-based contrast agents (GBCAs) but also through the use of endogenous sources of signal such as oxygen concentration or arterial spin labeling. As with any organ system, perfusion images are acquired repetitively in a single slice position to visualize the changes in signal generation as the contrast agent transits through the tissue of interest. Unique to the heart is that the image acquisition must be electrocardiographically gated to mitigate the impact of cardiac motion on image quality.

IMAGE ACQUISITION

The most commonly used pulse sequences for visualizing perfusion imaging in the heart is a saturation recovery preparation with either a gradient recalled echo or a steady-state free precession readout.[1] Typically, within a single heartbeat, three to five complete images are acquired during different parts of the cardiac cycle at different slice positions each. Additional images are then acquired repetitively for each slice position during the same portion of the cardiac cycle as in the prior heartbeat to generate a video that seems to show the contrast agent dynamically perfusing through the cardiac tissue of interest.

MYOCARDIAL INFARCTION

The classical example of the usefulness of perfusion imaging for the heart is in the setting of an acute myocardial infarction. Here, the coronary supply to a region of myocardium is significantly disrupted due to complete occlusion of a coronary artery often resulting in myocardial necrosis and destruction of the microvasculature. During perfusion imaging, there is decreased uptake of contrast agent into the infarcted myocardium

---

[a] Department of Medicine, From the Cardiovascular Division, University of Virginia Health, 1215 Lee Street, Box 800158, Charlottesville, VA 22908, USA; [b] Department of Radiology and Medical Imaging, From the Cardiovascular Division, University of Virginia Health, 1215 Lee Street, Box 800158, Charlottesville, VA 22908, USA
* Corresponding author.
E-mail address: apatel@virginia.edu

Magn Reson Imaging Clin N Am 32 (2024) 125–134
https://doi.org/10.1016/j.mric.2023.09.005

and thus no signal is generated within the infarcted myocardium as the contrast passes through the heart.[2] In distinction, contrast agent can readily perfuse into neighboring non-infarcted myocardium allowing for normal signal generation on dynamic T1-weighted imaging (**Fig. 1**). Resting perfusion defects may also occur in regions of myocardium impacted by a chronic myocardial infarction. However, in the presence of smaller subendocardial myocardial infarctions, the perfusion defect can be subtle (**Fig. 2**) limiting the clinical applicability of resting perfusion imaging as a sole modality for the detection of chronic myocardial infarction.[3]

MYOCARDIAL ISCHEMIA

The most common use of perfusion imaging of the heart is for the detection of myocardial ischemia and is recommended by the American College of Cardiology/American Heart Association[4] and the European Society of Cardiology[5] for the evaluation of patients with chest pain. Myocardial ischemia occurs when there is inadequate blood flow to meet the oxygen demands of the myocardium. The most common cause of myocardial ischemia is obstructive coronary artery disease, although abnormalities in the coronary microvasculature are increasingly recognized as an alternative cause of ischemia.[6] During resting conditions, myocardial blood flow (MBF) in healthy myocardium is approximately 1 mL/g/min and is expected to at least double in response to stress conditions as induced by exercise or following the administration of an inotropic or vasodilator medication. However, this ability of MBF to increase is blunted (ie, decreased myocardial perfusion reserve [MPR]) when the myocardium is ischemic. These physiologic variations in MBF

can be detected with the use of first-pass contrast imaging. Here, a GBCA is used as a blood flow tracer. In the absence of an underlying myocardial infarction or an obstructive coronary artery stenosis, the GBCA will result in homogenous increase in signal intensity of the myocardium as it perfuses though it during both resting and stress conditions. However, in myocardium supplied by an obstructive coronary artery stenosis (ischemic myocardium), the GBCA will perfuse into it more slowly and at lower concentrations than regions of myocardium supplied by an unobstructed coronary artery. This differential perfusion will appear as a perfusion defect characterized by regions of relatively lower signal intensity as the GBCA transits through the ischemic myocardium when compared with nonischemic myocardium (**Fig. 3**).

INTERPRETATION OF STRESS MYOCARDIAL PERFUSION IMAGES

The interpretation of stress myocardial perfusion images must be made in the context of both the resting myocardial perfusion images and late gadolinium enhancement (LGE) images acquired 10 to 20 minutes after the first-pass perfusion acquisition.[7] A true stress-induced perfusion defect is located along the subendocardium of the left ventricle (LV) myocardium in a coronary artery distribution and is typically greater than 1 pixel wide. When viewed as a video of first-pass perfusion, the defect typically is most pronounced after peak contrast enhancement of the LV cavity and lasts for several heartbeats after the contrast starts to wash out of the cavity (see **Fig. 3**). A perfusion defect due to ischemia is typically present only during stress and not during resting conditions. This is in contrast to

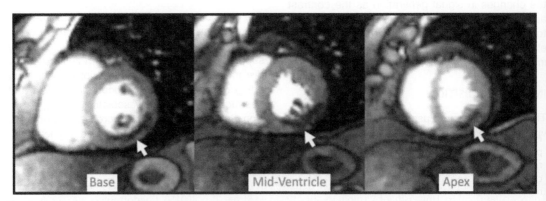

Base   Mid-Ventricle   Apex

Fig. 1. Resting perfusion defect and acute myocardial infarction. Selected T1-weighted images are shown from peak myocardial enhancement during dynamic first pass perfusion imaging using a gadolinium-based contrast agent. Arrows point to a resting perfusion defect in the inferior and inferolateral segments corresponding to the territory of recently infarcted myocardium.

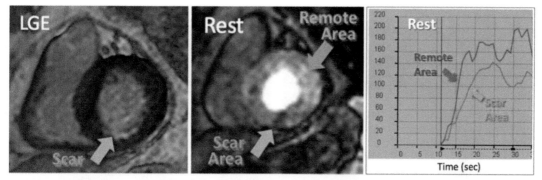

Fig. 2. Resting perfusion defect and chronic myocardial infarction. The panel on the left shows a region of late gadolinium enhancement (LGE) representing a prior subendocardial myocardial infarction. The center panel represents a subtle perfusion defect in the same territory. The right panel represents a time–intensity curve demonstrating the decreased rate of enhancement and overall signal intensity within the myocardial territory that has evidence of a prior myocardial infarction. (*From* Patel MB, Mor-Avi V, Kawaji K, et al. Role of Perfusion at Rest in the Diagnosis of Myocardial Infarction Using Vasodilator Stress Cardiovascular Magnetic Resonance. Am J Cardiol. Apr 1 2016;117(7):1072-7. doi:10.1016/j.amjcard.2015.12.054 [Figure 3 and 4].)

a dark rim artifact (**Fig. 4**) which is a subtle hypo-intensity often less than 1 pixel wide, present during both stress and resting conditions, and most pronounced before maximal contrast enhancement of the LV cavity and often fade rapidly thereafter.[8] The underlying cause of dark rim artifacts is often attributed to Gibbs ringing and exacerbated at lower temporal and spatial resolutions.[9] Stress-induced perfusion defects can also be seen in the setting of chronic myocardial infarction; thus, interpretation of stress perfusion images must be made together with LGE images (**Fig. 5**). Only stress-induced perfusion defects that either (1) occur in the absence of LGE or (2) extend beyond the region of LGE are attributed as ischemic perfusion defects. In addition to describing the presence or absence of perfusion defects due to ischemia, the number of American Heart Association myocardial segments that are involved and the persistence of the defects should be described as a metric of extent and severity of the ischemia.[10]

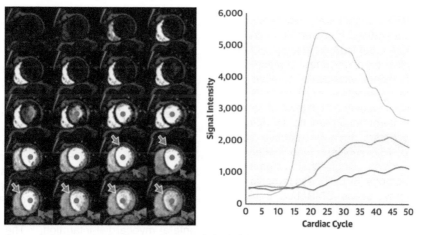

Fig. 3. The left panel shows a single short axis slice of the left ventricle as a gadolinium-based contrast agent perfuses through the myocardium. The gray arrow represents ischemic myocardium and the red arrow represents nonischemic myocardium. The graph on the right represents the change in signal intensity as the contrast perfuses through the myocardium in the ischemic (*gray line*) and in the nonischemic (*red line*) segments of the heart. The blue dot and blue line represent the change in signal intensity that occurs as the contrast agent transits through the left ventricular cavity. Stress-induced perfusion defect. (*From* Patel AR, Salerno M, Kwong RY, Singh A, Heydari B, Kramer CM. Stress Cardiac Magnetic Resonance Myocardial Perfusion Imaging: JACC Review Topic of the Week. J Am Coll Cardiol. Oct 19 2021;78(16):1655-1668. doi:10.1016/j.jacc.2021.08.022.)[56]

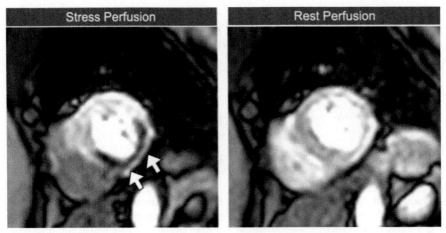

Fig. 4. The left image represents a large, severe stress-induced perfusion defect in the inferoseptal, inferior, and inferior segments, which is not present during resting conditions (*right image*). A faint circumferential hypointensity that is less than 1 pixel wide is seen along the entire subendocardial border on the rest perfusion image. This finding most likely represents a dark rim artifact. Stress-induced perfusion defect. (*From* Patel AR, Salerno M, Kwong RY, Singh A, Heydari B, Kramer CM. Stress Cardiac Magnetic Resonance Myocardial Perfusion Imaging: JACC Review Topic of the Week. J Am Coll Cardiol. Oct 19 2021;78(16):1655-1668. doi:10.1016/j.jacc.2021.08.022.)[56]

DIAGNOSTIC PERFORMANCE AND PROGNOSIS OF STRESS CARDIAC MAGNETIC RESONANCE

The diagnostic performance of stress cardiac magnetic resonance (CMR) has been extensively studied. A recent meta-analysis[11] identified 33 studies composed of a total of 7814 individuals demonstrated that stress CMR had a sensitivity of 81% (95% CI 68%–89%), a specificity of 86% (95% CI 75%–93%), and an area under the curve of the receiver operating characteristics curve of 0.84 (95% CI 0.77–0.89) for the detection of functionally obstructive coronary artery disease. The diagnostic performance was similar to what was observed in the prospective, multicenter Gada-CAD study, which revealed a high level of consistency in image interpretation among six different stress CMR readers.[12] In a prospective study which included 752 subjects who underwent stress CMR, stress single-photon emission computed tomography (SPECT), and invasive coronary angiography, stress CMR had a higher sensitivity and overall diagnostic performance than SPECT for the detection of obstructive coronary artery disease.[13] When compared with a reference standard of invasive fractional flow reserve (FFR) analysis, stress CMR outperformed stress echocardiography and stress SPECT and had a similar diagnostic performance as stress PET for the detection of hemodynamically significant coronary artery stenoses.[14] As a consequence of its higher diagnostic accuracy, the use

of stress CMR has been shown to result in a significant reduction of unnecessary invasive coronary angiograms when compared with standard of care.[15] Furthermore, in a randomized controlled trial testing invasive FFR versus stress CMR to guide coronary revascularization, the use of stress CMR resulted in fewer patients requiring invasive coronary angiography and coronary revascularization without a negative impact on patient outcomes.[16] These data explain why stress CMR has been shown to be cost-minimizing for the evaluation of chest pain when compared with invasive coronary angiography.[17]

In addition to its excellent diagnostic performance, a recent meta-analysis[11] composed of 31 prognostic studies and 67,080 individuals revealed that the presence of stress-induced ischemia as determined using stress CMR was associated with an increased risk of all-cause mortality (odds ratio [OR] 1.97), cardiovascular death (OR 6.40), and major adverse cardiovascular events (OR 5.33). In addition, as the burden of ischemia measured using stress CMR increases so does the risk of cardiovascular death and nonfatal myocardial infarction.[18] The prognostic performance of stress CMR persists irrespective of gender,[19,20] in the elderly,[21] in obese patients,[22,23] and in patients with challenging situations such as left ventricular dysfunction,[24,25] heart failure with preserved ejection fraction,[26] atrial fibrillation,[27] known coronary artery disease,[28,29] prior coronary revascularization,[30] or prior myocardial infarction.[31,32]

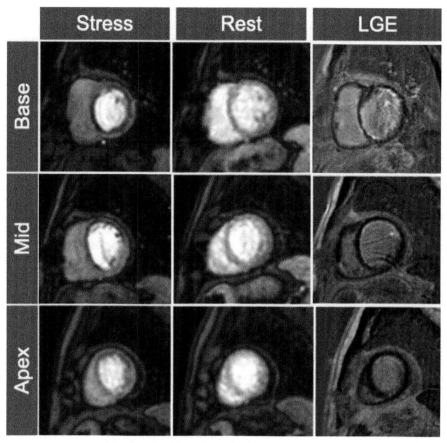

Fig. 5. The rows represent matching basal, mid, and apical left ventricular slices. The columns (from left to right) represent stress perfusion, rest perfusion, and late gadolinium enhancement (LGE) images. A large nearly circumferential perfusion defect is noted at stress but not rest. The stress-induced perfusion defect extends beyond the regions of subendocardial late gadolinium enhancement. These findings would be interpreted as myocardial infarction with evidence of peri-infarct ischemia. Example of peri-infarct ischemia. (*From* Patel AR, Salerno M, Kwong RY, Singh A, Heydari B, Kramer CM. Stress Cardiac Magnetic Resonance Myocardial Perfusion Imaging: ACC Review Topic of the Week. J Am Coll Cardiol. Oct 19 2021;78(16):1655-1668. doi:10.1016/j.jacc.2021.08.022.)[56]

QUANTITATIVE MYOCARDIAL BLOOD FLOW ANALYSIS

One of the major advancements in stress CMR is the ability to quantify global and regional absolute MBF in terms of mL/g/min during both resting and stress conditions and MPR. These values can be derived by using the myocardial time–intensity curves (tissue perfusion curves) and LV cavity time–intensity curve (arterial input function) as depicted in **Fig. 3**. The upslope of the time–intensity curve and the peak signal intensity are most closely associated to the MBF. These parameters are more strongly related to MBF when they are corrected for the arterial input function. The actual MBF can be accurately calculated using well-described mathematical tissue models such as deconvolution combined with a Fermi function fit[33] or the blood tissue exchange

model.[34] The calculation of the MBF requires an accurate determination of the AIF which is typically misrepresented due to T2* losses that occur in the setting of high gadolinium concentrations as the contrast agent transits the LV. Inaccurate representation of the AIF can be overcome by using the dual-bolus technique,[35] in which a low concentration of the GBCA is used to correctly depict the AIF and is followed by a higher concentration bolus of the GBCA to provide a high-quality representation of the tissue perfusion. Alternatively, the AIF can be accurately depicted by using a dual-sequence approach[36] in which a low-resolution image that accurately represents the AIF precedes several slices of high-resolution tissue perfusion images during each heartbeat of the perfusion sequence. In addition, several technical sources of error such as surface coil sensitivity correction, Bloch simulation-based look-up table correction, and in the case of the AIF measurement, correction of T2* losses must be accounted for.[37]

CLINICAL APPLICATIONS OF QUANTITATIVE MYOCARDIAL BLOOD FLOW ANALYSIS

MBF assessment can be used to create color-encoded maps that quantitatively depict changes in MBF that occur during resting and stress conditions. As seen in **Fig. 6**, stress MBF values are significantly decreased in myocardium supplied by a severely stenosed coronary artery.[38] The use of these color-encoded MBF maps can improve the diagnostic performance of less experienced interpreters.[39] The quantification of MBF additionally allows for a more accurate assessment of the ischemic burden in patient with multivessel coronary artery disease, which can be underestimated by visual assessment.[40,41] A distinct advantage of quantitative MBF and MPR is the ability to assess coronary microvascular disease in addition to epicardial coronary artery disease. Individuals of coronary microvascular disease have MBF values that are typically in between those seen in individuals with triple-vessel coronary disease and nonobstructive coronary artery disease.[42] The interpretation of stress MBF values must be made in the context of the resting MBF values. The

quantification of myocardial perfusion can be divided into two groups: (1) classical types and (2) endogen types.[43] Within the classical types, resting MBF is normal. When the stress MBF is also normal, the MPR too is normal and would be consistent with normal coronary microvascular function. However, if the stress MBF is reduced, the MPR would be reduced and diagnostic of abnormal coronary microvascular function. A normal variant of the endogen type occurs when the calculated MPR is greater than 2 despite both the resting and stress MBF being reduced. This finding is caused by low arterial blood pressures or heart rate with lower myocardial metabolic and oxygen demand. In contrast, an abnormal variant of the endogen type is present when the stress MBF is normal but associated with an elevated resting MBF resulting in a reduced MPR and is typically related to arterial hypertension, tachycardia, left ventricular hypertrophy, or obesity.

ALTERNATIVE CONTRAST AGENTS

Although GBCAs are the most commonly used contrast agent for perfusion imaging of the heart, other exogenous contrast agents such as ferumoxytol,[44,45] manganese,[46] and hyperpolarized [1–13C]pyruvate[47,48] are increasingly being evaluated

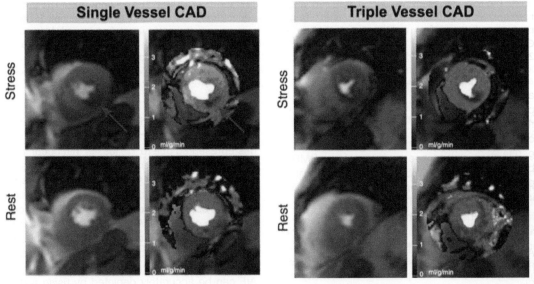

Fig. 6. The panels on the left represent perfusion images and myocardial blood flow maps during stress and resting conditions in a patient with single-vessel coronary artery disease. A stress-induced perfusion defect and region of reduced stress myocardial blood flow values are seen in the inferolateral segment. The panels on the right are from a patient with multivessel coronary artery disease. A global stress-induced perfusion defect along with diffusely reduced stress-induced blood flow values are seen. Myocardial blood flow quantification. (*From* Hsu LY, Jacobs M, Benovoy M, et al. Diagnostic Performance of Fully Automated Pixel-Wise Quantitative Myocardial Perfusion Imaging by Cardiovascular Magnetic Resonance. JACC Cardiovasc Imaging. May 2018;11(5):697-707. doi:10.1016/j.jcmg.2018.01.005.)

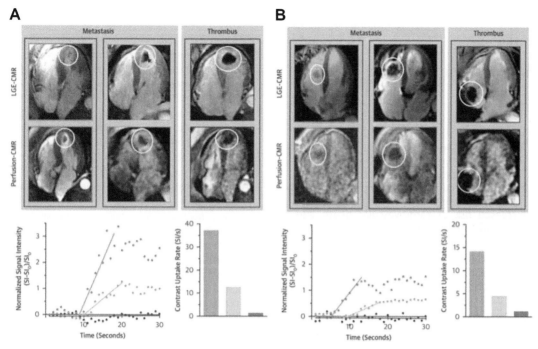

Fig. 7. Representative examples of left-sided (*A*) and right-sided (*B*) cardiac metastasis (CMET) and cardiac thrombus (CTHR) as, respectively, assessed by late gadolinium enhancement (LGE) and perfusion cardiac magnetic resonance (CMR) (top) as well as corresponding perfusion analyses to measure contrast kinetics (bottom). In brief, regions of interest were placed over lesions and tracked throughout the cardiac cycle so as to measure slope (contrast uptake rate) and plateau enhancement (contrast enhancement ratio). Note that for both examples, CMET (*pink and green*) demonstrated higher contrast enhancement than did CTHR (*blue*), consistent with presence of vascular supply. However, a range of vascularity was evident among CMET cases for which lesions with minimal enhancement on LGE-CMR (center; green outline) demonstrated a lower magnitude of semiquantitative perfusion than did diffusely enhancing lesions (left; pink outline), corresponding to lesser differentiation from CTHR. First-pass perfusion in cardiac masses. (*From* Chan AT, Maya TR, Park C, et al. Incremental Utility of First-Pass Perfusion CMR for Prognostic Risk Stratification of Cancer-Associated Cardiac Masses. JACC Cardiovasc Imaging. Jul 5 2023;doi:10.1016/j.jcmg.2023.05.007.)

as alternative agents for assessment of myocardial perfusion. In addition, there is increased interest in the use of endogenous contrast agents such as change in native myocardial T1 times,[49] blood oxygen level dependent signal,[50] and arterial spin labeling,[51] which hold the potential of performing perfusion imaging without the need to inject an intravenous contrast agent.

CARDIAC MASSES

Another important use of perfusion imaging in the heart is for the evaluation of the vascularity of cardiac masses.[52] In particular, a thrombus is typically avascular relative to most other masses and thus would not expect to enhance during first-pass perfusion (**Fig. 7**). Another important goal of first-pass perfusion is to better differentiate benign masses from malignant masses. Malignant tumors are much more likely (>70%) to demonstrate enhancement during first-pass perfusion than

benign tumors (~33%).[53,54] Although evidence of vascularity based on the presence of perfusion is a marker of malignant tumors, relative hypoperfusion suggests the presence of tumor necrosis and is associated with worse outcomes.[55]

SUMMARY

Perfusion imaging of the heart is an integral part of the CMR examination. The presence of a perfusion defect during resting conditions often indicates a recent myocardial infarction, whereas the presence of a stress-induced perfusion defect in the absence of an underlying myocardial scar indicates the presence of myocardial ischemia. Quantification of absolute MBF using perfusion images not only improves the assessment of ischemic burden in patients with multivessel coronary artery disease but also allows for the detection of coronary microvascular disease. In addition to the assessment of ischemic heart disease, cardiac perfusion imaging is an important tool for the evaluation of cardiac masses and other structures within the heart.

CLINICS CARE POINTS

- The most common use of perfusion imaging in the heart is for the assessment of myocardial ischemia during infusion of a vasodilator. There are extensive data supporting a high diagnostic accuracy that guides decision-making and helps identify patients at an increased risk of cardiovascular death and myocardial infarction.

- Quantification of myocardial blood flow using myocardial perfusion imaging allows for the assessment of both epicardial coronary artery disease and coronary microvascular disease.

- Perfusion imaging of the heart can be used as an adjunctive tool to differentiate benign from malignant tumors of the heart.

DISCLOSURES

AR Patel has a research grant from GE Healthcare, United States and receives research support from Siemens Healthineers, Germany, CircleCVI, and Neosoft. CM Kramer has a research grant from Eli Lilly and consults for Eli Lilly and Xencor.

REFERENCES

1. Patel AR, Epstein FH, Kramer CM. Evaluation of the microcirculation: advances in cardiac magnetic resonance perfusion imaging. J Nucl Cardiol 2008; 15(5):698–708.

2. Taylor AJ, Al-Saadi N, Abdel-Aty H, et al. Detection of acutely impaired microvascular reperfusion after infarct angioplasty with magnetic resonance imaging. Circulation 2004;109(17):2080–5.

3. Patel MB, Mor-Avi V, Kawaji K, et al. Role of perfusion at rest in the diagnosis of myocardial infarction using vasodilator stress cardiovascular magnetic resonance. Am J Cardiol 2016;117(7):1072–7.

4. Writing Committee M, Gulati M, Levy PD, et al. AHA/ACC/ASE/CHEST/SAEM/SCCT/SCMR guideline for the evaluation and diagnosis of chest pain: A Report of the American College of Cardiology/American Heart Association Joint Committee on Clinical Practice Guidelines. J Cardiovasc Comput Tomogr 2022; 16(1):54–122.

5. Knuuti J, Wijns W, Saraste A, et al. 2019 ESC Guidelines for the diagnosis and management of chronic coronary syndromes. Eur Heart J 2020;41(3): 407–77.

6. Taqueti VR, Di Carli MF. Coronary Microvascular Disease Pathogenic Mechanisms and Therapeutic Options: JACC State-of-the-Art Review. J Am Coll Cardiol 2018;72(21):2625–41.

7. Klem I, Heitner JF, Shah DJ, et al. Improved detection of coronary artery disease by stress perfusion cardiovascular magnetic resonance with the use of delayed enhancement infarction imaging. J Am Coll Cardiol 2006;47(8):1630–8.

8. Ta AD, Hsu LY, Conn HM, et al. Fully quantitative pixel-wise analysis of cardiovascular magnetic resonance perfusion improves discrimination of dark rim artifact from perfusion defects associated with epicardial coronary stenosis. J Cardiovasc Magn Reson 2018;20(1):16.

9. Ferreira P, Gatehouse P, Kellman P, et al. Variability of myocardial perfusion dark rim Gibbs artifacts due to sub-pixel shifts. J Cardiovasc Magn Reson 2009;11(1):17.

10. Hundley WG, Bluemke DA, Bogaert J, et al. Society for cardiovascular magnetic resonance (SCMR) guidelines for reporting cardiovascular magnetic resonance examinations. J Cardiovasc Magn Reson 2022;24(1):29.

11. Ricci F, Khanji MY, Bisaccia G, et al. Diagnostic and prognostic value of stress cardiovascular magnetic resonance imaging in patients with known or suspected coronary artery disease: a systematic review and meta-analysis. JAMA Cardiol 2023;8(7):662–73.

12. Arai AE, Schulz-Menger J, Berman D, et al. Gadobutrol-enhanced cardiac magnetic resonance imaging for detection of coronary artery disease. J Am Coll Cardiol 2020;76(13):1536–47.

13. Greenwood JP, Maredia N, Younger JF, et al. Cardiovascular magnetic resonance and single-photon emission computed tomography for diagnosis of coronary heart disease (CE-MARC): a prospective trial. Lancet 2012;379(9814):453–60.

14. Takx RA, Blomberg BA, El Aidi H, et al. Diagnostic accuracy of stress myocardial perfusion imaging compared to invasive coronary angiography with fractional flow reserve meta-analysis. Circ Cardiovasc Imaging 2015;8(1).

15. Greenwood JP, Ripley DP, Berry C, et al. Effect of Care Guided by Cardiovascular Magnetic Resonance, Myocardial Perfusion Scintigraphy, or NICE Guidelines on Subsequent Unnecessary Angiography Rates: The CE-MARC 2 Randomized Clinical Trial. JAMA 2016;316(10):1051–60.

16. Nagel E, Greenwood JP, McCann GP, et al. Magnetic Resonance Perfusion or Fractional Flow Reserve in Coronary Disease. N Engl J Med 2019; 380(25):2418–28.

17. Moschetti K, Kwong RY, Petersen SE, et al. Cost-minimization analysis for cardiac revascularization

in 12 health care systems based on the euroCMR/SPINS registries. JACC Cardiovasc Imaging 2022; 15(4):607–25.

18. Kwong RY, Ge Y, Steel K, et al. Cardiac magnetic resonance stress perfusion imaging for evaluation of patients with chest pain. J Am Coll Cardiol 2019;74(14):1741–55.

19. Heydari B, Ge Y, Antiochos P, et al. Sex-specific stress perfusion cardiac magnetic resonance imaging in suspected ischemic heart disease: insights from SPINS retrospective registry. JACC Cardiovasc Imaging 2023;16(6):749–64.

20. Pezel T, Garot P, Kinnel M, et al. Long-term prognostic value of ischaemia and cardiovascular magnetic resonance-related revascularization for stable coronary disease, irrespective of patient's sex: a large retrospective study. Eur Heart J Cardiovasc Imaging 2021;22(11):1321–31.

21. Pezel T, Sanguineti F, Kinnel M, et al. Prognostic value of dipyridamole stress perfusion cardiovascular magnetic resonance in elderly patients >75 years with suspected coronary artery disease. Eur Heart J Cardiovasc Imaging 2021;22(8):904–11.

22. Ge Y, Steel K, Antiochos P, et al. Stress CMR in patients with obesity: insights from the Stress CMR Perfusion Imaging in the United States (SPINS) registry. Eur Heart J Cardiovasc Imaging 2021;22(5):518–27.

23. Kinnel M, Garot J, Pezel T, et al. Prognostic value of vasodilator stress perfusion CMR in morbidly obese patients (BMI >/=40 kg/m(2)) without known CAD. JACC Cardiovasc Imaging 2020;13(5):1276–7.

24. Ge Y, Antiochos P, Steel K, et al. Prognostic Value of Stress CMR Perfusion Imaging in Patients With Reduced Left Ventricular Function. JACC Cardiovasc Imaging 2020;13(10):2132–45.

25. Pezel T, Sanguineti F, Kinnel M, et al. Safety and prognostic value of vasodilator stress cardiovascular magnetic resonance in patients with heart failure and reduced ejection fraction. Circ Cardiovasc Imaging 2020;13(9):e010599.

26. Pezel T, Hovasse T, Sanguineti F, et al. Long-term prognostic value of stress CMR in patients with heart failure and preserved ejection fraction. JACC Cardiovasc Imaging 2021;14(12):2319–33.

27. Pezel T, Sanguineti F, Kinnel M, et al. Feasibility and prognostic value of vasodilator stress perfusion CMR in patients with atrial fibrillation. JACC Cardiovasc Imaging 2021;14(2):379–89.

28. Antiochos P, Ge Y, Heydari B, et al. Prognostic value of stress cardiac magnetic resonance in patients with known coronary artery disease. JACC Cardiovasc Imaging 2022;15(1):60–71.

29. Pezel T, Hovasse T, Lefevre T, et al. Prognostic value of stress CMR in symptomatic patients with coronary stenosis on CCTA. JACC Cardiovasc Imaging 2022; 15(8):1408–22.

30. Pezel T, Hovasse T, Kinnel M, et al. Long-term prognostic value of stress cardiovascular magnetic resonance in patients with history of percutaneous coronary intervention. Circ Cardiovasc Imaging 2021;14(6):e012374.

31. Pezel T, Garot P, Kinnel M, et al. Prognostic value of vasodilator stress perfusion cardiovascular magnetic resonance in patients with prior myocardial infarction. JACC Cardiovasc Imaging 2021;14(11):2138–51.

32. Heitner JF, Kim RJ, Kim HW, et al. Prognostic value of vasodilator stress cardiac magnetic resonance imaging: a multicenter study with 48 000 patient-years of follow-up. JAMA Cardiol 2019;4(3):256–64.

33. Jerosch-Herold M, Wilke N, Stillman AE. Magnetic resonance quantification of the myocardial perfusion reserve with a Fermi function model for constrained deconvolution. Med Phys 1998;25(1):73–84.

34. Bassingthwaighte JB, Wang CY, Chan IS. Blood-tissue exchange via transport and transformation by capillary endothelial cells. Circ Res 1989;65(4):997–1020.

35. Christian TF, Aletras AH, Arai AE. Estimation of absolute myocardial blood flow during first-pass MR perfusion imaging using a dual-bolus injection technique: comparison to single-bolus injection method. J Magn Reson Imaging 2008;27(6):1271–7.

36. Gatehouse PD, Elkington AG, Ablitt NA, et al. Accurate assessment of the arterial input function during high-dose myocardial perfusion cardiovascular magnetic resonance. J Magn Reson Imaging 2004; 20(1):39–45.

37. Kellman P, Hansen MS, Nielles-Vallespin S, et al. Myocardial perfusion cardiovascular magnetic resonance: optimized dual sequence and reconstruction for quantification. J Cardiovasc Magn Reson 2017; 19(1):43.

38. Hsu LY, Jacobs M, Benovoy M, et al. Diagnostic performance of fully automated pixel-wise quantitative myocardial perfusion imaging by cardiovascular magnetic resonance. JACC Cardiovasc Imaging 2018;11(5):697–707.

39. Villa ADM, Corsinovi L, Ntalas I, et al. Importance of operator training and rest perfusion on the diagnostic accuracy of stress perfusion cardiovascular magnetic resonance. J Cardiovasc Magn Reson 2018;20(1):74.

40. Patel AR, Antkowiak PF, Nandalur KR, et al. Assessment of advanced coronary artery disease: advantages of quantitative cardiac magnetic resonance perfusion analysis. J Am Coll Cardiol 2010;56(7):561–9.

41. Kotecha T, Chacko L, Chehab O, et al. Assessment of multivessel coronary artery disease using cardiovascular magnetic resonance pixelwise quantitative perfusion mapping. JACC Cardiovasc Imaging 2020;13(12):2546–57.

42. Kotecha T, Martinez-Naharro A, Boldrini M, et al. Automated pixel-wise quantitative myocardial perfusion mapping by CMR to detect obstructive coronary artery disease and coronary microvascular dysfunction: validation against invasive coronary physiology. JACC Cardiovasc Imaging 2019;12(10):1958–69.

43. Schindler TH, Fearon WF, Pelletier-Galarneau M, et al. Myocardial perfusion PET for the detection and reporting of coronary microvascular dysfunction: A JACC: cardiovascular imaging expert panel statement. JACC Cardiovasc Imaging 2023;16(4):536–48.

44. Colbert CM, Hollowed JJ, Nguyen DN, et al. Fractional myocardial blood volume by ferumoxytol-enhanced MRI: Estimation of ischemic burden. Magn Reson Med 2023;89(4):1557–66.

45. Nguyen KL, Shao J, Ghodrati VK, et al. Ferumoxytol-enhanced CMR for vasodilator stress testing: a feasibility study. JACC Cardiovasc Imaging 2019; 12(8 Pt 1):1582–4.

46. Eriksson R, Johansson L, Bjerner T, et al. Contrast enhancement of manganese-hydroxypropyl-tetraacetic acid, an MR contrast agent with potential for detecting differences in myocardial blood flow. J Magn Reson Imaging 2006;24(4):858–63.

47. Joergensen SH, Hansen ESS, Bogh N, et al. Detection of increased pyruvate dehydrogenase flux in the human heart during adenosine stress test using hyperpolarized [1-(13C)]pyruvate cardiovascular magnetic resonance imaging. J Cardiovasc Magn Reson 2022;24(1):34.

48. Fuetterer M, Busch J, Traechtler J, et al. Quantitative myocardial first-pass cardiovascular magnetic resonance perfusion imaging using hyperpolarized [1-(13C)] pyruvate. J Cardiovasc Magn Reson 2018; 20(1):73.

49. Burrage MK, Shanmuganathan M, Masi A, et al. Cardiovascular magnetic resonance stress and rest T1-mapping using regadenoson for detection of ischemic heart disease compared to healthy controls. Int J Cardiol 2021;333:239–45.

50. Fischer K, Guensch DP, Friedrich MG. Response of myocardial oxygenation to breathing manoeuvres and adenosine infusion. Eur Heart J Cardiovasc Imaging 2015;16(4):395–401.

51. Aramendia-Vidaurreta V, Echeverria-Chasco R, Vidorreta M, et al. Quantification of myocardial perfusion with vasodilation using arterial spin labeling at 1.5T. J Magn Reson Imaging 2021;53(3):777–88.

52. Motwani M, Kidambi A, Herzog BA, et al. MR imaging of cardiac tumors and masses: a review of methods and clinical applications. Radiology 2013; 268(1):26–43.

53. Mousavi N, Cheezum MK, Aghayev A, et al. Assessment of cardiac masses by cardiac magnetic resonance imaging: histological correlation and clinical outcomes. J Am Heart Assoc 2019;8(1):e007829.

54. Kassi M, Polsani V, Schutt RC, et al. Differentiating benign from malignant cardiac tumors with cardiac magnetic resonance imaging. J Thorac Cardiovasc Surg 2019;157(5):1912–1922 e2.

55. Chan AT, Maya TR, Park C, et al. Incremental utility of first-pass perfusion cmr for prognostic risk stratification of cancer-associated cardiac masses. JACC Cardiovasc Imaging 2023. https://doi.org/10.1016/j.jcmg.2023.05.007.

56. Patel AR, Salerno M, Kwong RY, et al. Stress cardiac magnetic resonance myocardial perfusion imaging: JACC review topic of the week. J Am Coll Cardiol 2021;78(16):1655–68.

Magnetic Resonance Perfusion Imaging for Breast Cancer

Durga Udayakumar, PhD*, Ananth J. Madhuranthakam, PhD,
Başak E. Doğan, MD

KEYWORDS

- Breast cancer • DCE-MRI • Ultrafast DCE-MRI • Perfusion imaging • Microvascular density
- Quantitative modeling

KEY POINTS

- Breast cancer is a global health concern, ranking as the most frequently diagnosed cancer in women, and it carries a substantial socioeconomic burden.
- Breast cancer is a complex disease with 4 major subtypes, each having distinct prognostic factors, treatment responses, and survival rates, highlighting the importance of personalized approaches to care.
- Advances in targeted therapies, coupled with widespread screening programs, have significantly improved the 5-year survival rates for primary breast cancer patients by enabling early detection and timely treatment.
- Imaging techniques, particularly mammography and MRI, are indispensable tools in diagnosing and managing breast cancer, with MRI playing a vital role in cases of inconclusive mammography results or dense breast tissue.
- Dynamic contrast-enhanced (DCE) MRI, which measures tumor perfusion and assesses angiogenesis, has become a cornerstone of breast cancer imaging, offering valuable clinical insights and high negative-predictive value, though its specificity may vary.

INTRODUCTION

Breast cancer is the most frequently diagnosed cancer among women globally, carrying a significant socioeconomic burden. In 2020, approximately 2.26 million new cases of breast cancer were identified worldwide.[1] Within the United States, an estimated 287,850 women received new diagnoses of invasive breast cancer in 2022, and roughly 43,250 women succumbed to the disease.[2] Breast cancer is a heterogeneous disease and detailed molecular profiling has classified breast cancer into 4 major subtypes—luminal-A, luminal-B, human epidermal growth factor receptor 2 (HER2)-enriched, and basal-like.[3–5] Each subtype exhibits distinct prognoses, risks of

progression, responses to treatment, and survival outcomes.[6] Over the past 2 decades, advancements in our understanding of breast cancer pathophysiology have led to the development of several targeted therapies. These therapies, tailored to specific breast cancer subtypes, have substantially improved survival rates.[7] For patients with primary breast cancer, the 5-year survival rate now exceeds 99%.[8] One major factor contributing to this increase in patient survival is the widespread adoption of breast cancer screening, which has facilitated early detection and subsequently led to timely intervention.[9]

Imaging plays a crucial role in the screening, diagnosis, staging, and management of breast cancer. While mammography remains the primary imaging

Department of Radiology, Advanced Imaging Research Center, UT Southwestern Medical Center, Dallas, TX 75390, USA
* Corresponding author.
E-mail address: Durga.Udayakumar@UTSouthwestern.edu

Magn Reson Imaging Clin N Am 32 (2024) 135–150
https://doi.org/10.1016/j.mric.2023.09.012
1064-9689/24/© 2023 Elsevier Inc. All rights reserved.

modality for breast cancer screening, ultrasound (US) or magnetic resonance imaging (MRI) are often employed in certain conditions, specifically for patients with dense breast tissue or when mammography results are inconclusive. Breast MRI has thus evolved into an indispensable tool for various applications, including pre-operative staging, therapy monitoring, detection of recurrence, and resolving ambiguous findings from mammography or US.[10] MRI offers high-resolution anatomic images that can be augmented with functional data, such as tumor perfusion and cellularity, to provide a comprehensive evaluation of breast cancer. This approach, known as multiparametric MRI (mpMRI), has become the standard clinical protocol for breast cancer imaging and is readily available on all major MR scanners.[11]

One of the most important breast tumor characteristics to consider is the angiogenesis, a key process in the development and progression of breast cancer.[12] Biologically, angiogenesis is triggered by hypoxic conditions within the tumor microenvironment, leading to the activation of hypoxia-inducible factors transcriptional activity. This activation results in the increased expression of vascular endothelial growth factor, which in turn initiates a series of events including endothelial cell proliferation, migration, tube formation, and the maturation of microvessels. These microvessels promote the delivery of oxygen and nutrients to the tumor. Clinically, elevated levels of angiogenesis are associated with poorer outcomes and a greater likelihood of distant metastasis in breast cancer patients.[13] Dynamic contrast-enhanced (DCE) MRI, a technique that measures tumor perfusion, serves as an imaging metric to quantify *in vivo* tumor angiogenesis. DCE-MRI has become the cornerstone of breast MRI protocols and is currently the most sensitive method for detecting breast cancer. DCE-MRI boasts a high negative-predictive value (NPV; ability to correctly predict the absence of disease at final pathologic examination) that ranges between 89% and 99%, although its specificity can vary, ranging from 47% to 97%.[14–16] Additionally, DCE-MRI plays a well-established role in evaluating therapy response.[17]

This review offers a comprehensive overview of MR perfusion imaging in breast cancer with a particular focus on DCE-MRI, its role in clinical applications, and delves into emerging perfusion imaging techniques for breast cancer.

DYNAMIC CONTRAST-ENHANCED MRI
Principles of Dynamic Contrast-enhanced-MRI

Contrast-enhanced MRI (CE-MRI) is an imaging technique that utilizes T1-weighted MR images,

captured after the intravenous (i.v.) administration of an exogenous gadolinium-based contrast agent (GBCA). The paramagnetic properties of these low-molecular-weight GBCAs shorten the T1 relaxation times in both blood and tissues, thereby increasing their signal intensity in T1-weighted images. Compared to a T1-weighted image acquired before the administration of GBCA, areas where the contrast agent has extravasated appear brighter on CE-MRI. This brightness is typically proportional to the concentration of the GBCA. Tumors acquire increased vascularity due to angiogenesis, creating an environment conducive for a higher concentration of GBCA. This results in an enhanced appearance of tumors, reflected by increased signal intensity on CE-MRI. Comparative studies indicate that these changes in signal intensity correlate with the microvascular density (MVD) within the tumors.[18] CE-MRI is routinely employed for various oncological applications, including breast cancer.

In standard CE-MRI, T1-weighted images are acquired both before and after the injection of GBCA to identify pathologies, including tumors, that exhibit increased signal intensity. However, a single CE-MRI image does not capture the dynamics of contrast flow through the tumor microenvironment. While the signal intensity on CE-MRI is directly proportional to both MVD and GBCA concentration, the rate of enhancement is influenced by factors such as vascular permeability and the characteristics of the tumor microenvironment. These factors affect the diffusion and temporal retention of the contrast agent. Understanding the temporal dynamics of contrast flow allows for the examination of physiologic parameters related to perfusion, microvascular permeability, and the fractional volume of the extravascular-extracellular space (EES). These insights can assist in characterizing the underlying pathology. Consequently, dynamic contrast-enhanced (DCE) MRI protocols have been developed and adopted for breast cancer imaging.[19] These protocols involve acquiring T1-weighted images before, during, and after the i.v. administration of GBCA.

Acquisition of Dynamic Contrast-enhanced MRI for Breast Imaging

Breast imaging, including DCE-MRI, is generally recommended to be performed on either a 1.5 Tesla (T) or 3 T MR scanner, using a dedicated breast receiver coil to achieve an adequate signal-to-noise ratio. Technological advancements over the years have led to the development of 7-channel and 16-channel breast coils, which are now standard in clinical practice.[20] Patients are positioned prone, feet first, in the scanner, with their breasts centrally located within the receiver coil. To minimize motion artifacts related to respiration or other movements, gentle support for the breasts is provided using soft materials. This is particularly beneficial for those patients with smaller breasts.

The breast imaging protocol should adhere to the guidelines established by the American College of Radiology (ACR) Breast MRI Accreditation Program.[21] A comprehensive breast MRI protocol includes a T2-weighted or bright fluid sequence, as well as a series of DCE-MRI scans. The optimal DCE-MRI acquisition should employ a T1-weighted fast radiofrequency (RF) spoiled gradient echo (SPGR) or fast field echo (FFE) sequence, designed for high sensitivity to the contrast agent and a wide dynamic range. The protocol should also include high spatial resolution, full breast coverage without any slice gaps, moderate (90–120 seconds) to high (10–30 seconds) temporal resolution, and uniform fat suppression throughout the imaging volume. DCE-MRI is ideally performed in an axial orientation with an in-plane resolution of at least 1 mm and a slice thickness of no more than 3 mm, all while ensuring continuous coverage (ie, without slice gaps). Due to these stringent requirements, DCE-MRI of the breast was initially performed using 2-dimensional (2D) acquisitions.[22] However, advancements in hardware such as faster gradients, combined with accelerated acquisition techniques like parallel imaging and compressed sensing, have made it possible to perform 3D acquisitions that meet the criteria for high spatial and moderate-to-high temporal resolution.[23,24]

The ACR recommends a temporal resolution of less than 4 minutes (240 seconds) for DCE-MRI of the breast. However, most current DCE-MRI protocols have even higher temporal resolutions. For semi-quantitative analysis (discussed further below), a moderate temporal resolution of 90 to 180 seconds should be acquired, comprising at least 4 phases as a minimum. Alternatively, for quantitative pharmacokinetic modeling (also elaborated below), a high temporal resolution of 10 to 30 seconds is preferable, and should be maintained for at least 6 minutes following the contrast injection. High temporal resolution can be achieved using time-resolved acquisition techniques such as time-resolved imaging of contrast kinetics (TRICKS)[25] or its alternatives (eg, time-resolved angiography with interleaved stochastic trajectories (TWIST) or differential subsampling with cartesian ordering [DISCO]).[23,26] The GBCA is typically administered as a bolus at a standard dose of 0.1 mmol/kg, injected at a rate of 2 mL/s,

and is followed by a saline flush of 10 to 15 mL at the same rate. At least 1 phase of the DCE-MRI should be acquired before GBCA injection, and a minimum of 3 phases should be acquired during and after the contrast injection. In the context of breast cancer, peak enhancement usually occurs within the first 2 minutes following GBCA injection and thus the first post-contrast image should be acquired within this time frame.[27]

Optimized contrast between the tumor and surrounding tissue is crucial in DCE-MRI. Therefore, fat suppression is recommended to enhance the visualization of contrast on post-contrast images.[28] The presence of increased B0 and B1 inhomogeneities within the breast's field of view (FOV) can sometimes result in poor fat suppression, an issue that is particularly challenging at 3 T.[29] To address this, spectrally selective adiabatic inversion (SPAIR) is often employed to achieve uniform fat suppression in DCE-MRI scans. In such cases, it is also recommended to include a single non-fat-suppressed pre-contrast T1-weighted acquisition to aid in evaluating fat-containing breast lesions. Alternative options include Dixon-based fat/water-separated acquisitions, which produce both fat-suppressed and non-fat-suppressed images in a single scan, albeit with slightly extended scan times.[30] Dixon acquisitions offer the advantage of uniform fat suppression due to their increased robustness against B0 inhomogeneities and should be considered when possible. Furthermore, subtracting pre-contrast images from post-contrast images can enhance the visibility of contrast uptake. However, motion misregistration will become an important issue that needs to be addressed. Implementing motion correction techniques can be beneficial in reducing artifacts that might arise during image subtraction.

An example of a DCE-MRI protocol for breast imaging at 3 T using a 16-channel breast coil is as follows[18]: 3D T1-weighted SPGR/FFE, fat suppression using SPAIR, axial orientation, FOV = 240 mm (A/P) × 360 mm (R/L) × 180 mm (F/H), spatial resolution = 0.5 × 0.5 × 1.3 mm^3, TR/TE = 5.9/3.0 ms, flip angle = 10°, acceleration factor = 2 (R/L) × 2 (F/H), number of signal averages = 1, scan time = 3:00 minute. Four phases are acquired with 1 phase acquired before contrast injection and 3 phases after contrast injection with first post-contrast scan starting at 30 second after contrast injection. This protocol can be adapted to meet the specifications of higher temporal resolution using higher acceleration factors or time-resolved acquisition methods for pharmacokinetic modeling. Subsequently, high spatial resolution post-contrast images are acquired at 2 to 3 phases. In such scenarios, a T1 mapping acquisition is also performed before contrast injection using variable flip angles (eg, 2°, 5°, and 10°) to enable accurate pharmacokinetic modeling.[31]

Analysis of Dynamic Contrast-Enhanced-MRI for Breast Imaging

Several methods are available for analyzing DCE-MRI data related to breast cancer. These include (i) simple visual inspection of all DCE phases; (ii) semi-quantitative analysis of signal intensity variations across different phases; (iii) pharmacokinetic modeling using multi-compartment analysis to generate parametric maps; and (iv) emerging techniques involving radiomics and deep-learning-based analysis. All these methods necessitate co-registering all DCE phases to extract information from the same region of interest (ROI).

Visual inspection
This involves a subjective assessment of contrast uptake and can be done either by comparing post-contrast DCE phases to a pre-contrast image or by performing subtraction between different phases. Additional qualitative evaluation can be based on the signal intensity time curve and categorized as follows (**Fig. 1**)[32]: Type I (persistent) refers to continuous signal intensity increase after contrast injection; Type II (plateau) refers to an initial signal increase followed by a relatively constant signal intensity (±5%); and Type III (washout) refers to an initial peak in contrast uptake followed by a decrease in signal intensity over time. A study that classified lesions as Type I for benign and Types II and III for malignant achieved a 91% sensitivity and 83% specificity in diagnosing breast cancer.[33] However, because qualitative assessment is inherently subjective, it has limitations in terms of repeatability and applicability in both diagnostic setting and in clinical trials.

Semi-quantitative analysis
Contrast kinetics can be evaluated by analyzing signal intensity variations across different phases and calculating several quantitative parameters. These parameters include (1) initial peak percentage enhancement (PE); (2) peak signal enhancement ratio (SER); (3) washout fraction (WF); and (4) functional tumor volume (FTV). Initial peak PE and peak SER are typically calculated on a voxel-by-voxel basis within the tumor. WF is calculated as the fraction of all tumor voxels that exhibit washout, defined as those with $PE \geq 50\%$ and $SER \geq 1.1$. Finally, FTV is calculated in cm^3 by summing volumes of all voxels within the tumor with initial $PE \geq 50\%$. Semi-quantitative analysis involves the direct calculation of these parameters from signal intensities without converting those values to GBCA concentration levels, making it less complex. However, these parameters can be influenced by factors such as the underlying image acquisition and contrast injection protocols.[27,34] This makes the comparison of results challenging when obtained at different time points, with different MR scanners, or at different sites. Despite these limitations, semi-quantitative analysis is relatively straightforward both in acquisition (requiring only 4 phases) and in processing, and hence is widely adopted for DCE-MRI analysis of breast cancer in current clinical practice and clinical trials.[35]

Quantitative modeling and analysis
Pharmacokinetic modeling of DCE-MRI offers the potential for noninvasive measurements and

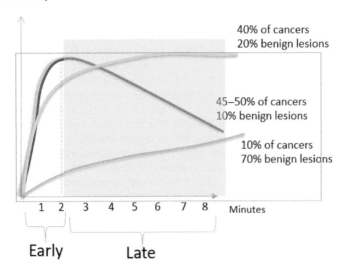

% Intensity

40% of cancers
20% benign lesions

45–50% of cancers
10% benign lesions

10% of cancers
70% benign lesions

1 2 3 4 5 6 7 8   Minutes

Early   Late

Fig. 1. The American College of Radiology Breast Imaging-Reporting and Data System (BI-RADS) time intensity curve classifications and their prevalence in benign versus malignant lesions. Red: early upslope and washout; Yellow: early upslope and plateau; Green: delayed and persistent curves.

functional characterization of tissue microvasculature. Among various pharmacokinetic models, Toft's model is the most widely used model for DCE-MRI of the breast. This model includes 2 tissue compartments: an intravascular space and an EES. Upon entering the tumor microvasculature, low molecular weight GBCAs diffuse from the capillaries into the EES. This diffusion depends on blood flow and vessel permeability. As the GBCA concentration in the EES increases, it eventually diffuses back into the capillaries, reaching equilibrium. The Toft's model can be expressed as follows:[36,37]

$$C_t(t) = K^{trans} \int_0^t C_p(\tau).e^{-k_{ep}(t-\tau)}.d\tau + v_e.C_p(\tau)$$

(Equation 1)

Here, C_t represents GBCA concentration in the tissue, C_p represents the GBCA concentration in the arterial blood plasma, K^{trans} is the transfer constant characterizing GBCA diffusion from the intravascular volume to EES, and k_{ep} is the rate constant for GBCA diffusion back to blood plasma from EES. K^{trans} and k_{ep} are related through the EES fractional volume (v_e): $k_{ep} = K^{trans}/v_e$. DCE-MRI measures signal intensities, whereas pharmacokinetic analysis models the GBCA concentration in various compartments. The first step, therefore, is to convert MRI signal intensities into GBCA concentration using known contrast agent relaxivity (r_1) and the image acquisition parameters. The MRI signal intensity for each dynamic time point t in a T1-weighted SPGR sequence is given by:[38]

$$S(t) = M_0.sin(\alpha).\frac{1 - e^{-TR/T_1(t)}}{1 - cos(\alpha).e^{-TR/T_1(t)}}$$

(Equation 2)

where M_0 is the equilibrium signal intensity, which depends on proton density and other scanner scaling factors, α is the flip angle, TR is the repetition time, and $T_1(t)$ is the longitudinal relaxation time that depends on the pre-contrast baseline T_1 ($T_{1,0}$) and C_t, which can be expressed as follows:[39]

$$\frac{1}{T_1(t)} = \frac{1}{T_{1,0}} + r_1.C_t(t)$$

(Equation 3)

r_1 is the longitudinal relaxivity of the GBCA and depends upon the temperature and field strength. $T_{1,0}$ can be estimated from variable flip angle T1 mapping acquisition. By using equations [2] and [3], MRI signal intensities are converted into GBCA concentrations in the tissue (C_t). A similar method can be applied to estimate the GBCA concentration

in the arterial blood plasma (C_p), commonly referred to as arterial input function (AIF). Measuring a true AIF from the vessel feeding the tumor might not be practical due to issues like small vessel size or localization difficulties. In such cases, the AIF can be measured in a large vessel within the DCE-MRI imaging volume, or population-based AIFs can be used as an alternative.[40] Various groups have successfully utilized pharmacokinetic modeling to derive parameter maps (eg, **Fig. 2**), achieving high sensitivity and specificity in distinguishing between benign and malignant lesions.[34,41]

Emerging radiomics and deep learning–based analysis

Radiomics is an emerging field that transforms voxel intensities from medical images into higher-dimensional data for improved decision making.[42] Radiomics has made major advancements in the field of oncology including breast cancer. Image features for radiomics can be extracted from entire tumors or from specific sub-volumes within tumors, referred to as "habitats".[43,44] Radiomic analyses can be performed using open-source software platforms like 3-dimensional (3D) Slicer,[45,46] integrated with the PyRadiomics library.[47,48] For DCE-MRI analysis of the breast, each phase must first be normalized to 0 mean and unit variance. Radiomics features can then be extracted from the tumor ROIs for statistical analyses across various categories. Xiao and colleagues demonstrated that several radiomic features extracted from DCE-MRI of the breast were promising for predicting increased MVD, achieving a maximum area under the curve (AUC) of 0.84 (P = .002).[18] This suggests that DCE-MRI is a viable non-invasive imaging method for assessing in vivo angiogenesis in breast cancer. Furthermore, Lyu and colleagues developed and trained an artificial neural network to differentiate benign from malignant lesions among Breast Imaging-Reporting and Data System (BI-RADS) 4 breast lesions, achieving a diagnostic performance with an AUC ranging from 0.915 to 0.956.[49]

CLINICAL APPLICATIONS OF DYNAMIC CONTRAST-ENHANCED-MRI IN BREAST CANCER

DCE-MRI is the backbone of any breast MRI protocol and has an excellent sensitivity and good specificity for breast cancer detection. DCE-MRI provides high-resolution morphologic information, as well as functional information about tumor neoangiogenesis. As discussed in the introduction, tumor neoangiogenesis is a key hallmark of cancer development and metastatic potential, that is,

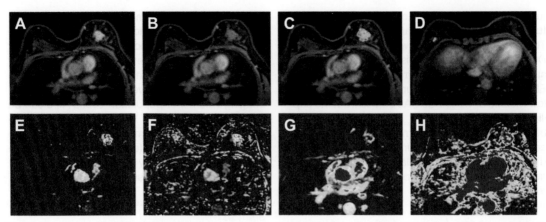

Fig. 2. Assessment of BI-RADS 4 breast lesions in a 51-year-old female using high-temporal resolution ultrafast dynamic contrast-enhanced (DCE)-MRI: A mass was clearly identified in the left breast on enhanced T1-weighted imaging (*A–D*), K_{ep} (*E*), V_p (*F*), K^{trans} (*G*), and K^{trans} map (*H*) from high–temporal resolution DCE-MRI. All region of interests (ROIs) were manually drawn to cover the intralesional area (B, red color), perilesional area (C, green color), and background parenchymal enhancement area (D, yellow color). The pathologic result was breast invasive ductal carcinoma (grade III). (*Adapted from* Mann RM, Mus RD, van Zelst J, Geppert C, Karssemeijer N, Platel B. A novel approach to contrast-enhanced breast magnetic resonance imaging for screening: high-resolution ultrafast dynamic imaging. Invest Radiol. Sep 2014;49(9):579-85. https://doi.org/10.1097/RLI. 0000000000000057.)

the development of a dedicated vasculature with abnormal vessel permeability that supports the high metabolic demand for oxygen and nutrients, especially in aggressive tumors.[50] Specific peptide hormones released by cancer cells promote cancer angiogenesis as soon as they exceed 2 mm in size.[51,52] DCE-MRI is able to depict and characterize this abnormal vasculature and permeability as a tumor-specific feature through the assessment of breast kinetic enhancement features, after the i.v. application of GBCA.[53]

Breast Cancer Screening with Breast MRI— Who Are the Best Candidates?

Women at high lifetime risk of developing breast cancer

Women with a calculated lifetime risk of breast cancer of 20% or more, based primarily on family history, are considered at high risk.[54] The decrease in mammographic sensitivity is exacerbated in younger women with dense breast tissue and in women at high risk for the development of breast cancer, particularly BRCA1 and BRCA2 mutation carriers.[55,56] Failure to detect these biologically aggressive tumors results in the development of interval cancers: that is, cancers that become clinically apparent between 2 rounds of routine screening with mammography. The addition of supplemental screening modalities to mammography, including breast US and digital breast tomosynthesis, has been shown to increase the cancer detection rate (CDR) in women with

dense breast tissue.[57] The addition of breast US to mammography in women with dense breast tissue detects an additional 3.7 cancers per 1000 patients screened.[58,59] While US is more likely to identify small, node negative, invasive cancers, it is time consuming to perform, even with automated breast US methods, with scanning times that range upwards of 20 minutes for hand held devices.[60] More importantly, US has a much lower positive predictive value of biopsy (PPV3 = 0.11) compared to mammography (PPV3 = 0.29), resulting in many more biopsies being performed for benign disease.[58,61]

Currently, DCE-MRI is the most sensitive imaging method for breast cancer detection. Numerous studies have shown DCE-MRI to be superior to mammography and US in identifying breast cancer at a significantly earlier stage in high-risk screening populations.[62–64] Not only does screening with breast MRI result in a higher sensitivity (71%– 100%) than mammography (13%–59%) and US (13%–65%), a significant number of MRI-detected cancers (43%) are less than 1 cm in size when compared with those detected by mammography and US ($P < .001$).[62–65] Furthermore, the sensitivity of MRI in detecting these additional cancers is unaffected by the age of the patient, their breast density, or their genetic mutation status.[66]

MRI-detected breast cancers have the advantage of being less frequently associated with axillary nodal metastases (21.4%) when compared with mammography-detected cancers (54.6% $P < .001$).[62] In patients with BRCA mutations, MRI

method of screening over traditional screening modalities, translates into improved overall survival. Evans and colleagues used the prospective MRI breast screening study (Magnetic Resonance Imaging in Breast Screening [MARIBS]) patient survival data on 649 women aged 35 to 55 years who received annual MRI screening based on the presence of a proven or likely BRCA1, BRCA2, or TP53 mutation in addition to 338 patients who underwent screening MRI after the implementation of the National Institutes for Health and Care Guidance (NICE) criteria endorsing MRI screening.[67] Ten-year overall survival (OS) rate for patients screened with MRI in addition to mammography was 95.3% compared to 87.7% in patients screened with mammography alone. In light of compelling evidence that supports MRI's superior sensitivity, the ACR and the American Cancer Society currently recommend intensive imaging screening with DCE-MRI for women with BRCA1 and BRCA2 mutations or women at a greater than 20% lifetime risk for the development of breast cancer using computer-based risk assessment models.[68,69] Carriers of other gene mutations associated with breast cancer risk who would benefit from breast MRI screening are summarized in **Table 1**.

Breast cancer survivors and average risk women with dense breasts

The ACR recently updated their guidelines to broaden the scope of women recommended for breast MRI screening. Women diagnosed with breast cancer prior to age 50, or those with a personal history of breast cancer, and dense breasts regardless of age are recommended to have annual supplemental breast MRI.[70] In addition, women diagnosed with atypia or lobular carcinoma in situ are encouraged to consider supplemental surveillance with MRI, especially if other risk factors are present.[70] There is mounting evidence that average risk women with extremely dense breasts benefit from breast MRI screening. For women with dense breast tissue, and no other risk factors, the Dense Tissue and Early Breast Neoplasm Screening (DENS)trial reported that the incremental CDR by MRI exceeded 16 cancers per 1000 examinations.[71] The Eastern Cooperative Oncology Group-American College of Radiology Imaging Network 1141 (EA1141)trial was a multicenter trial that included 1444 women with dense breasts at average breast cancer risk who had both abbreviated MRI and tomosynthesis mammography on the same day interpreted by different radiologists.[72] The prevalent CDR by MRI was reported to be 15.2 per 1000 examinations (22/1444), whereas the CDR by mammography was only 6.2

Table 1
Hereditary gene mutations associated with increased lifetime risk for breast cancer

Gene	Associated Syndrome	Lifetime Risk for Breast Cancer, %
ATM	Ataxia–telangiectasia	20–40
BRCA1, BRCA2		>60
BARD1		20–40
CDH1	Hereditary diffuse gastric cancer	41–60
CHEK2		20–40
NF1	Neurofibromatosis type 1	20–40
PALB2	Fanconi anemia	41–60
PTEN	Cowden syndrome and Bannayan–Riley–Ruvalcaba syndrome	40–60
RAD51C, RAD51D		20–40
STK11	Peutz–Jeghers syndrome	32–54
TP53	Li–Fraumeni syndrome	>60

per 1000 examinations (9/1444). Only abbreviated MRI was able to detect all 3 high-grade invasive cancers in the study, and the detection rate of invasive cancers by MRI was higher than that by tomosynthesis. Therefore, MRI facilitates early detection of biologically aggressive cancers in average risk women, which is prevalent at the same rate as in mutation carriers, and can help save more lives.

Application of Ultrafast Dynamic Contrast-Enhanced MRI in Clinical Applications

Standard DCE-MRI entails a high-spatial and high-temporal-resolution protocol to optimize sensitivity and specificity. DCE acquisition comprises at least 1 pre-contrast and multiple post contrast phases. Spatial and temporal resolutions are competing demands for dynamic sequence, and there are inherent tradeoffs between these 2 properties. In the last decade, the emphasis has been on higher spatial resolution to obtain better morphologic evaluation. The high sensitivity of breast MRI depends on the fact that most breast cancers show early enhancement that peaks in 2 minutes or less. However, so do most benign lesions. Typically, cancers tend to lose contrast due to "leaky" irregular vasculature, leading to "washout" in signal after 2 minutes, which can be captured on time intensity curve (**Fig. 3**). However, some benign lesions also demonstrate early washout, and up to 40% of cancers show sustained enhancement, or "plateau" curve which overlaps with benign lesion enhancements on MRI. However, cancers wash-in period can be more distinctive. Most breast cancers start to enhance within 10 seconds after the arrival of contrast material in the major vessels, whereas benign lesions, on average, enhance later (after 15 seconds).

Over the last decade, there has been a lot of interest in developing temporal acceleration techniques. Scan acceleration is achieved by omitting some of the data that are normally acquired (ie, by undersampling). This missing information can be recovered in majority of the cases, since temporally resolved images demonstrate predictable patterns. Compressed sensing utilizes the observation that the compressed signals stand well above the diffuse undersampling artifacts. As a result, the reconstruction can separate true signals from the artifacts in an iterative manner, and in doing so, recovers the missing data and

improves reconstruction accuracy. The net effect is the ability to achieve previously unachievable scan speeds while having acceptable spatial resolution. The benefit of this method is tracking *inflow* of contrast in breast lesions more precisely and capture early arterial enhancement (**Fig. 4**).

The key metrics are related to how fast contrast arrives within the lesion, such as time to enhance and maximum slope (MS) of the kinetic enhancement curve, defined as slope of the relative enhancement versus time curve, expressed in percent per second, and reflects how rapidly a lesion enhances (eg, **Table 2**). The ultrafast (UF) sequences used today can achieve a diagnostic spatial resolution (under $1 \times 1 \times 2.5$ mm) acceptable according to international standards. However, in-plane resolution is not sufficient for multiplanar reconstruction. UF MRI can be integrated in standard MRI protocol (**Fig. 5**) as demonstrated by Mann and colleagues.[73] They analyzed 95 benign and 104 malignant lesions and tested the value of MS in distinguishing benign vs malignant disease. Using MS threshold >6.4%/s to categorize malignant lesions, yielded 90% sensitivity and 67% specificity. The discriminating power of the MS (AUC of

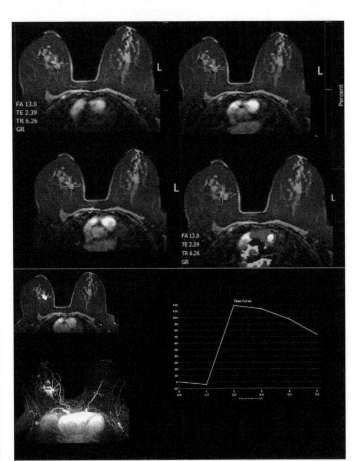

Fig. 3. A 57-year-old patient with multifocal right invasive lobular cancer. Top: Ultrafast DCE-MRI scans obtained at 12-s intervals with full breast coverage using Time-resolved angiography With Interleaved Stochastic Trajectories (TWIST) (view sharing). Bottom: Standard dynamic image of the same patient with a timing of 90 second per phase, maximum intensity project, and time-intensity curve of the cancer, all obtained during the same examination as the ultrafast, show enhancing medial breast mass and sampling site within the tumor. Time-intensity curve shows typical wash out pattern after the third dynamic phase.

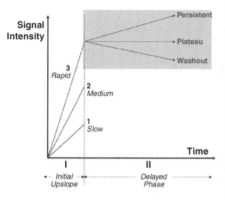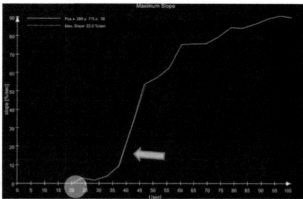

Fig. 4. Differences in time-intensity curve interpretation of standard dynamic (left) versus ultrafast MRI sequences (right). In the classic BI-RADS curve classification, emphasis is on the contrast behavior in the delayed phase since washout is so specific to cancer, as seen on the left. On the right, kinetic curve obtained with ultrafast MRI in the first 100 seconds of contrast injection, showing variation in the contrast uptake.

0.83) was significantly better than that of the BIR-ADS curve types, which achieved an AUC of 0.692 (P = .0036). Mounting evidence suggests improved specificity with UF-MRI. In a recent study,[74] pooled sensitivity of all radiologists was similar for UF-MRI and the full diagnostic protocol (0.84; 95% CI, 0.78–0.88 vs 0.86; 95% CI, 0.81–0.90, respectively; P = .50), specificity of UF-MRI was higher for all radiologists individually and significantly higher when pooled over all breast radiologists (0.82; 95% CI, 0.79–0.84 vs 0.76; 95% CI, 0.74–0.79, respectively; P = .002) and inter-reader agreement was better for UF-MRI (κ = 0.730 vs κ = 0.665). Therefore, kinetic information provided by UF-MRI outperformed the classic BI-RADS-based information.[75] Adding UFMRI to standard dynamic breast MRI may increase regular diagnostic performance by increasing its specificity and decreasing unnecessary needle biopsies of benign lesions.

Application of Breast MRI for Extent of Disease Evaluation in Newly Diagnosed Breast Cancer

Published series over the last decade consistently show that MRI identifies clinically and radiologically occult foci of malignancy. The median prevalence of detecting additional foci of cancer is 16% (range, 10%–34%). In approximately 1300 women who were deemed eligible for breast cancer surgery, MRI altered the surgical management in favor of wider excision or mastectomy in a median of 16% (range, 6%–26%) of breast cancer patients.[76] MRI has been shown to correlate with pathologic disease extent better than other imaging modalities (**Fig. 6**). It is particularly sensitive in the assessment of pectoralis muscle invasion, for which it has a sensitivity of 95% and specificity 65% to 93%.[77] In order to optimally assess pectoral muscle involvement, thin sectioning, and obtaining multiplanar imaging is important (**Fig. 7**). A pitfall in diagnosis is disruption of the retromammary fat plane which may be confused with involvement. Pectoral muscle enhancement is highly specific to anterior chest wall invasion and should be the primary criteria used to determine pectoral involvement.

In evaluating the axillary nodal metastasis, MRI is more sensitive compared to US, however, it is less specific. Smaller volume metastases are better identified with MRI compared to US. However, the sensitivity is below that of surgical staging (ie, sentinel lymph node biopsy [SLNB]). Therefore, SLNB continues to be standard of care for all patients with benign-appearing axillae.

Table 2			
Ultrafast DCE-MRI metrics tested to distinguish benign vs malignant breast lesions			
Functional Value	**Malignant Lesions**	**Benign Lesions**	**P-Value**
Time to Enhance (s)	7–12.9	12–12.9	<.001
Maximum Slope (%/s)	13–29	6–18	<.001
Initial Enhancement Rate	183 ± 45	142 ± 60	.0014
Arterial-Venous Interval (s)	8.14–11.84	12.95–19.61	.006

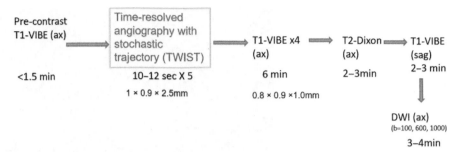

Fig. 5. An example breast imaging MRI protocol integrating ultrafast DCE-MRI using TWIST, along with pre-contrast and post-contrast DCE-MRI phases using T1-VIBE, followed by T2-Dixon, high-resolution T1-VIBE, and diffusion-weighted MR imaging (DWI) in a standard of care dynamic protocol.

Application of Dynamic Contrast-enhanced-MRI for the Assessment of Neoadjuvant Chemotherapy

There are several benefits of neoadjuvant therapy. If the tumor is responsive, reducing its size before surgery could potentially convert an inoperable breast cancer to a resectable one or convert from complete mastectomy to partial mastectomy. Another potential benefit of neoadjuvant therapy is that the extent of axillary surgery could be reduced. Another important advantage is the ability to directly observe therapeutic efficacy when systemic therapy is given in the neoadjuvant setting; whereas there is no measurable disease to follow when therapy is given after surgery. This observation has led to the use of neoadjuvant therapy in clinical trials as a platform for accelerated approval of new drugs by the US Food and Drug Administration. Tumor response to neoadjuvant therapy can also provide prognostic information. The attainment of pathologic complete response (pCR) after completion of neoadjuvant therapy and surgical resection is associated with improved disease-free survival.

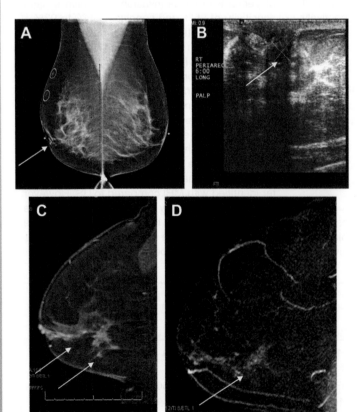

Fig. 6. A 64-year-old woman with palpable right subareolar mass on mammogram (A, *arrow*). Ultrasound showed a 1.5 cm suspicious mass (B) biopsy confirmed evidence of invasive lobular cancer, Grade 1. Breast MRI early dynamic T1-weighted performed for disease extent showed 11 cm segmental enhancement including the subareolar region (C) better seen on subtraction maximum intensity projection image (D) substantially increasing disease stage, and altering management for the patient. MRI-guided needle biopsy confirmed evidence of additional disease more posteriorly, which was also verified on mastectomy specimen.

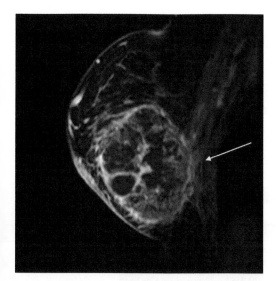

Fig. 7. Sagittal delayed contrast-enhanced dynamic breast magnetic resonance (MR) image in a woman with locally advanced breast cancer. Interpectoral/prepectoral edema and partial thickness enhancement in pectoral fascia and muscle are seen in keeping with anterior chest wall involvement.

Breast MR imaging is the most sensitive modality for assessment of tumor response to neoadjuvant therapy. The PPV (ability to correctly predict the presence of residual disease at final pathologic examination) was high at 93%.[78–81] The NPV was only moderate at 65%, which decreased the overall diagnostic accuracy to 84%. Overall pooled sensitivity range is 63% to 88%, and specificity 55% to 93%. MR imaging has better accuracy compared with mammography, US, or clinical breast examination. Despite these promising data, MR imaging is not currently reliable enough to allow patients to avoid surgical resection after complete imaging response (**Fig. 8**). A prospective, multi-institutional trial that validated the accuracy of breast MR imaging for assessment of neoadjuvant therapy response is the American College of Radiology Imaging Network (ACRIN) 6657 study, which was performed in conjunction with the multi-institutional Investigation of Serial Studies to Predict Your Therapeutic Response with Imaging And moLecular Analysis (I-SPY TRIAL).[82,83] This study involved 216 women with stage II or stage III breast cancer treated with neoadjuvant chemotherapy. The highest predictive value for predicting pathologic response after neoadjuvant chemotherapy was achieved by using both MR imaging and clinical measurements of tumor size. MR imaging tumor size estimates by using volume measurements were superior to measurements of the longest diameter for predicting therapy response. Furthermore, MR imaging metrics such as functional tumor volume and voxel-based signal intensities comparing pre-, early, and late postcontrast images, correctly predict the absence of disease at final pathologic examination.

NEXT-GENERATION MAGNETIC RESONANCE PERFUSION IMAGING METHODS FOR BREAST CANCER

DCE-MRI is the most sensitive imaging method for identifying and characterizing breast cancer, but it comes with its own set of challenges. The main concern had been the development of nephrogenic systemic fibrosis (NSF) in patients with compromised renal function with the use of linear GBCAs.[84] While the risk of NSF has been largely mitigated with the use of macrocyclic GBCAs,[85] new concerns have arisen about gadolinium deposition in various organs, including the brain, especially in patients with repeated GBCA exposure.[86,87] These challenges, along with the additional personnel costs due to i.v. injection, the cost of the contrast agent, and patient discomfort,[88] have fueled interest in alternative, non-contrast agent-based MR perfusion imaging methods.

Intravoxel Incoherent Motion

Diffusion-weighted MR imaging (DWI) is routinely performed in breast imaging protocols to improve lesion characterization and specificity.[89,90] DWI probes tissue structure at a microscopic level, based on the diffusion of water molecules. When diffusion gradients are applied, blood microcirculation in capillary networks (ie, perfusion) also contributes to the diffusion MRI signal. This effect, known as intravoxel incoherent motion (IVIM), can be modeled as follows:[91]

$$S(b) = S_{b0} \cdot \left[f_p \cdot e^{-bD_p} + (1 - f_p) \cdot e^{-bD_t} \right]$$

(Equation 4)

where S(b) represents the DWI signal at different b-values, S_{b0} is the DWI signal at b = 0 s/mm^2, f_p is the perfusion fraction, D_p is the pseudo-diffusion coefficient attributed to perfusion, and D_t is the diffusion coefficient of tissue water. The perfusion effect is only observed at low b-values since D_p is substantially higher than D_t and decreases more rapidly with higher b-values. IVIM is gaining traction in cancer imaging due to its ability to evaluate neovascularization and treatment effects.[92] A study by Dijkstra and colleagues found that IVIM achieved a sensitivity of 92.2%, a specificity of 52.2%, and an NPV of 57.1% in differentiating benign from malignant lesions, compared to

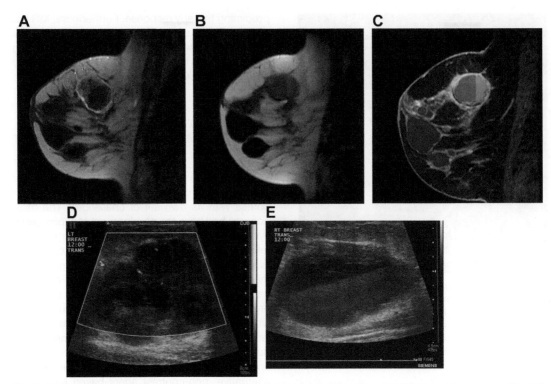

Fig. 8. Right sagittal DCE-MRI without fat saturation (non-fat-sat) images of a 54-year-old woman with right breast cancer before (*A*) and after (*B*) neoadjuvant chemotherapy. Increase in internal necrosis and absence of residual enhancement are evident on post chemotherapy image. T2-weighted fat-suppressed image (*C*) shows fluid/fluid level confirming internal necrosis and hemorrhage as the residual abnormality. On pre therapy (*D*) and post therapy ultrasound images (*E*) the measurable disease appears increased in size, while internal necrosis is evident. Sonographically, it was not feasible to assess residual invasive cancer component, and the tumor was reported as stable to progressive disease. The patient underwent surgical excision, pathology demonstrating only necrosis without viable invasive disease, assessed as complete pathologic response.

DCE-MRI's 100% sensitivity, 30.4% specificity, and 100% NPV.[93]

Arterial Spin Labeling

Arterial spin labeling (ASL) is an advanced non-contrast MRI method that generates perfusion images by magnetically labeling the water protons in the blood. In ASL, 2 images are acquired: a label image with magnetically labeled inflowing blood, and a control image with inflowing blood at its full magnetization. The subtraction between the label and the control image cancels out the static tissue signals and generates a perfusion "map" where the signal intensity is proportional to the amount of labeled blood. ASL has been well-established for brain applications and is currently supported by major MR scanner vendors.[94] Outside brain applications, it is still an emerging method and a variety of ASL methods are currently being developed for a broad range of applications.[95] However, ASL applications for breast imaging have been limited due to intrinsic challenges such as the difficulty in identifying feeding vessels and relatively slower blood flow in these feeding vessels.[96] However, ongoing advancements aim to make ASL a viable option for breast imaging.[97]

SUMMARY

Perfusion is crucial in the neovascularization of breast tumors, facilitating their rapid growth and proliferation. Over the years, MRI specifically DCE-MRI has become an indispensable imaging modality for measuring perfusion. It is widely used in the screening, diagnosis, prognosis, and management of breast cancer patients. DCE-MRI is now a standard component of clinical breast imaging protocols and clinical trials, mandated by both the ACR accreditation and the BI-RADS classification. Various analytical methods are available for processing DCE-MRI data with semi-quantitative analysis using 4 DCE phases being the most commonly employed technique. DCE-MRI has proven to be highly valuable in several aspects including differentiating benign from malignant lesions, classifying molecular subtypes, and most importantly, offering a non-invasive way to assess treatment response.

CLINICS CARE POINTS

- DCE-MRI has become the cornerstone of breast MRI protocols and is currently the most sensitive method for detecting breast cancer with a high NPV of 89% to 99%.

- DCE-MRI is superior to mammography and US in identifying breast cancer at a significantly earlier stage in high-risk screening populations.

- MRI-detected breast cancers have the advantage of being less frequently associated with axillary nodal metastases (21.4%) when compared with mammography-detected cancers (54.6% $P < .001$).

- Ten-year overall survival rate for breast cancer patients screened with MRI in addition to mammography was 95.3% compared to 87.7% in patients screened with mammography alone.

- Breast MR imaging is the most sensitive modality for assessment of tumor response to neoadjuvant therapy with a PPV as high as 93%.

REFERENCES

1. World Cancer Research Fund International (WCRF). Breast Cancer Statistics. Available at: https://www.wcrf.org/cancer-trends/breast-cancer-statistics. Accessed Septmber 06, 2023.

2. American Cancer Society. Breast Cancer Facts and Figures. Available at: https://www.cancer.org/research/cancer-facts-statistics/breast-cancer-facts-figures.html. Accessed Septmber 06, 2023.

3. Coates AS, Winer EP, Goldhirsch A, et al. Tailoring therapies–improving the management of early breast cancer: St Gallen International Expert Consensus on the Primary Therapy of Early Breast Cancer 2015. Ann Oncol 2015;26(8):1533–46.

4. Cancer Genome Atlas Network. Comprehensive molecular portraits of human breast tumours. Nature 2012;490(7418):61–70. https://doi.org/10.1038/nature11412.

5. Sorlie T, Perou CM, Tibshirani R, et al. Gene expression patterns of breast carcinomas distinguish tumor subclasses with clinical implications. Proc Natl Acad Sci U S A 2001;98(19):10869–74.

6. Goldhirsch A, Winer EP, Coates AS, et al. Personalizing the treatment of women with early breast cancer: highlights of the St Gallen International Expert Consensus on the Primary Therapy of Early Breast Cancer 2013. Ann Oncol 2013;24(9):2206–23.

7. Waks AG, Winer EP. Breast Cancer Treatment: A Review. JAMA. Jan 22 2019;321(3):288–300.

8. Chavez-MacGregor M, Mittendorf EA, Clarke CA, et al. Incorporating Tumor Characteristics to the American Joint Committee on Cancer Breast Cancer Staging System. Oncologist. Nov 2017;22(11):1292–300.

9. Duffy SW, Tabar L, Yen AM, et al. Mammography screening reduces rates of advanced and fatal breast cancers: Results in 549,091 women. Cancer 2020;126(13):2971–9.

10. Bitencourt A, lima M, Langs G, et al. Editorial: Impact of Breast MRI on Breast Cancer Treatment and Prognosis. Front Oncol 2022;12:825101.

11. Marino MA, Helbich T, Baltzer P, et al. Multiparametric MRI of the breast: A review. J Magn Reson Imaging. Feb 2018;47(2):301–15.

12. Schneider BP, Miller KD. Angiogenesis of breast cancer. J Clin Oncol. Mar 10 2005;23(8):1782–90.

13. Uzzan B, Nicolas P, Cucherat M, et al. Microvessel density as a prognostic factor in women with breast cancer: a systematic review of the literature and meta-analysis. Cancer Res 2004;64(9):2941–55.

14. Bennani-Baiti B, Bennani-Baiti N, Baltzer PA. Diagnostic Performance of Breast Magnetic Resonance Imaging in Non-Calcified Equivocal Breast Findings: Results from a Systematic Review and Meta-Analysis. PLoS One 2016;11(8):e0160346.

15. Mann RM, Cho N, Moy L. Breast MRI: State of the Art. Radiology. Sep 2019;292(3):520–36.

16. Peters NH, Borel Rinkes IH, Zuithoff NP, et al. Meta-analysis of MR imaging in the diagnosis of breast lesions. Radiology. Jan 2008;246(1):116–24.

17. Jun W, Cong W, Xianxin X, et al. Meta-Analysis of Quantitative Dynamic Contrast-Enhanced MRI for the Assessment of Neoadjuvant Chemotherapy in Breast Cancer. Am Surg 2019;85(6):645–53.

18. Xiao J, Rahbar H, Hippe DS, et al. Dynamic contrast-enhanced breast MRI features correlate with invasive breast cancer angiogenesis. NPJ Breast Cancer 2021;7(1):42.

19. Turnbull LW. Dynamic contrast-enhanced MRI in the diagnosis and management of breast cancer. NMR Biomed. Jan 2009;22(1):28–39.

20. Nnewihe AN, Grafendorfer T, Daniel BL, et al. Custom-fitted 16-channel bilateral breast coil for bidirectional parallel imaging. Magn Reson Med 2011;66(1):281–9.

21. American College of Radiology (ACR). ACR Breast Accreditation Program: Modalities. Available at: https://www.acraccreditation.org/modalities/mri. Accessed September 06, 2023.

22. Kuhl CK, Schild HH, Morakkabati N. Dynamic bilateral contrast-enhanced MR imaging of the breast: trade-off between spatial and temporal resolution. Radiology. Sep 2005;236(3):789–800.

23. Saranathan M, Rettmann DW, Hargreaves BA, et al. Variable spatiotemporal resolution three-dimensional Dixon sequence for rapid dynamic contrast-enhanced breast MRI. J Magn Reson Imag 2014;40(6):1392–9.

24. Benkert T, Block KT, Heller S, et al. Comprehensive Dynamic Contrast-Enhanced 3D Magnetic Resonance Imaging of the Breast With Fat/Water Separation and High Spatiotemporal Resolution Using Radial Sampling, Compressed Sensing, and Parallel Imaging. Invest Radiol. Oct 2017;52(10):583–9.

25. Korosec FR, Frayne R, Grist TM, et al. Time-resolved contrast-enhanced 3D MR angiography. Magn Reson Med. Sep 1996;36(3):345–51.

26. Tudorica LA, Oh KY, Roy N, et al. A feasible high spatiotemporal resolution breast DCE-MRI protocol for clinical settings. Magn Reson Imaging 2012; 30(9):1257–67.

27. Partridge SC, Stone KM, Strigel RM, et al. Breast DCE-MRI: influence of postcontrast timing on automated lesion kinetics assessments and discrimination of benign and malignant lesions. Acad Radiol. Sep 2014;21(9):1195–203.

28. Miyazaki M, Wheaton A, Kitane S. Enhanced fat suppression technique for breast imaging. J Magn Reson Imag 2013;38(4):981–6.

29. Lin C, Rogers C, Majidi S. Fat suppression techniques in breast magnetic resonance imaging: a critical comparison and state of the art. Rep Med Imag 2015;8:37–49.

30. Madhuranthakam AJ, Yu H, Shimakawa A, et al. T_2-weighted 3D fast spin echo imaging with water-fat separation in a single acquisition. J Magn Reson Imag 2010;32(3):745–51.

31. Madhuranthakam AJ, Yuan Q, Pedrosa I. Quantitative Methods in Abdominal MRI: Perfusion Imaging. Top Magn Reson Imag 2017;26(6):251–8.

32. Macchini M, Ponziani M, Iamurri AP, et al. Role of DCE-MR in predicting breast cancer subtypes. Radiol Med. Oct 2018;123(10):753–64.

33. Kuhl CK, Mielcareck P, Klaschik S, et al. Dynamic breast MR imaging: are signal intensity time course data useful for differential diagnosis of enhancing lesions? Radiology 1999;211(1):101–10.

34. Sorace AG, Partridge SC, Li X, et al. Distinguishing benign and malignant breast tumors: preliminary comparison of kinetic modeling approaches using multi-institutional dynamic contrast-enhanced MRI data from the International Breast MR Consortium 6883 trial. J Med Imaging 2018;5(1):011019.

35. Arasu VA, Kim P, Li W, et al. Predictive Value of Breast MRI Background Parenchymal Enhancement for Neoadjuvant Treatment Response among HER2-Patients. J Breast Imaging 2020;2(4):352–60.

36. Tofts PS, Kermode AG. Measurement of the blood-brain barrier permeability and leakage space using dynamic MR imaging. 1. Fundamental concepts. Magn Reson Med. Feb 1991;17(2):357–67.

37. Tofts PS, Brix G, Buckley DL, et al. Estimating kinetic parameters from dynamic contrast-enhanced T(1)-weighted MRI of a diffusable tracer: standardized quantities and symbols. J Magn Reson Imag 1999; 10(3):223–32.

38. Bernstein MA, King KF, Zhou XJ. Handbook of MRI pulse sequences. New York: Elsevier; 2004. p. 1017.

39. Shen Y, Goerner FL, Snyder C, et al. T1 relaxivities of gadolinium-based magnetic resonance contrast agents in human whole blood at 1.5, 3, and 7 T. Invest Radiol. May 2015;50(5):330–8.

40. Xiu Z, Muzi M, Huang J, et al. Patient-Adaptive Population-Based Modeling of Arterial Input Functions. IEEE Trans Med Imaging. Jan 2023;42(1):132–47.

41. Li K, Machireddy A, Tudorica A, et al. Discrimination of Malignant and Benign Breast Lesions Using Quantitative Multiparametric MRI: A Preliminary Study. Tomography 2020;6(2):148–59.

42. Gillies RJ, Kinahan PE, Hricak H. Radiomics: Images Are More than Pictures, They Are Data. Radiology. Feb 2016;278(2):563–77.

43. Gillies RJ, Balagurunathan Y. Perfusion MR Imaging of Breast Cancer: Insights Using "Habitat Imaging". Radiology. Jul 2018;288(1):36–7.

44. Cho HH, Kim H, Nam SY, et al. Measurement of Perfusion Heterogeneity within Tumor Habitats on Magnetic Resonance Imaging and Its Association with Prognosis in Breast Cancer Patients. Cancers 2022; 14(8). https://doi.org/10.3390/cancers14081858.

45. 3D Slicer Image Computing Platform. Updated Nov. 22, 2022. Available at: https://www.slicer.org/. Accessed September 08, 2023.

46. Fedorov A, Beichel R, Kalpathy-Cramer J, et al. 3D Slicer as an image computing platform for the Quantitative Imaging Network. Magn Reson Imaging. Nov 2012;30(9):1323–41.

47. van Griethuysen JJM, Fedorov A, Parmar C, et al. Computational Radiomics System to Decode the Radiographic Phenotype. Cancer Res. Nov 1 2017; 77(21):e104–7.

48. Zwanenburg A, Vallieres M, Abdalah MA, et al. The Image Biomarker Standardization Initiative: Standardized Quantitative Radiomics for High-Throughput Image-based Phenotyping. Radiology 2020;295(2): 328–38.

49. Lyu Y, Chen Y, Meng L, et al. Combination of ultrafast dynamic contrast-enhanced MRI-based radiomics and artificial neural network in assessing BI-RADS 4 breast lesions: Potential to avoid unnecessary biopsies. Front Oncol 2023;13:1074060.

50. Weidner N, Semple JP, Welch WR, et al. Tumor angiogenesis and metastasis—correlation in invasive breast carcinoma. N Engl J Med. Jan 3 1991;324(1):1–8.

51. Folkman J. Role of angiogenesis in tumor growth and metastasis. Semin Oncol 2002;29(6 Suppl 16): 15–8.

52. Senger DR, Galli SJ, Dvorak AM, et al. Tumor cells secrete a vascular permeability factor that promotes accumulation of ascites fluid. Science. Feb 25 1983; 219(4587):983–5.

53. Mootz AR, Madhuranthakam AJ, Dogan B. Changing Paradigms in Breast Cancer Screening: Abbreviated Breast MRI. Eur J Breast Health 2019;15(1): 1–6.

54. Daly MB, Pal T, Berry MP, et al. Genetic/Familial High-Risk Assessment: Breast, Ovarian, and Pancreatic, Version 2.2021, NCCN Clinical Practice Guidelines in Oncology. J Natl Compr Canc Netw. Jan 6 2021;19(1):77–102.

55. Lord SJ, Lei W, Craft P, et al. A systematic review of the effectiveness of magnetic resonance imaging (MRI) as an addition to mammography and ultrasound in screening young women at high risk of breast cancer. Eur J Cancer. Sep 2007;43(13):1905–17.

56. Warner E, Messersmith H, Causer P, et al. Systematic review: using magnetic resonance imaging to screen women at high risk for breast cancer. Ann Intern Med 2008;148(9):671–9.

57. Yi A, Jang MJ, Yim D, et al. Addition of Screening Breast US to Digital Mammography and Digital Breast Tomosynthesis for Breast Cancer Screening in Women at Average Risk. Radiology. Mar 2021; 298(3):568–75.

58. Berg WA, Zhang Z, Lehrer D, et al. Detection of breast cancer with addition of annual screening ultrasound or a single screening MRI to mammography in women with elevated breast cancer risk. JAMA. Apr 4 2012;307(13):1394–404.

59. Berg WA. Current Status of Supplemental Screening in Dense Breasts. J Clin Oncol 2016;34(16):1840–3.

60. Zanotel M, Bednarova I, Londero V, et al. Automated breast ultrasound: basic principles and emerging clinical applications. Radiol Med. Jan 2018;123(1): 1–12.

61. Brem RF, Tabar L, Duffy SW, et al. Assessing improvement in detection of breast cancer with three-dimensional automated breast US in women with dense breast tissue: the SomoInsight Study. Radiology. Mar 2015;274(3):663–73.

62. Kriege M, Brekelmans CT, Boetes C, et al. Efficacy of MRI and mammography for breast-cancer screening in women with a familial or genetic predisposition. N Engl J Med 2004;351(5):427–37.

63. Leach MO, Boggis CR, Dixon AK, et al. Screening with magnetic resonance imaging and mammography of a UK population at high familial risk of breast cancer: a prospective multicentre cohort study (MARIBS). Lancet May 21-27 2005;365(9473):1769–78.

64. Sardanelli F, Podo F. Breast MR imaging in women at high-risk of breast cancer. Is something changing in early breast cancer detection? Eur Radiol. Apr 2007; 17(4):873–87.

65. Warner E, Plewes DB, Shumak RS, et al. Comparison of breast magnetic resonance imaging, mammography, and ultrasound for surveillance of women at high risk for hereditary breast cancer. J Clin Oncol 2001;19(15):3524–31.

66. Riedl CC, Luft N, Bernhart C, et al. Triple-modality screening trial for familial breast cancer underlines the importance of magnetic resonance imaging and questions the role of mammography and ultrasound regardless of patient mutation status, age, and breast density. J Clin Oncol 2015;33(10):1128–35.

67. Evans DG, Kesavan N, Lim Y, et al. MRI breast screening in high-risk women: cancer detection and survival analysis. Breast Cancer Res Treat. Jun 2014;145(3):663–72.

68. Monticciolo DL, Newell MS, Moy L, et al. Breast Cancer Screening in Women at Higher-Than-Average Risk: Recommendations From the ACR. J Am Coll Radiol. Mar 2018;15(3 Pt A):408–14.

69. Saslow D, Boetes C, Burke W, et al. American Cancer Society guidelines for breast screening with MRI as an adjunct to mammography. CA Cancer J Clin. Mar-Apr 2007;57(2):75–89.

70. Monticciolo DL, Newell MS, Moy L, et al. Breast Cancer Screening for Women at Higher-Than-Average Risk: Updated Recommendations From the ACR. J Am Coll Radiol 2023. https://doi.org/10.1016/j.jacr.2023.04.002.

71. Bakker MF, de Lange SV, Pijnappel RM, et al. Supplemental MRI Screening for Women with Extremely Dense Breast Tissue. N Engl J Med. Nov 28 2019; 381(22):2091–102.

72. Kuhl CK. Abbreviated breast MRI for screening women with dense breast: the EA1141 trial. Br J Radiol 2018;91(1090):20170441.

73. Mann RM, Mus RD, van Zelst J, et al. A novel approach to contrast-enhanced breast magnetic resonance imaging for screening: high-resolution ultrafast dynamic imaging. Invest Radiol. Sep 2014; 49(9):579–85.

74. van Zelst JCM, Vreemann S, Witt HJ, et al. Multireader Study on the Diagnostic Accuracy of Ultrafast Breast Magnetic Resonance Imaging for Breast Cancer Screening. Invest Radiol. Oct 2018; 53(10):579–86.

75. Liu Y, Wang S, Qu J, et al. High-temporal resolution DCE-MRI improves assessment of intra- and peri-breast lesions categorized as BI-RADS 4. BMC Med Imaging 2023;23(1):58.

76. Pettit K, Swatske ME, Gao F, et al. The impact of breast MRI on surgical decision-making: are patients at risk for mastectomy? J Surg Oncol 2009; 100(7):553–8.

77. Myers KS, Stern E, Ambinder EB, et al. Breast cancer abutting the pectoralis major muscle on breast

MRI: what are the clinical implications? Br J Radiol. Mar 1 2021;94(1119):20201202.

78. Marinovich ML, Houssami N, Macaskill P, et al. Meta-analysis of magnetic resonance imaging in detecting residual breast cancer after neoadjuvant therapy. J Natl Cancer Inst. Mar 6 2013;105(5):321–33.

79. Sheikhbahaei S, Trahan TJ, Xiao J, et al. FDG-PET/CT and MRI for Evaluation of Pathologic Response to Neoadjuvant Chemotherapy in Patients With Breast Cancer: A Meta-Analysis of Diagnostic Accuracy Studies. Oncol 2016;21(8):931–9.

80. Wu LM, Hu JN, Gu HY, et al. Can diffusion-weighted MR imaging and contrast-enhanced MR imaging precisely evaluate and predict pathological response to neoadjuvant chemotherapy in patients with breast cancer? Breast Cancer Res Treat. Aug 2012;135(1):17–28.

81. Yuan Y, Chen XS, Liu SY, et al. Accuracy of MRI in prediction of pathologic complete remission in breast cancer after preoperative therapy: a meta-analysis. AJR Am J Roentgenol. Jul 2010;195(1):260–8.

82. Hylton NM, Blume JD, Bernreuter WK, et al. Locally advanced breast cancer: MR imaging for prediction of response to neoadjuvant chemotherapy–results from ACRIN 6657/I-SPY TRIAL. Radiology. Jun 2012;263(3):663–72.

83. Hylton NM, Gatsonis CA, Rosen MA, et al. Neoadjuvant Chemotherapy for Breast Cancer: Functional Tumor Volume by MR Imaging Predicts Recurrence-free Survival-Results from the ACRIN 6657/CALGB 150007 I-SPY 1 TRIAL. Radiology 2016;279(1):44–55.

84. Alabousi M, Davenport MS. Use of Intravenous Gadolinium-based Contrast Media in Patients with Kidney Disease and the Risk of Nephrogenic Systemic Fibrosis: Radiology In Training. Radiology. Aug 2021;300(2):279–84.

85. ACR. American College of Radiology Manual on Contrast Media Version 2023. https://www.acr.org/-/media/ACR/Files/Clinical-Resources/Contrast_Media.pdf. Accessed Sep. 06, 2023.

86. Lenkinski RE. Gadolinium Retention and Deposition Revisited: How the Chemical Properties of Gadolinium-based Contrast Agents and the Use of Animal Models Inform Us about the Behavior of These Agents in the Human Brain. Radiology. Dec 2017;285(3):721–4.

87. McDonald RJ, Levine D, Weinreb J, et al. Gadolinium Retention: A Research Roadmap from the 2018 NIH/ACR/RSNA Workshop on Gadolinium Chelates. Radiology. Nov 2018;289(2):517–34.

88. Iyad N, M SA, Alkhatib SG, et al. Gadolinium contrast agents- challenges and opportunities of a multidisciplinary approach: Literature review. Eur J Radiol Open 2023;11:100503.

89. Baltzer P, Mann RM, Iima M, et al. Diffusion-weighted imaging of the breast-a consensus and mission statement from the EUSOBI International Breast Diffusion-Weighted Imaging working group. Eur Radiol. Mar 2020;30(3):1436–50.

90. Iima M, Honda M, Sigmund EE, et al. Diffusion MRI of the breast: Current status and future directions. J Magn Reson Imag 2020;52(1):70–90.

91. Iima M, Le Bihan D. The road to breast cancer screening with diffusion MRI. Front Oncol 2023;13:993540.

92. Arian A, Seyed-Kolbadi FZ, Yaghoobpoor S, et al. Diagnostic accuracy of intravoxel incoherent motion (IVIM) and dynamic contrast-enhanced (DCE) MRI to differentiate benign from malignant breast lesions: A systematic review and meta-analysis. Eur J Radiol 2023;167:111051.

93. Dijkstra H, Dorrius MD, Wielema M, et al. Quantitative DWI implemented after DCE-MRI yields increased specificity for BI-RADS 3 and 4 breast lesions. J Magn Reson Imag 2016;44(6):1642–9.

94. Hernandez-Garcia L, Aramendia-Vidaurreta V, Bolar DS, et al. Recent Technical Developments in ASL: A Review of the State of the Art. Magn Reson Med. Nov 2022;88(5):2021–42.

95. Taso M, Aramendia-Vidaurreta V, Englund EK, et al. Update on state-of-the-art for arterial spin labeling (ASL) human perfusion imaging outside of the brain. Magn Reson Med 2023;89(5):1754–76.

96. Kawashima M, Katada Y, Shukuya T, et al. MR perfusion imaging using the arterial spin labeling technique for breast cancer. J Magn Reson Imag 2012;35(2):436–40.

97. Franklin SL, Voormolen N, Bones IK, et al. Feasibility of Velocity-Selective Arterial Spin Labeling in Breast Cancer Patients for Noncontrast-Enhanced Perfusion Imaging. J Magn Reson Imag 2021;54(4):1282–91.

Perfusion MR Imaging of Liver
Principles and Clinical Applications

Anupama Ramachandran, MD[a,b], Hero Hussain, MD[b],
Nicole Seiberlich, PhD[b], Vikas Gulani, MD, PhD[b,*]

KEYWORDS

- Perfusion • Dynamic contrast-enhanced imaging • DCE MR Imaging • Liver perfusion • Liver
- Compartment modeling

KEY POINTS

- Perfusion can be quantified using dynamic T_{1w} imaging after the injection of contrast agent (dynamic contrast-enhanced MR imaging [DCE MR imaging]).
- The liver is challenging for perfusion imaging because of its dual afferent blood supply, rapid contrast dynamics, requirement for high-resolution coverage of a large organ, and movement with respiration.
- Rapid imaging techniques for high spatiotemporal resolution 3D DCE MR imaging enable measurement of perfusion parameters.
- Several groups have applied quantitative perfusion modeling for understanding normal liver, diffuse liver disease, and focal lesions.
- Standardization of data acquisition and analysis methods remains a challenge.

INTRODUCTION

Each organ has a microcirculatory network (arterioles, capillaries, and venules) with unique characteristics. The term perfusion refers to the movement of blood through this microcirculation. Perfusion MR imaging is a family of techniques used to characterize the microvascular environment by modeling the MR signal using parameters reflecting blood flow and tissue permeability and parameter measurement from an MR experiment. These parameters offer insight into physiologic and pathologic processes. For example, inflammation and neoplasms each have effects on blood flow and/or tissue permeability, and understanding these changes offers a better understanding of pathology.

Arterial spin labeling (ASL) and intravoxel incoherent motion (IVIM) require no injected material.

Dynamic contrast-enhanced (DCE) MR imaging techniques use gadolinium-based contrast agents (GBCAs). When measuring liver perfusion, the dual hepatic blood supply (arterial and portal) must be taken into consideration in the model applied. In ASL experiments, protons are labeled in a vessel proximal to the organ of interest by applying radiofrequency (RF) pulses, and their movement into tissue spaces is modeled quantitatively to obtain perfusion-related parameters. IVIM is an offshoot of diffusion imaging.[1] It is hypothesized in IVIM that the microvascular contributions to diffusion and true tissue diffusion can be separated by using very small or short motion sensitivity gradients to characterize the relatively fast incoherent motion of perfusion while using larger or longer gradients to characterize true diffusion. The labeling and perfusion quantification for both techniques are very difficult in liver due to dual inflow and motion.

Prior publication: Nil.

[a] Brigham and Women's Hospital, Harvard University, Boston, MA, USA; [b] Department of Radiology, University of Michigan, AnnArbor, MI, USA

* Corresponding author. Department of Radiology, University of Michigan, Ann Arbor, 1500 East Medical Center Drive, B1G503, Ann Arbor, MI 48109-5030.

E-mail address: vikasgulani@med.umich.edu

Magn Reson Imaging Clin N Am 32 (2024) 151–160
https://doi.org/10.1016/j.mric.2023.09.003

A detailed discussion of these non-contrast methods is out of scope of this article.

The most widely explored techniques for perfusion imaging in the abdomen use DCE MR imaging, in which intravenous injection of a GBCA serves as an extrinsic label, and perfusion properties are modeled based on signal changes observed over time. This idea follows logically from routine clinical practice, where the appearance of tissues on pre-contrast and multiple timed post-contrast T1-weighted images have long been used to characterize pathologies. The feasibility of MR perfusion using DCE was described in pig livers in 1999.[2] The utility of DCE MR imaging has been widely explored in the literature. The authors review the principles, clinical applications, recent advances, and challenges in hepatic DCE perfusion imaging.

PHYSIOLOGY OF PERFUSION OF NORMAL LIVER

The liver represents a unique biological system because of its dual afferent blood supply. Of the total hepatic blood flow ($\sim$100–130 mL/min per 100 g), approximately one-fourth to one-third is via the hepatic artery (HA), and the rest via the portal vein (PV).[3,4] Blood from the terminal hepatic arterioles and portal venules mixes in the sinusoids, which represent the hepatic capillary bed. These sinusoids are lined by fenestrated endothelial cells without a basement membrane, allowing easy movement of solutes to and from the perisinusoidal space of Disse, termed the interstitial or the extravascular extracellular space (EES) in liver models.[5]

The main mechanism by which hepatic blood flow remains constant is by modulation of hepatic arterial flow through the hepatic arterial buffer response,[6] mediated by local concentration of the vasodilator adenosine.[7] When blood flow in the PV is reduced, the HA dilates, and increasing flow into the sinusoids. This process reverses when portal flow is increased. Unlike arterial flow, portal venous flow cannot be controlled. The ratio of portal venous to hepatic arterial flow can be altered in various diseases and such alterations can be quantified using DCE MR imaging.

GENERAL PRINCIPLES OF DYNAMIC CONTRAST-ENHANCED MR IMAGING

DCE MR imaging involves sequential acquisition of T_1-weighted (T_{1w}) images during and after the administration of a GBCA. Both extracellular and hepatobiliary contrast agents shorten the T_1-relaxation time and have been used for DCE MR imaging.[8,9] The changes in signal intensity (SI) on serial T_{1w} images occur because the GBCA moves into, through, or out from the tissue and are observed using a SI time curve. Such curves can then be analyzed using three approaches: qualitative, semiquantitative, and quantitative.

In qualitative assessment, the shape of SI–time curves is studied and categorized as one of three types: Type 1: rapid enhancement followed by rapid washout (malignant); Type 2: rapid enhancement with a plateau (may be malignant); and Type 3: slow rising enhancement (may be malignant, eg, cholangiocarcinoma).[10] Qualitative assessment is used broadly in routine clinical practice, but clearly does not provide measurements that reflect liver perfusion.

The semiquantitative approach uses various ratios, timings, and slopes calculated from SI–time curves, which are indicative of various perfusion parameters, as summarized in **Table 1**.[11]

Although simple to perform, semiquantitative analyses also have important drawbacks. Because the true concentration of GBCA in tissues is not estimated, the perfusion parameters obtained cannot be reliably reproduced. Also, the shape of the SI–time curve is affected by the volume and injection rate of the GBCA, plus cardiac physiology.

Quantitative models provide metrics to describe the flow of blood and tissue perfusion and are technically demanding. Quantitative DCE MR imaging perfusion modeling is described below.

QUANTITATIVE DYNAMIC CONTRAST-ENHANCED PERFUSION MR IMAGING: A STEPWISE OVERVIEW
Tracer Kinetic Models and Perfusion Parameters for Hepatic Dynamic Contrast-Enhanced MR Imaging

The first step in perfusion imaging is model selection. There is no consensus on the best model for hepatic perfusion MR imaging, as each has a physiologic rationale and may be suitable in some circumstances. When describing perfusion measurements, it is important to describe the type of model and reason for selection.

The simplest model is a single vascular input, single-compartment Tofts model.[12,13] Although convenient because it is widely available in commercial software packages, *it should be avoided in liver* because the dual blood supply is not reflected in the model. The remaining models reflect the dual vascular input. In most tissue types, extracellular GBCA can move into two compartments, specifically the vascular and EES, which can be described via a dual-compartment model.[14,15]

Table 1
Perfusion parameters in semiquantitative analysis

Perfusion Parameter	Definition
Maximum SI or peak enhancement ratio	The ratio of difference between the maximum signal intensity (SI) and baseline SI to the baseline SI. $SI_{maximum} - SI_{baseline}/SI_{baseline}$
Time to peak	The time from baseline to peak of the SI–time curve
Wash-in slope	Indicates the velocity of enhancement and determined by the slope of the SI–time curve from baseline to peak
Wash-out slope	Indicates the velocity of washout and determined by the slope of the SI–time curve from peak to the end of the curve
Initial area under the gadolinium curve (IAUGC)	Indicates the amount of enhancement over a defined period, usually from the start of the upslope to 60 or 90 s
Hepatic perfusion index (HPI)	Indicates the ratio of arterial perfusion to the total (arterial + portal) liver perfusion. Arterial and portal perfusion in the liver can be distinguished using peak splenic enhancement relative to peak aortic enhancement.[12] Arterial perfusion = $$\frac{\text{Maximum slope in the liver enhancement curve before splenic peak}}{\text{peak aortic enhancement}}$$ Portal perfusion = $$\frac{\text{Maximum slope in the liver enhancement curve after splenic peak}}{\text{peak aortic enhancement}}$$

In the normal liver, there is instantaneous free passage of contrast between the vascular and EES through fenestrations. Thus, the dual-compartment model can be effectively reduced to a single-compartment model (**Fig. 1A**), the compartment being a combination of the sinusoids and the space of Disse, illustrated as deep purple in the cartoon. Because this model is computationally simpler, it is often applied as an approximation of normal liver.[16] We explain this

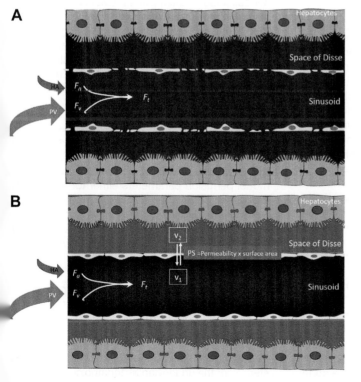

Fig. 1. Various commonly used dual vascular input compartment models for the liver. (*A*) Dual vascular input, single-tissue compartment model.[18–21] The vascular space and space of Disse (EES) is combined into one compartment, shown as deep purple. Key parameters include HBF or F_t, absolute total liver blood flow (ml/min/100 mL); F_a, absolute arterial blood flow (ml/min/100 mL) or arterial fraction of total flow; F_p, absolute portal venous blood flow (ml/min/100 mL) or portal fraction of total flow; DV, distribution volume (%); MTT, mean transit time (seconds). (*B*) The dual-input dual-compartment model, illustrated for the cirrhotic liver.[28] The two compartments are separated functionally due to collagen deposition. Key parameters include F, total hepatic perfusion (ml/min/100 mL); F_A, arterial perfusion (ml/min/100 mL); F_{pv}, portal venous perfusion (ml/min/100 mL), α, arterial fraction (%); v_2, fractional extracellular volume (dimensionless); v_1, fractional intracellular volume (dimensionless).

dual-input single-compartment model[17,18] as an exemplar of possible approaches to signal modeling. The model is described as follows:

$$\frac{dC_L(t)}{dt} = k_{1a}C_a(t-\tau_a) + k_{1p}C_p(t-\tau_b) - k_2C_L(t)$$

$C_L(t)$, $C_a(t)$, and $C_p(t)$ are contrast concentrations in liver tissue, aorta, and PV, respectively. k_{1a} is the aortic inflow rate constant, k_{1p} the portal venous inflow rate constant, and k_2 the outflow rate constant. τ_a and τ_b represent the transit time contrast to arrive to the aorta and PV, respectively. Liver perfusion parameters can be calculated, including arterial fraction (AF: $k_{1a}/(k_{1a} + k_{1p})$), distribution volume (DV: $(k_{1a} + k_{1p})/k_2$), and mean transit time (MTT: $1/k_2$). Portal fraction is 1-AF.

In a dual-compartment model, the space of Disse and the vascular compartment are t assumed separate. This is physiologically important in a cirrhotic liver (**Fig. 1B**), where the transport between the vascular and the interstitial compartment is hampered by collagen deposition. A discussion of the mathematics behind this model is omitted for brevity. A more complex variant, termed a dual-input dual-compartment distributed parameter model, allows for a concentration gradient between the vascular space and the EES. The measured and calculated parameters vary according to model.

Data Acquisition and Analysis

For quantitative DCE perfusion MR imaging, a pre-contrast T_1 map is first obtained and reflects the intrinsic T_1 values in the tissue. This is typically acquired using variable flip angle gradient-recalled echo (GRE) sequence.[19] Dynamic high spatiotemporal resolution T_{1w} images are then collected using 3D T_{1w} GRE. These images should include the aorta proximal to the HA and PV. Imaging is started before contrast injection (baseline) and continued for several minutes through contrast passage. 0.1 mmol/kg GBCA is injected at 2 to 5 mL/sec, followed by a saline flush. The aortic (arterial) enhancement is very rapid during the first pass of the bolus, and the enhancement of the liver and particularly arterial-enhancing lesions is similarly fast. To capture these dynamics, a temporal resolution of less than 2 seconds per imaged volume is ideal.[20,21] Spatial resolution is optimized to allow characterization of small lesions.

The SI at each timepoint is converted into gadolinium concentration using pre-contrast T_1 maps and known relaxivity of the GBCA. The arterial input function, which describes the concentration of the contrast agent through the arterial system into the liver, is typically obtained from the aorta[22] due to the small size of the HA and bulk motion. The venous input function is measured from the PV. The SI measurements in both vessels are converted into gadolinium concentration time curves.

Motion Correction

The liver exhibits significant motion during respiration, both in the anterior–posterior and craniocaudal directions and also nonrigid deformation due to contact with adjacent, differently moving structures. Tracer kinetic models function with the assumption that signal changes arise from the same volume of tissue throughout the time course. Thus, motion and tissue deformation must be accounted for. The three strategies used include (1) performing the acquisition over multiple breathholds, (2) using respiratory triggering and collecting data at the same time of each respiratory cycle, and (3) performing free breathing acquisitions with retrospective removal of motion effects.[23–26] The requirement of multiple sequential breathholds is technically simplest, but associated with patient discomfort and misregistration between different breathholds,[27,28] limiting the ability to characterize small foci. Respiratory triggering significantly lowers the temporal resolution and adversely affects quantitative modeling. Thus, the third approach, while the most challenging, is the most desirable.

A promising approach starts with the observation that 20% to 25% of images in a free-breathing data set collected at a temporal resolution of less than 2 sec/volume are preregistered to one another and do not require registration.[24] Leaving these images unaltered, the remainder of the images in the data set are registered to the temporally nearest "non-moving" neighbor image, allowing use of the full data set to obtain perfusion maps.

Model Fitting

Finally, the obtained vascular and tissue gadolinium concentration–time curves are used with the tracer kinetic model of choice to quantify the model perfusion parameters either for a region of interest or pixel-by-pixel (maps). Model parameters can be obtained via multivariate fitting or dictionary-based approaches.[29,30] The workflow for perfusion analysis in the liver is summarized in **Fig. 2**.

CLINICAL APPLICATIONS OF HEPATIC DYNAMIC CONTRAST-ENHANCED MR IMAGING
Evaluation of Chronic Liver Disease

Perfusion changes in liver fibrosis and cirrhosis stem from the underlying histopathologic changes,

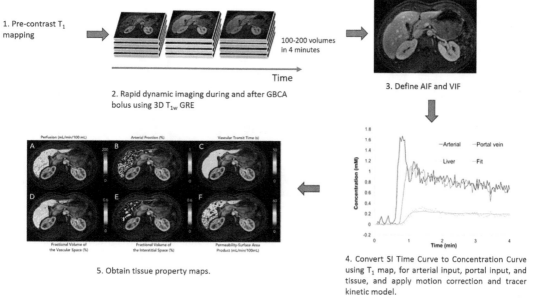

1. Pre-contrast T_1 mapping

100-200 volumes in 4 minutes

Time

2. Rapid dynamic imaging during and after GBCA bolus using 3D T_{1w} GRE

3. Define AIF and VIF

4. Convert SI Time Curve to Concentration Curve using T_1 map, for arterial input, portal input, and tissue, and apply motion correction and tracer kinetic model.

5. Obtain tissue property maps.

Fig. 2. Data acquisition and analysis workflow for liver perfusion MR imaging. (Panes 4 and 5 are *adapted from* Ghodasara and colleagues[29])

especially collagen deposition in the space of Disse and loss of endothelial fenestrations. Studies using a dual-input single-compartment kinetic model found a reduction in the total hepatic flow[31,32] primarily due to decrease in the portal venous flow[31,33–35] with compensatory increase in the arterial flow and elevation of the AF.[25,31,33–36] Using instead a dual-compartment model,[25] the relative volume of the interstitial space increased and the volume of the vascular space decreased in the cirrhotic liver. The finding of increased interstitial volume explains the increase in MTT and DV observed in the studies performed using single-compartment model. The increase in DV was reported to be the parameter that showed the best performance for the diagnosis of advanced fibrosis.[33,34] Advanced liver fibrosis can be diagnosed by using a DV of GBCA of at least 21%, with a sensitivity of 77%, specificity of 79%, and area under the receiver opertor characteristic (AUROC) of 0.82.[33] However, in studies performed using a hepatobiliary contrast agent, the DV was reported to be *decreased* in fibrotic liver, as the hepatobiliary contrast is taken up by hepatocytes.[35] In such studies, DV can be used as an indicator of the fraction of functioning hepatocytes, thus indirectly reflecting liver function. Perfusion parameters also correlate with the severity of fibrosis. For example, the absolute arterial flow has been shown to be the best predictor of mild fibrosis (AUROC: 0.70).[35] In summary, perfusion parameters derived via DCE MR imaging show promise as biomarkers of advanced liver fibrosis, and for follow-up of patients with chronic liver disease, as the parameters correlate with the severity of fibrosis.

Evaluation of Liver Tumors

Characterization: The microcirculation of liver tumors differs significantly from the normal liver parenchyma. Neoangiogenensis is the hallmark of primary (hepatocellular carcinoma [HCC]) and secondary (metastatic) malignant liver tumors. As these new blood vessels are generated from hepatic arterial circulation, DCE MR imaging shows an increase in arterial flow with reduction in portal flow compared with normal liver[9,37,38] and expected significant increase in AF in both metastases[9,10,24,39,40] and HCC.[27,37,38] **Fig. 3** shows representative property maps from a dual-input dual-compartment model for a metastatic lung adenocarcinoma lesion (3D spiral GRAPPA fat-sat GRE acquisition).

Although most studies showed significantly higher AF,[9,10,24,27,37–40] several groups have highlighted that portal perfusion in HCC[22,41] and metastases[9] is still significant, with one group reporting that HCC portal perfusion was *higher* than AF.[41] The proposed reason was that they analyzed early HCCs. Studies show that portal perfusion progressively decreases parallel to progression from dysplastic nodule to HCC.[42,43] The determination of relative HA and PV contribution to tumors has implications for treatment. For example, hepatic arterial embolization can be used to treat metastases that are predominantly

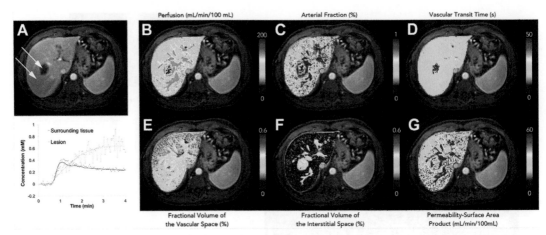

Fig. 3. Representative property maps for lung adenocarcinoma metastasis using a dual-input dual-compartment model showing quantitative differentiation of neoplastic from liver tissue. (*A*) A T1-weighted image and single-voxel contrast concentration curves from both the lesion (*white arrow*) and surrounding liver tissue (*yellow arrow*). Fitted data using the dual-input two-compartment model. (*B–G*) Corresponding perfusion maps for various parameters. (*Reproduced from* Ghodasara and colleagues[29])

supplied by the HA. Also, perfusion parameters can be used to assess response of such tumors to transarterial chemoembolization (TACE) or transarterial embolization.[44]

A comparison of perfusion characteristics of HCC and metastases[23,25,41] using three tracer kinetic models shows that metastases had higher fractional interstitial volume,[25] DV,[23] and longer MTT[23,41] compared with HCC. The common contributing factor could be the increased interstitial space volume in metastases compared with HCC. Nonzero extravasation parameters have been measured in liver metastases, indicating the presence of interstitial space.[9] The presence of larger EES in metastases also accounts for the slower and continuously increasing enhancement in metastases, in contrast to the early enhancement followed by washout of HCC, which is a hypervascular tumor, and where GBCA remains largely confined to the vascular space. **Fig. 4** compares the hypothesized differences in microcirculation of metastases and HCC.[44]

Early detection: Micrometastases are a reason for disease recurrence after surgical resection of malignant liver tumors. DCE MR imaging, via detecting perfusion changes (increase in hepatic perfusion index [HPI] and decrease in portal venous perfusion[39,45–47]) can help with identification of micrometastases. Higher HPI and a higher AF have been reported in the apparently normal liver adjacent to metastases, suggesting the potential of occult neoplastic tissue.[23,48]

Prognosis: Increase in HA fraction of blood supply correlates with increasing aggressive behavior of HCC and metastases.[38,49] Thus, perfusion parameters could be used as prognostic biomarkers and could help tailor chemotherapy regimens.

Treatment response assessment and prediction of survival outcome: Changes in the perfusion characteristics are important indicators in the assessment of response of advanced HCC to targeted therapies such as TACE and radiofrequency ablation, because these therapies do not result in tumor shrinkage. DCE-MR imaging has been used to demonstrate the effects of antiangiogenic drugs such as bevacizumab[50,51] and sorafenib.[52] The expected response after antiangiogenic therapy is a paradoxic *increase* in blood flow and normalization or decreased capillary permeability, indicated by reduction in K^{trans}.[53] For example, patients receiving bevacizumab and folinic acid, fluorouracil and irinotecan (FOLFIRI) regimen for colorectal carcinoma metastases had a decrease in K^{trans} and k_{ep} that correlated with treatment response as early as 1 week after therapy.[51] In addition, studies have shown that the presence of high $IAUGC_{180}$,[54] high slope,[55] high K_{ep},[55] and high K^{trans}[52] on pretreatment DCE MR imaging of HCC was associated with longer survival or stable disease, indicating the value of DCE MR imaging as a prognostic indicator. Perfusion properties are potential biomarkers for monitoring response and predicting survival outcome, as they were noted to consistently reduce after therapy in most of the clinical trials.[51,52,54,56–62]

CHALLENGES AND RECENT ADVANCES

The requirement of high spatiotemporal resolution has been a major challenge. Golden-angle RAdial

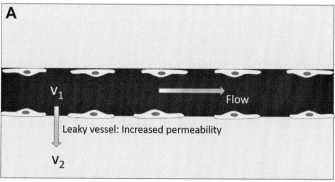

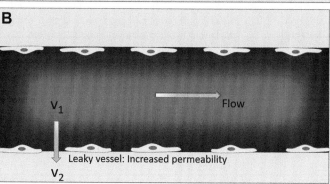

Fig. 4. Illustration of the proposed microcirculatory differences between metastases and HCC using a dual compartment model. Metastases (e.g. colorectal carcinoma metastases) (*A*) shows higher interstitial volume (v_2) and lower intravascular volume (v_1)[9,44] whereas HCC (*B*), a hypervascular tumor, has higher intravascular volume (v_1) and lower interstitial volume (v_2)[25,44]

Sparse Parallel imaging[63,64] and spiral GRAPPA-based DCE MR imaging[23–25,29] are techniques that have enabled hepatic DCE MR imaging with high spatiotemporal resolution. The latter has been used for the quantitative analysis discussed above. Such technologies could enable clinically useable motion-robust DCE MR imaging because they could provide both current standard anatomic images and quantitative maps.[65]

Another major limitation of DCE MR imaging is that data acquisition and analysis methods vary across vendors, institutions, and field strengths.[66] For DCE-MR imaging to be implemented in routine practice, these methods must be standardized, which requires validation and reproducibility studies. Recommendations for standardization of DCE MR imaging published in 2019 by the Quantitative Imaging Biomarker Alliance committee[66] is a step in the direction of incorporating DCE MR imaging into routine practice.

SUMMARY

Perfusion MR imaging technologies could improve the diagnostic and prognostic value of imaging. Current fast MR imaging techniques have enabled quantitative 3D DCE MR imaging with high spatio-temporal resolution, but further testing and standardization is still needed for widespread clinical utilization.

CONFLICTS OF INTEREST

The authors receive research support from Siemens Healthineers. VG and NES have intellectual property licensed by Siemens Healthineers.

DISCLOSURES

Financial support: Nil.

REFERENCES

1. Le Bihan D, Breton E, Lallemand D, et al. MR imaging of intravoxel incoherent motions: application to diffusion and perfusion in neurologic disorders. Radiology 1986;161:401–7.
2. Scharf J, Zapletal C, Hess T, et al. Assessment of hepatic perfusion in pigs by pharmacokinetic analysis of dynamic MR images. J Magn Reson Imaging 1999;9:568–72.
3. Lautt WW, Greenway CV. Conceptual review of the hepatic vascular bed. Hepatol Baltim Md 1987;7: 952–63.
4. Greenway CV, Stark RD. Hepatic vascular bed. Physiol Rev 1971;51:23–65.
5. Feldman M, Friedman LS, Brandt LJ. Sleisenger and Fordtran's gastrointestinal and liver disease: Pathophysiology, diagnosis, management. Elsevier Health Sciences; 2020.

6. Gülberg V, Haag K, Rössle M, et al. Hepatic arterial buffer response in patients with advanced cirrhosis. Hepatology 2002;35:630–4.

7. Lautt WW, Legare DJ, Ezzat WR. Quantitation of the hepatic arterial buffer response to graded changes in portal blood flow. Gastroenterology 1990;98:1024–8.

8. Sourbron S, Sommer WH, Reiser MF, et al. Combined quantification of liver perfusion and function with dynamic gadoxetic acid–enhanced MR imaging. Radiology 2012;263:874–83.

9. Koh TS, Thng CH, Lee PS, et al. Hepatic metastases: in vivo assessment of perfusion parameters at dynamic contrast-enhanced mr imaging with dual-input two-compartment tracer kinetics model. Radiology 2008;249:307–20.

10. Koh TS, Thng CH, Hartono S, et al. Dynamic contrast-enhanced MRI of neuroendocrine hepatic metastases: A feasibility study using a dual-input two-compartment model: DCE MRI of Neuroendocrine Hepatic Metastases. Magn Reson Med 2011;65:250–60.

11. Madhuranthakam AJ, Yuan Q, Pedrosa I. Quantitative methods in abdominal MRI: perfusion imaging. Top Magn Reson Imaging TMRI 2017;26:251.

12. Tofts PS. Modeling tracer kinetics in dynamic Gd-DTPA MR imaging. J Magn Reson Imaging JMRI 1997;7:91–101.

13. Tofts PS, Brix G, Buckley DL, et al. Estimating kinetic parameters from dynamic contrast-enhanced T1-weighted MRI of a diffusable tracer: Standardized quantities and symbols. J Magn Reson Imaging 1999;10:223–32.

14. Sourbron SP, Buckley DL. On the scope and interpretation of the Tofts models for DCE-MRI. Magn Reson Med 2011;66:735–45.

15. Sourbron S. Technical aspects of MR perfusion. Eur J Radiol 2010;76:304–13.

16. Kim SH, Kamaya A, Willmann JK. CT perfusion of the liver: principles and applications in oncology. Radiology 2014;272:322–44.

17. Materne R, Van Beers BE, Smith AM, et al. Non-invasive quantification of liver perfusion with dynamic computed tomography and a dual-input one-compartmental model. Clin Sci Lond Engl 1979 2000;99:517–25.

18. Materne R, Smith Am, Peeters F, et al. Assessment of hepatic perfusion parameters with dynamic MRI. Magn Reson Med 2002;47:135–42.

19. Wang HZ, Riederer SJ, Lee JN. Optimizing the precision in T1 relaxation estimation using limited flip angles. Magn Reson Med 1987;5:399–416.

20. Ingrisch M, Sourbron S. Tracer-kinetic modeling of dynamic contrast-enhanced MRI and CT: a primer. J Pharmacokinet Pharmacodyn 2013;40:281–300.

21. Pandharipande PV, Krinsky GA, Rusinek H, et al. Perfusion imaging of the liver: current challenges and future goals. Radiology 2005;234:661–73.

22. Yang JF, Zhao ZH, Zhang Y, et al. Dual-input two-compartment pharmacokinetic model of dynamic contrast-enhanced magnetic resonance imaging in hepatocellular carcinoma. World J Gastroenterol 2016;22:3652–62.

23. Pahwa S, Liu H, Chen Y, et al. Quantitative perfusion imaging of neoplastic liver lesions: A multi-institution study. Sci Rep 2018;8:4990.

24. Chen Y, Lee GR, Wright KL, et al. Free-breathing liver perfusion imaging using 3d through-time spiral GRAPPA acceleration. Invest Radiol 2015;50:367–75.

25. Ghodasara S, Pahwa S, Dastmalchian S, et al. Free-breathing 3D liver perfusion quantification using a dual-input two-compartment model. Sci Rep 2017;7:17502.

26. Zheng X, Xiao L, Fan X, et al. Free breathing DCE-MRI with motion correction and its values for benign and malignant liver tumor differentiation. Radiol Infect Dis 2015;2:65–71.

27. Bultman EM, Brodsky EK, Horng DE, et al. Quantitative hepatic perfusion modeling using DCE-MRI with sequential breathholds. J Magn Reson Imaging 2014;39:853–65.

28. Wang J, Chen LT, Tsang YM, et al. Dynamic contrast-enhanced MRI analysis of perfusion changes in advanced hepatocellular carcinoma treated with an antiangiogenic agent: a preliminary study. Am J Roentgenol 2004;183:713–9.

29. Ghodasara S, Chen Y, Pahwa S, et al. Quantifying perfusion properties with DCE-MRI using a dictionary matching approach. Sci Rep 2020;10:10210.

30. Martinez-Hernandez A. The hepatic extracellular matrix. II. Electron immunohistochemical studies in rats with CCl4-induced cirrhosis. Lab Investig J Tech Methods Pathol 1985;53:166–86.

31. Annet L, Materne R, Danse E, et al. Hepatic flow parameters measured with MR imaging and Doppler US: correlations with degree of cirrhosis and portal hypertension. Radiology 2003;229:409–14.

32. Van Beers BE, Materne R, Annet L, et al. Capillarization of the sinusoids in liver fibrosis: Noninvasive assessment with contrast-enhanced MRI in the rabbit. Magn Reson Med 2003;49:692–9.

33. Hagiwara M, Rusinek H, Lee VS, et al. Advanced liver fibrosis: diagnosis with 3D whole-liver perfusion MR imaging—initial experience. Radiology 2008;246:926–34.

34. Patel J, Sigmund EE, Rusinek H, et al. Diagnosis of cirrhosis with intravoxel incoherent motion diffusion MRI and dynamic contrast-enhanced MRI alone and in combination: Preliminary experience. J Magn Reson Imaging 2010;31:589–600.

35. Chen BB, Hsu CY, Yu CW, et al. Dynamic contrast-enhanced magnetic resonance imaging with Gd-EOB-DTPA for the evaluation of liver fibrosis in

chronic hepatitis patients. Eur Radiol 2012;22: 171–80.

36. Baxter S, Wang ZJ, Joe BN, et al. Timing bolus dynamic contrast-enhanced (DCE) MRI assessment of hepatic perfusion: Initial experience. J Magn Reson Imaging 2009;29:1317–22.

37. Taouli B, Johnson RS, Hajdu CH, et al. Hepatocellular carcinoma: perfusion quantification with dynamic contrast-enhanced MRI. Am J Roentgenol 2013;201: 795–800.

38. Chen BB, Hsu CY, Yu CW, et al. Dynamic contrast-enhanced MR imaging of advanced hepatocellular carcinoma: comparison with the liver parenchyma and correlation with the survival of patients receiving systemic therapy. Radiology 2017;283:923.

39. Totman JJ, O'gorman RL, Kane PA, et al. Comparison of the hepatic perfusion index measured with gadolinium-enhanced volumetric MRI in controls and in patients with colorectal cancer. Br J Radiol 2005;78:105–9.

40. Miyazaki K, Collins DJ, Walker-Samuel S, et al. Quantitative mapping of hepatic perfusion index using MR imaging: a potential reproducible tool for assessing tumour response to treatment with the antiangiogenic compound BIBF 1120, a potent triple angiokinase inhibitor. Eur Radiol 2008;18:1414–21.

41. Abdullah SS, Pialat JB, Wiart M, et al. Characterization of hepatocellular carcinoma and colorectal liver metastasis by means of perfusion MRI. J Magn Reson Imaging 2008;28:390–5.

42. Liu Y, Matsui O. Changes of intratumoral microvessels and blood perfusion during establishment of hepatic metastases in mice. Radiology 2007;243: 386–95.

43. Hayashi N, Masumoto T, Abe O, et al. Accuracy of abnormal paraspinal muscle findings on contrast-enhanced MR images as indirect signs of unilateral cervical root-avulsion injury. Radiology 2002;223: 397–402.

44. Thng CH, Koh TS, Collins D, et al. Perfusion imaging in liver MRI. Magn Reson Imaging Clin N Am 2014; 22:417–32.

45. Leggett DA, Kelley BB, Bunce IH, et al. Colorectal cancer: diagnostic potential of CT measurements of hepatic perfusion and implications for contrast enhancement protocols. Radiology 1997;205: 716–20.

46. Blomley MJ, Coulden R, Dawson P, et al. Liver perfusion studied with ultrafast CT. J Comput Assist Tomogr 1995;19:424–33.

47. Miles KA, Leggett DA, Kelley BB, et al. In vivo assessment of neovascularization of liver metastases using perfusion CT. Br J Radiol 1998;71:276–81.

48. White MJ, O'Gorman RL, Charles-Edwards EM, et al. Parametric mapping of the hepatic perfusion index with gadolinium-enhanced volumetric MRI. Br J Radiol 2007;80:113–20.

49. Lin G, Lunderquist A, Hägerstrand I, et al. Postmortem examination of the blood supply and vascular pattern of small liver metastases in man. Surgery 1984;96:517–26.

50. Ferl GZ, O'Connor JPB, Parker GJM, et al. Mixed-effects modeling of clinical DCE-MRI data: Application to colorectal liver metastases treated with bevacizumab. J Magn Reson Imaging 2015;41:132–41.

51. Hirashima Y, Yamada Y, Tateishi U, et al. Pharmacokinetic parameters from 3-Tesla DCE-MRI as surrogate biomarkers of antitumor effects of bevacizumab plus FOLFIRI in colorectal cancer with liver metastasis. Int J Cancer 2012;130: 2359–65.

52. Hsu CY, Shen YC, Yu CW, et al. Dynamic contrast-enhanced magnetic resonance imaging biomarkers predict survival and response in hepatocellular carcinoma patients treated with sorafenib and metronomic tegafur/uracil. J Hepatol 2011;55:858–65.

53. Jain RK. Normalization of tumor vasculature: an emerging concept in antiangiogenic therapy. Science 2005;307:58–62.

54. Jarnagin WR, Schwartz LH, Gultekin DH, et al. Regional chemotherapy for unresectable primary liver cancer: results of a phase II clinical trial and assessment of DCE-MRI as a biomarker of survival. Ann Oncol 2009;20:1589–95.

55. Chen BB, Shao YY, Lin ZZ, et al. Dynamic contrast-enhanced and intravoxel incoherent motion MRI biomarkers are correlated to survival outcome in advanced hepatocellular carcinoma. Diagnostics 2021;11:1340.

56. Yopp AC, Schwartz LH, Kemeny N, et al. Antiangiogenic therapy for primary liver cancer: correlation of changes in dynamic contrast-enhanced magnetic resonance imaging with tissue hypoxia markers and clinical response. Ann Surg Oncol 2011;18: 2192–9.

57. De Bruyne S, Van Damme N, Smeets P, et al. Value of DCE-MRI and FDG-PET/CT in the prediction of response to preoperative chemotherapy with bevacizumab for colorectal liver metastases. Br J Cancer 2012;106:1926–33.

58. Zhu AX, Sahani DV, Duda DG, et al. Efficacy, safety, and potential biomarkers of sunitinib monotherapy in advanced hepatocellular carcinoma: a phase II study. J Clin Oncol 2009;27:3027–35.

59. Vriens D, van Laarhoven HWM, van Asten JJA, et al. Chemotherapy response monitoring of colorectal liver metastases by dynamic Gd-DTPA-enhanced MRI perfusion parameters and 18F-FDG PET metabolic rate. J Nucl Med Off Publ Soc Nucl Med 2009;50:1777–84.

60. Rata M, Khan K, Collins DJ, et al. DCE-MRI is more sensitive than IVIM-DWI for assessing antiangiogenic treatment-induced changes in colorectal liver metastases. Cancer Imag 2021;21:67.

61. Pokuri VK, Tomaszewski GM, Ait-Oudhia S, et al. Efficacy, safety, and potential biomarkers of sunitinib and transarterial chemoembolization (TACE) combination in advanced hepatocellular carcinoma (HCC): Phase II Trial. Am J Clin Oncol 2018;41:332.

62. Saito K, Ledsam J, Sugimoto K, et al. DCE-MRI for early prediction of response in hepatocellular carcinoma after TACE and sorafenib therapy: a pilot study. J Belg Soc Radiol 2018;102:40.

63. Feng L, Grimm R, Block KT, et al. Golden-angle radial sparse parallel MRI: Combination of compressed sensing, parallel imaging, and golden-angle radial sampling for fast and flexible dynamic volumetric MRI. Magn Reson Med 2014;72:707–17.

64. Feng L, Axel L, Chandarana H, et al. XD-GRASP: Golden-angle radial MRI with reconstruction of extra motion-state dimensions using compressed sensing. Magn Reson Med 2016;75:775–88.

65. Luna A, Pahwa S, Bonini C, et al. Multiparametric MR Imaging in Abdominal Malignancies. Magn Reson Imaging Clin N Am 2016;24:157–86.

66. Shukla-Dave A, Obuchowski NA, Chenevert TL, et al. Quantitative imaging biomarkers alliance (QIBA) recommendations for improved precision of DWI and DCE-MRI derived biomarkers in multicenter oncology trials. J Magn Reson Imaging 2019;49:e101–21.

MR Perfusion Imaging for Kidney Disease

Mingyan Wu, MD, PhD[a,b], Jeff L. Zhang, PhD[c,*]

KEYWORDS

• MR imaging • Perfusion • Blood flow • Kidney disease

KEY POINTS

- Compared with GFR, renal perfusion could be more sensitive to functional impairment.
- For renal tumors, DCE MR imaging can provide measurement of multiple physiologic parameters with high signal-to-noise ratio and spatial resolution.
- ASL and IVIM do not use exogenous contrast medium, and are ideal options for repeated follow-up assessments for CKD or renal transplants.

INTRODUCTION

Different from most other organs, the kidneys receive arterial blood not merely for consuming the delivered oxygen, but more importantly for filtering the blood.[1] Blood flow of a healthy kidney is about one-tenth of the entire cardiac output, or a perfusion of about 600 mL/min/100 g when normalized to tissue volume or weight. In this article, we use the terms "renal blood flow" (RBF) and "perfusion" interchangeably. Numerous studies found decreased perfusion in kidneys with chronic kidney disease (CKD) or acute kidney injury.[2–5] Although glomerular filtration rate (GFR) is conventionally regarded as the indicator of renal function, renal perfusion has several advantages for renal functional assessment. First, GFR is preserved by multiple mechanisms, including the renin-angiotensin system, so that early injury or impairment would not affect GFR. Renal perfusion was found to correlate with capillary density, so might be sensitive to early stage of functional impairment. Second, different from GFR that is typically reported for each or both kidneys, renal perfusion is measured for each tissue voxels within the imaging field of view. Perfusion of different intrarenal regions is evaluated separately. For example, cortical perfusion mostly reflects glomerular blood flow and medullary perfusion may indicate hypoperfusion and thus hypoxic state of renal medulla.[6]

Using a variety of MR imaging methods, quantitative mapping of renal perfusion has been extensively investigated in the past two decades. Dynamic contrast-enhanced (DCE) MR imaging measures perfusion of kidney tissue for the purpose of functional assessment, and in patients with renal tumors can provide measurements of tumor perfusion that may guide antiangiogenic therapy.[7] For patients with CKD or transplanted kidney, injection of contrast agent is avoided by instead using arterial spin labeling (ASL) method, in which renal arterial blood is temporarily "magnetized" to measure renal tissue perfusion.[8] Diffusion-weighted imaging provides yet another option of quantifying tissue perfusion, termed "intravoxel incoherent motion (IVIM)" analysis. Recently renal MR imaging research has reached the consensus that, after decades of development and applications, the renal MR imaging tools are technically ready for large-scale clinical trials.[8,9]

In this review, we present a concise introduction of the principles of the perfusion imaging methods and then a summary of recent applications, with

[a] Central Research Institute, UIH Group, Shanghai, China; [b] School of Biomedical Engineering Building, Room 409, 393 Huaxia Middle Road, Shanghai 201210, China; [c] School of Biomedical Engineering, ShanghaiTech University, Room 409, School of Biomedical Engineering Building, 393 Huaxia Middle Road, Shanghai 201210, China
* Corresponding author.
E-mail address: zhanglei2@shanghaitech.edu.cn

Magn Reson Imaging Clin N Am 32 (2024) 161–170
https://doi.org/10.1016/j.mric.2023.09.004
1064-9689/24/© 2023 Elsevier Inc. All rights reserved.

the hope of accelerating the clinical adoption of MR perfusion imaging methods. For literature review, we searched PubMed (pubmed.gov) with the following combination of keywords: "(kidney [title] or renal[title]) and (arterial spin labeling)," or "(kidney [title] or renal[title]) and (IVIM)," or "(kidney [title] or renal[title]) and (DCE-MR imaging)," and set the range of years to be 2017 to 2023. Among the resulted 173 articles, we excluded 97 reviews, case reports, or articles in which kidney is not the primary focus, so included the remaining 76 articles for this review. The 76 articles were further classified into two categories: 34 articles of technical developments, and 42 of clinical applications on CKD, renal tumors, or kidney transplants. **Fig. 1** graphically shows the MR imaging methods and the renal diseases that are covered in this review.

TECHNICAL PRINCIPLES AND RECENT DEVELOPMENTS

This section briefly introduces the principles of ASL, IVIM, and DCE, followed by a summary of recent technical developments or improvements on these methods for renal perfusion measurement.

Arterial Spin Labeling

ASL is a noncontrast MR imaging method that does not use any exogenous contrast agent. Instead, arterial blood is magnetically inverted or labeled; after some postlabeling delay (PLD) for the labeled blood to perfuse into tissue of interest, imaging of the tissue is performed. Because the image would contain signals from the labeled blood and stationary tissue, the imaging process is typically performed twice, with the arterial labeling process and without the process, and difference of the two images (termed as "the difference image")

would be the amount of labeled blood in the tissue of interest at the time instant of PLD. Quantification of tissue perfusion based on the difference image should consider multiple factors, such as proton density, tissue and blood relaxation rates, and bolus shape of blood labeling.

A recent paper published by a multinational group of renal MR imaging investigators provides consensus-based recommendations on how renal ASL can be performed, from image acquisition to data analysis.[10] Major recommendations by the paper include: either pseudocontinuous method or flow-sensitive alternating inversion recovery (a pulsed method) for blood labeling; single-slice single-shot echo planar sequence or single-shot turbo spin echo for tissue imaging; for extended coverage, preference of multiple two-dimensional slices over three-dimensional (3D) volume imaging; repeated acquisitions with a same PLD for simple data analysis[11]; using background suppression in imaging[12–14]; and retrospective image registration for eliminating motion artifact.

Recent technical developments for renal ASL have been focused on mitigating the impact of respiratory motion or variable arterial transit time (ATT) for the estimated perfusion. The developments were made to the labeling, imaging, or analysis step of renal ASL. For the labeling step, Echeverria-Chasco and coworkers[15] optimized the gradient parameters (average gradient and the ratio of maximal and average gradients) for pseudocontinuous labeling at the abdominal aorta, to improve the robustness of blood labeling to variable flow velocity or ATT. To properly consider variable ATT, one straightforward option is to repeat image acquisitions with different PLDs, but it increases acquisition time accordingly.[16] Using a technique termed as saturated

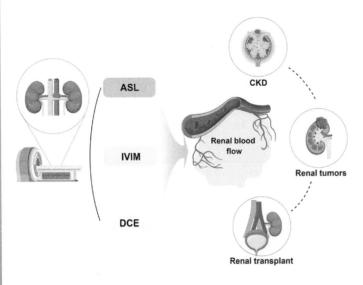

Fig. 1. MR imaging provides multiple methods (ASL, DCE, IVIM) that can measure renal perfusion or blood flow. (by Figdraw)

ASL

CKD

IVIM

Renal blood flow

Renal tumors

DCE

Renal transplant

multidelay renal arterial spin labeling, Ning and colleagues[17] performed multiple image acquisitions of different PLDs after a single labeling, substantially reducing time for acquiring multi-PLD data. Yet another innovative approach for addressing the variable ATT issue was to use velocity-selective labeling,[18–20] instead of the spatially selective labeling as the pseudocontinuous or pulsed methods. The velocity-selective labeling was also found to be robust to respiratory motion artifact. For the imaging step, Zhang and colleagues[21] integrated a navigator-base method into free-breathing two-dimensional ASL imaging to prospectively compensate respiratory motion of kidneys, and improved signal precision by about 20%. 3D volume imaging would not only provide extended coverage for entire kidneys, but also make image registration in postprocessing easier. The feasibility of 3D ASL was recently tested in adult[22] and pediatric[23] patients with CKD. For the analysis step, Zhou and colleagues[24] proposed a "quantitative transport mapping" method for analyzing multiple-PLD data. Without forcing a same arterial input function for all the different tissue voxels, the method could potentially quantify tissue perfusion with higher accuracy than conventional tracer kinetic models. Further evaluation based on the perfusion map often requires segmentation of renal cortex and medulla. Bones and colleagues[25] used a deep-learning approach for automatically segmenting renal cortex in ASL images, and achieved comparable accuracy of RBF as manual segmentation.

Intravoxel Incoherent Motion Analysis

IVIM is a model that considers water diffusion and capillary perfusion in analyzing diffusion-weighted images.[26] For diffusion-weighted imaging, magnetic field gradients are applied toward multiple different directions, so that water diffusion along the gradients results in magnetization dephasing and thus signal decay. A parameter termed as "b value" is used to combine the overall effect of the magnitude and duration of the gradients and diffusion time. Diffusion-weighted images acquired with high b values are generally darker than those of low b values. In practice, multiple images of a same field of view are acquired with different b values; using a simple exponential-decay function to characterize water diffusion, signals of different b values are fitted for each tissue voxel to obtain estimate of diffusivity (D or apparent diffusion coefficient [ADC]) for the voxel, or diffusivity map for the entire field of view. To account for the potential effect of capillary perfusion, in addition to water diffusion,

IVIM analysis uses a sum of two exponential functions to fit diffusion-weighted signals, resulting in two diffusivity coefficients. The higher coefficient (often termed as pseudodiffusivity or D*) corresponds to presumably faster capillary perfusion along the applied field gradients. The relative weight factor of the pseudodiffusion component or perfusion fraction (f_p) can also be determined in the signal fitting. Both the parameters D* and f_p are believed to reflect renal tissue perfusion.[27]

Recent technical studies were aimed to improve precision of IVIM-estimated renal perfusion. With diffusion-weighted imaging using conventional bipolar gradients, Sigmund and colleagues[28] found that renal pseudodiffusivity measured at different cardiac-cycle phases were significantly different, indicating the sensitivity of IVIM-quantified renal perfusion to variation of upstream blood velocity and/or pressure. Using a deep-learning-based segmentation method, Lv and colleagues[29] registered renal diffusion-weighted imaging images acquired during free breathing of subjects, and improved precision of the quantified perfusion parameters. In fitting the diffusion-weighted decay signals, Stabinska and colleagues[30] used a nonnegative least-squares approach to further distinguish the slower capillary blood flow and the faster blood flow in larger vessels.

Dynamic Contrast-Enhanced MR Imaging

DCE MR imaging for the kidneys has been mainly used for measuring single-kidney GFR, RBF, and mean transit times, but the vascular phase (eg, the initial 30–60 seconds after contrast injection) of the acquired dynamic images can also be used to perform voxel-wise analysis for mapping renal perfusion. For image acquisition, a low dose of contrast agent is intravenously injected, and as the contrast agent transits through the kidneys, dynamic imaging is performed to record the process. Fast T1-weighted sequence is typically used for the imaging, in which contrast agent enhances signal intensity. In postprocessing of the images, tracer kinetic model is applied to each voxel's contrast concentration versus time curve to estimate its perfusion.

Recent studies on image acquisition of renal DCE MR imaging focused on accelerating image acquisition, to improve temporal resolution of the acquired dynamic images. Using time-resolved imaging of contrast kinetics, Jiang and colleagues[31] proposed a rapid multislice T1 measurement method, which imaged eight axial slices in 1.23 seconds. Using differential subsampling with Cartesian ordering and fat suppression,

Yamada and colleagues[32] achieved temporal resolution of about 2 seconds for 3D coverage of human kidneys.

For postprocessing of renal DCE MR imaging, one focus of technical development was to reduce respiratory motion artifact in the acquired dynamic images. De Boer and colleagues[33] proposed to reconstruct fat-only images from the acquired dynamic images, and used the fat-only images to facilitate image registration thus obtaining more accurate estimates of renal perfusion. To improve image registration, Coll-Font and coworkers[34] used a linear time invariant model to create a motion-free version of dynamic template volumes, and registered each real volume to its template with matched contrast and interpolated the outlier volumes corrupted by motion. Segmentation of renal parenchyma and between renal cortex and medulla are necessary steps in the postprocessing of DCE MR imaging. Haghighi and colleagues[35] used a cascade network that involved two 3D convolutional neural networks to segment renal parenchyma in DCE MR imaging images, and achieved high segmentation accuracy for healthy and diseased kidneys. Klepaczko and colleagues[36] used U-Net convolutional neural networks to segment kidneys from background region, with accuracy of 94%, and then classified the intrarenal voxels into renal cortex and medulla based on features of the voxels' dynamic signals, with accuracy of 90% to 93%. Huang and colleagues[37] segmented renal cortex, medulla, and renal pelvis in DCE images by classifying voxels based on their time-intensity signals and their spatial position relative to predefined seeds.

In summary, all three MR imaging methods (ASL, IVIM, and DCE) are capable of measuring renal perfusion. We already have a recommended protocol for performing renal ASL, and the technique has been continuously improved, particularly in its labeling for resolving variable ATT issue and in achieving coverage of entire kidneys. IVIM for renal perfusion is straightforward to implement, but further effort might be needed to precisely extract renal capillary perfusion from the acquired images. DCE has well-established protocol for image acquisition analysis. The method requires injection of low dose of contrast agent, but measures multiple physiologically meaningful parameters besides renal perfusion. Recent technical developments for renal DCE focused on reducing the impact of respiratory motion, by either accelerating imaging or better registering the acquired dynamic images in postprocessing. All three methods would benefit from reliable segmentation of renal cortex and medulla with deep learning approaches.

RECENT APPLICATIONS IN KIDNEY DISEASES

Multiple recent studies have applied the previously discussed MR imaging perfusion methods for various kidney-related diseases. In this section, we classified the studies based on the disease categories in the following order: CKD, renal tumor, and renal transplant. Under each disease category, we review the three MR imaging methods' findings. **Table 1** summarizes the specific aims of the applications achieved by each MR imaging method.

Chronic Kidney Disease

CKD affects more than 10% of the general population worldwide, with even higher prevalence in older individuals, or patients with diabetes or hypertension. CKD is diagnosed as reduced GFR, often estimated from serum creatinine, and if needed, a biopsy is used for examining pathologic injury. Renal perfusion was also found to decrease with CKD, which may be caused by renal capillary rarefaction.[68] DCE MR imaging is capable of measuring single-kidney GFR and renal perfusion in a single scan.[69] Risk of nephrogenic systemic fibrosis associated with the use of gadolinium-based contrast agent was a concern; however, it was proven to be extremely low

Table 1 Potential capabilities of renal MR imaging perfusion methods as demonstrated in recent applications	
MR Imaging Method	**Specific Aim of Application**
ASL	Evaluation of renal perfusion and function in CKD[38–44]
	Differentiation between different types of renal tumors[45]
	Assessment of renal tumor response to antiangiogenic therapies[46]
	Assessment of renal perfusion in transplanted kidneys[47–51]
IVIM	Assessment of early stage CKD[52–57]
	Subtyping and grading of renal tumors[58–61]
	Assessment of renal perfusion in transplanted kidneys[62–64]
DCE	Subtyping and grading of renal tumors[65,66]
	Assessment of renal tumor response to antiangiogenic therapies[67]

particularly with the use of macrocyclic types.[70] Hence, it is expected that recent applications of DCE for patients with CKD were still scarce, except for one study on evaluating the method's repeatability.[71] Most applications of MR perfusion for CKD in the past 5 years have used either ASL or IVIM.

Recent studies focused on correlating ASL-measured renal perfusion against serum-based GFR or biopsy results that are clinically used for CKD diagnosis. A few studies found significant correlation between ASL-measured perfusion and GFR for patients with CKD.[38–41] In a cohort of 80 patients with CKD, Mao and colleagues[44] found a significant correlation between ASL-measured RBF and increased interstitial fibrosis. Pi and colleagues[42] found that ASL-measured RBF was able to discriminate CKD with mild pathologic injury against healthy control subjects. Because repeated follow-up measurements are necessary for patients with CKD, Li and colleagues[43] tested the reproducibility of a renal ASL protocol in healthy subjects, and found good consistency between the measurements over 18 months.

Similar to ASL, IVIM was applied to patients with CKD, to explore its potential relationship with estimated GFR, urinary, or histopathologic results. In adult and children patients with CKD, Liang and colleagues[55,57] found that cortical and medullary f_p were capable of differentiating healthy subjects and early stage CKD. Mao and colleagues[52–54] found that all IVIM parameters were significantly lower in the patients with CKD than in the healthy control subjects and that the IVIM parameters exhibited significant correlation with serum creatinine level, 24-hour urinary protein level, and histopathologic fibrosis scores. Sułkowska and colleagues[56] found moderate but not significant correlation between IVIM-measured f_p and a histopathologic index that reflects glomerular sclerosis and mesangial matrix increase. It was speculated that the correlation might be lowered because of high estimation error in the parameter f_p, with up to 40% to 60% coefficient of variance measured in the study.

In summary, the recent applications on CKD focused on exploring the potential correlation between the noncontrast perfusion imaging methods (ie, ASL and IVIM) and the clinical indices of CKD (ie, estimated GFR, biopsy, and urinary protein level). Promising correlations were found. Despite the low precision in measurement, IVIM has been popular for kidney applications, probably because of its easy implementation and the additionally measured water diffusion, which may reflect renal fibrosis.

Renal Tumor

Renal tumor is not functional impairment as in CKD that involves an entire kidney, but typically affects only a part of a kidney. Because of their different properties from healthy kidney tissue, most renal tumors are detected by some morphologic imaging methods. After initial diagnosis, a biopsy is often prescribed to determine the mass's malignancy and subtype. Perfusion imaging would allow assessment of functional status of the nontumor kidney tissue and more importantly of vascularity (eg, vascular volume and permeability) of renal tumors,[72] and these measurements are valuable in the pretreatment and posttreatment stages of managing renal tumors.

DCE MR imaging for renal tumors recently focused on assessing intratumor heterogeneity of renal tumors. For heterogeneous tumors, limited tissue samples from clinical biopsies would provide biased information on some properties of tumor, thus leading to possible treatment failure. Using an analysis approach termed as radiomics, Dwivedi and colleagues[66] extracted features from DCE MR imaging images of clear cell renal cell carcinoma (RCC), to predict tumors of high-grade histology and to differentiate tumors with necrosis from those without necrosis. For both purposes, the predictive models based on the DCE image features performed significantly better than that based on tumor size. Using a vertically integrated radiogenomics approach, Udayakumar and colleagues[65] correlated DCE MR imaging features and RNA sequencing data acquired from spatially colocalized regions of clear cell RCCs, and then used the learned correlations to predict tumor angiogenesis and inflammation features based on DCE MR imaging. In an independent group of patients with metastatic RCC, the proposed method successfully identified phenotypes with better response to antiangiogenic therapy. One study[67] used conventional tracer kinetic modeling technique to estimate perfused tumor volume and mean transfer constant and extracellular volume for metastatic RCC, and found that early change (either 4 or 10 weeks) of these parameters after antiangiogenic treatment can predict disease progression at 6 months.

Without using exogenous contrast, ASL provides estimate for tumor perfusion only, but not tumor vascular or extracellular volume. Still, the measured perfusion is valuable in subtyping and treatment monitoring of renal tumors. Using ASL, Ye and colleagues[45] found that tumor perfusion in clear cell RCC was significantly higher than that in fat-poor angiomyolipoma. Tsai and colleagues[46] used ASL-measured perfusion to track changes in tumor vascularity of RCC metastases before and during antiangiogenic therapy. The measured tumor perfusion was shown to be promising in predicting responders and indicating disease progression for the metastases in various organs including lung, lymph nodes, and liver.

IVIM analysis provides measurements for water diffusion (D) and tissue perfusion (D*, f_p) of renal tumors. In most tumors, water diffusion is expected to be restricted because of increased cellularity and decreased interstitial space.[73] Zhu and colleagues[59] found that the IVIM parameters were capable of differentiating various types of renal tumors, including clear cell, chromophobe, and papillary RCCs. In 180 patients with renal tumors, Ding and colleagues[60] confirmed that the IVIM parameters performed better than ADC or diffusion kurtosis in discriminating between clear cell RCC, non–clear cell RCC, and benign renal tumor. To accurately grade clear cell RCC is also important for clinical management. In 107 patients with pathologically proven clear cell RCC, Zhu and colleagues[58] found progressively decreased D* and increased f_p as tumor grade increased (from I to IV). In a separate study with 146 clear cell RCCs, the group concluded that the IVIM parameters performed better than ADC in grading clear cell RCCs. Radiomics was also applied to renal IVIM in a study to differentiate minimal-fat angiomyolipoma and RCC.[61] For the differentiation, the radiomics model performed significantly better than a regular regression model, presumably because of the better discrimination ability of the texture features used in the former model.

In summary, imaging of renal tumor may cover heterogeneous intratumor regions, thus avoiding sampling bias of biopsy. All three MR imaging perfusion methods were shown to be promising in differentiating various subtypes, grading, and monitoring effects of antiangiogenic treatment of renal tumors. Besides tumor perfusion, DCE MR imaging also measures tumor vascular volume and extracellular volume, which may provide a more comprehensive characterization for renal tumors.

Renal Transplant

As a recent review summarized, MR imaging of renal transplant is valuable in detecting posttransplant renal dysfunction, differentiating between different causes of dysfunction, and monitoring renal function during and after therapeutic interventions.[74] Of the three MR imaging perfusion methods, DCE has been investigated much less frequently for renal transplants because of its usage of gadolinium-based contrast medium, despite the recent consensus that the macrocyclic

type is safe.[70] In the following section, we review recent studies that tested ASL or IVIM on renal transplants.

Similar to CKD studies, applications of ASL for renal transplants focused on exploring the potential correlation between renal perfusion and clinical indices, such as estimated GFR and histopathology results. In a group of patients with stable allograft function, Radovic and colleagues[48] found significant correlation between estimated GFR and cortical RBF measured with a pulsed ASL method. Wang and colleagues[47] found that ASL-measured cortical perfusion was capable of differentiating renal transplants with normal function and those with subclinical pathology, and that the differentiation capability is further improved when taking proteinuria into consideration. Yu and colleagues[50] and Wang and colleagues[51] found ASL-measured perfusion to significantly correlate with interstitial fibrosis and peritubular capillary density, respectively. For the purpose of posttransplantation monitoring, precision of perfusion measurement is important. Echeverria-Chasco and coworkers[49] tested the reproducibility of a pseudocontinuous ASL method with a group of 20 kidney transplants with stable function, and found within-subject coefficient of variance of cortical blood flow to be low (10.73%) and that of medullary blood flow to be high (16.41%).

Similar to ASL, IVIM-measured perfusion of renal transplant was also correlated to pathology results,[63] by comparing cortical and medullary f_p and D* against a composite pathologic score from biopsy. Delayed graft function (DGF) happens within the first week after transplantation,[75] and its timely detection and characterization is critical for the graft's long-term outcome. In a group of 50 patients that received renal transplant within 3 to 10 days, Hashim and colleagues[62] performed IVIM, and found that cortical and medullary f_p were significantly lower in the cases with DGF than functioning ones; it was also found that whole-parenchyma f_p had the potential of predicting time to recovery from DGF (Spearman correlation of −0.65). In an independent study, Chang and colleagues[64] reached a similar conclusion that cortical and medullary f_p differentiated DGF and functioning transplants, and also found that the DGF kidneys with some complications (eg, acute tubular necrosis, acute rejection) had significantly lower cortical f_p than those without complication. Low reproducibility is a major problem with the IVIM-derived flow parameters. As Echeverria-Chasco and coworkers[49] measured, coefficient of variance computed from two separate measurements were all higher than 15% for parameters f_p and D* for either renal cortex or medulla.

SUMMARY

Renal perfusion or RBF reflects overall function of a kidney, and as the recent studies suggested, showed significant correlation with estimated GFR in either CKD or renal transplants. Renal perfusion can also be measured for each tissue voxel, and when used for heterogeneous tumor, would characterize renal tumor with less sampling bias than clinical biopsy. Further effort is needed to determine potential association between renal perfusion and the various histopathologic findings, such as tubulointerstitial fibrosis and nephritis. Of the three MR imaging methods discussed in this review, DCE provides tumor perfusion with the best signal-to-noise ratio and spatial resolution and additional measures, such as vascular and extracellular volumes, and therefore is widely used for radiomics analysis of renal tumor. ASL and IVIM are good options for assessing CKD and renal transplants, for which repeated follow-up examinations are usually required.

CLINICS CARE POINTS

- Renal perfusion measured with noncontrast ASL or IVIM shows much promise in replacing estimated GFR and biopsy in diagnosing and characterizing CKD and renal transplant.
- DCE MR imaging measures multiple important parameters including tumor perfusion for entire tumor and kidney, so is ideal for radiomic analysis of renal tumors and may assist in optimizing therapeutic regimens.

DISCLOSURE

The authors have nothing to disclose.

REFERENCES

1. Edwards A, Kurtcuoglu V. Renal blood flow and oxygenation. Pflugers Arch 2022;474(8):759–70.
2. Evans RG, Ince C, Joles JA, et al. Haemodynamic influences on kidney oxygenation: clinical implications of integrative physiology. Clin Exp Pharmacol Physiol 2013;40(2):106–22.
3. Gomez H, Ince C, De Backer D, et al. A unified theory of sepsis-induced acute kidney injury: inflammation, microcirculatory dysfunction, bioenergetics, and the tubular cell adaptation to injury. Shock 2014;41(1):3–11.
4. Ow CPC, Ngo JP, Ullah MM, et al. Renal hypoxia in kidney disease: cause or consequence? Acta Physiol (Oxf) 2018;222(4):e12999.
5. Chawla LS, Eggers PW, Star RA, et al. Acute kidney injury and chronic kidney disease as interconnected syndromes. N Engl J Med 2014;371(1):58–66.
6. Wang B, Li ZL, Zhang YL, et al. Hypoxia and chronic kidney disease. EBioMedicine. Mar 2022;77:103942.
7. Rosen MA, Schnall MD. Dynamic contrast-enhanced magnetic resonance imaging for assessing tumor vascularity and vascular effects of targeted therapies in renal cell carcinoma. Clin Cancer Res 2007;13(2 Pt 2):770s–6s.
8. Odudu A, Nery F, Harteveld AA, et al. Arterial spin labelling MRI to measure renal perfusion: a systematic review and statement paper. Nephrol Dial Transplant 2018;33(suppl_2):ii15–21.
9. Caroli A, Schneider M, Friedli I, et al. Diffusion-weighted magnetic resonance imaging to assess diffuse renal pathology: a systematic review and statement paper. Nephrol Dial Transplant 2018;33(suppl_2):ii29–40.
10. Nery F, Buchanan CE, Harteveld AA, et al. Consensus-based technical recommendations for clinical translation of renal ASL MRI. MAGMA 2020;33(1):141–61.
11. Shirvani S, Tokarczuk P, Statton B, et al. Motion-corrected multiparametric renal arterial spin labelling at 3 T: reproducibility and effect of vasodilator challenge. Eur Radiol 2019;29(1):232–40.
12. Taso M, Guidon A, Alsop DC. Influence of background suppression and retrospective realignment on free-breathing renal perfusion measurement using pseudo-continuous ASL. Magn Reson Med 2019;81(4):2439–49.
13. Bones IK, Harteveld AA, Franklin SL, et al. Enabling free-breathing background suppressed renal pCASL using fat imaging and retrospective motion correction. Magn Reson Med 2019;82(1):276–88.
14. Ahn HS, Yu HC, Kwak HS, et al. Assessment of renal perfusion in transplanted kidney patients using pseudo-continuous arterial spin labeling with multiple post-labeling delays. Eur J Radiol 2020;130:109200.
15. Echeverria-Chasco R, Vidorreta M, Aramendia-Vidaurreta V, et al. Optimization of pseudo-continuous arterial spin labeling for renal perfusion imaging. Magn Reson Med 2021;85(3):1507–21.
16. Conlin CC, Oesingmann N, Bolster B Jr, et al. Renal plasma flow (RPF) measured with multiple-inversion-time arterial spin labeling (ASL) and tracer kinetic analysis: validation against a dynamic contrast-enhancement method. Magn Reson Imaging 2016;37:51–5.
17. Ning Z, Chen S, Chen Z, et al. Saturated multi-delay renal arterial spin labeling technique for simultaneous perfusion and T(1) quantification in kidneys. Magn Reson Med 2022;88(3):1055–67.
18. Franklin SL, Bones IK, Harteveld AA, et al. Multi-organ comparison of flow-based arterial spin labeling

techniques: spatially non-selective labeling for cerebral and renal perfusion imaging. Magn Reson Med 2021;85(5):2580–94.

19. Bones IK, Franklin SL, Harteveld AA, et al. Influence of labeling parameters and respiratory motion on velocity-selective arterial spin labeling for renal perfusion imaging. Magn Reson Med 2020;84(4): 1919–32.

20. Bones IK, Franklin SL, Harteveld AA, et al. Exploring label dynamics of velocity-selective arterial spin labeling in the kidney. Magn Reson Med 2021;86(1): 131–42.

21. Zhang K, Triphan SMF, Ziener CH, et al. Navigator-based slice tracking for kidney pCASL using spin-echo EPI acquisition. Magn Reson Med 2023. https://doi.org/10.1002/mrm.29621.

22. Lu F, Yang J, Yang S, et al. Use of three-dimensional arterial spin labeling to evaluate renal perfusion in patients with chronic kidney disease. J Magn Reson Imag 2021;54(4):1152–63.

23. Nery F, De Vita E, Clark CA, et al. Robust kidney perfusion mapping in pediatric chronic kidney disease using single-shot 3D-GRASE ASL with optimized retrospective motion correction. Magn Reson Med 2019;81(5):2972–84.

24. Zhou L, Zhang Q, Spincemaille P, et al. Quantitative transport mapping (QTM) of the kidney with an approximate microvascular network. Magn Reson Med 2021;85(4):2247–62.

25. Bones IK, Bos C, Moonen C, et al. Workflow for automatic renal perfusion quantification using ASL-MRI and machine learning. Magn Reson Med 2022; 87(2):800–9.

26. Le Bihan D, Breton E, Lallemand D, et al. MR imaging of intravoxel incoherent motions: application to diffusion and perfusion in neurologic disorders. Radiology 1986;161(2):401–7.

27. Zhang JL, Sigmund EE, Chandarana H, et al. Variability of renal apparent diffusion coefficients: limitations of the monoexponential model for diffusion quantification. Meta-Analysis. Radiology 2010;254(3):783–92.

28. Sigmund EE, Mikheev A, Brinkmann IM, et al. Cardiac phase and flow compensation effects on renal flow and microstructure anisotropy MRI in healthy human kidney. J Magn Reson Imag 2022. https://doi.org/10.1002/jmri.28517.

29. Lv J, Huang W, Zhang J, et al. Performance of U-net based pyramidal lucas-kanade registration on free-breathing multi-b-value diffusion MRI of the kidney. Br J Radiol 2018;91(1086):20170813.

30. Stabinska J, Ljimani A, Zollner HJ, et al. Spectral diffusion analysis of kidney intravoxel incoherent motion MRI in healthy volunteers and patients with renal pathologies. Magn Reson Med 2021;85(6): 3085–95.

31. Jiang K, Tang H, Mishra PK, et al. Measurement of murine kidney functional biomarkers using DCE-MRI: a multi-slice TRICKS technique and semi-automated image processing algorithm. Magn Reson Imaging 2019;63:226–34.

32. Yamada T, Masui T, Sasaki M, et al. Time resolved DCE-MRI of the kidneys: evaluation of the renal vasculatures and tumors using F-DISCO with and without compressed sensing in normal and wide-bore 3T systems. Medicine (Baltim) 2022;101(31): e29971.

33. de Boer A, Leiner T, Vink EE, et al. Modified Dixon-based renal dynamic contrast-enhanced MRI facilitates automated registration and perfusion analysis. Magn Reson Med 2018;80(1):66–76.

34. Coll-Font J, Afacan O, Chow JS, et al. Modeling dynamic radial contrast enhanced MRI with linear time invariant systems for motion correction in quantitative assessment of kidney function. Med Image Anal 2021;67:101880.

35. Haghighi M, Warfield SK, Kurugol S. Automatic renal segmentation in DCE-MRI using convolutional neural networks. Presented at: 2018 IEEE 15th international symposium on biomedical imaging (ISBI 2018); 2018.

36. Klepaczko A, Eikefjord E, Lundervold A. Healthy kidney segmentation in the DCE-MR images using a convolutional neural network and temporal signal characteristics. Sensors 2021;21(20). https://doi.org/10.3390/s21206714.

37. Huang W, Li H, Wang R, et al. A self-supervised strategy for fully automatic segmentation of renal dynamic contrast-enhanced magnetic resonance images. Med Phys 2019;46(10):4417–30.

38. Kannenkeril D, Janka R, Bosch A, et al. Detection of changes in renal blood flow using arterial spin labeling MRI. Am J Nephrol 2021;52(1):69–75.

39. Gillis KA, McComb C, Patel RK, et al. Non-contrast renal magnetic resonance imaging to assess perfusion and corticomedullary differentiation in health and chronic kidney disease. Nephron 2016;133(3): 183–92.

40. Mora-Gutiérrez JM, Garcia-Fernandez N, Slon Roblero MF, et al. Arterial spin labeling MRI is able to detect early hemodynamic changes in diabetic nephropathy. J Magn Reson Imag 2017;46(6):1810–7.

41. Li LP, Tan H, Thacker JM, et al. Evaluation of renal blood flow in chronic kidney disease using arterial spin labeling perfusion magnetic resonance imaging. Kidney Int Rep 2017;2(1):36–43.

42. Pi S, Li Y, Lin C, et al. Arterial spin labeling and diffusion-weighted MR imaging: quantitative assessment of renal pathological injury in chronic kidney disease. Abdom Radiol (NY) 2023;48(3):999–1010.

43. Li LP, Thacker J, Li W, et al. Consistency of multiple renal functional MRI measurements over 18 months. J Magn Reson Imag 2018;48(2):514–21.

44. Mao W, Ding X, Ding Y, et al. Evaluation of interstitial fibrosis in chronic kidney disease by multiparametric

functional MRI and histopathologic analysis. Eur Radiol 2022. https://doi.org/10.1007/s00330-022-09329-7.

45. Ye J, Xu Q, Wang SA, et al. Differentiation between fat-poor angiomyolipoma and clear cell renal cell carcinoma: qualitative and quantitative analysis using arterial spin labeling MR imaging. Abdom Radiol (NY) 2020;45(2):512–9.

46. Tsai LL, Bhatt RS, Strob MF, et al. Arterial spin labeled perfusion MRI for the evaluation of response to tyrosine kinase inhibition therapy in metastatic renal cell carcinoma. Radiology 2021;298(2):332–40.

47. Wang W, Yu Y, Li X, et al. Early detection of subclinical pathology in patients with stable kidney graft function by arterial spin labeling. Eur Radiol 2021; 31(5):2687–95.

48. Radovic T, Jankovic MM, Stevic R, et al. Detection of impaired renal allograft function in paediatric and young adult patients using arterial spin labelling MRI (ASL-MRI). Sci Rep 2022;12(1):828.

49. Echeverria-Chasco R, Martin-Moreno PL, Garcia-Fernandez N, et al. Multiparametric renal magnetic resonance imaging: a reproducibility study in renal allografts with stable function. NMR Biomed 2023; 36(2):e4832.

50. Yu YM, Wang W, Wen J, et al. Detection of renal allograft fibrosis with MRI: arterial spin labeling outperforms reduced field-of-view IVIM. Eur Radiol 2021; 31(9):6696–707.

51. Wang W, Yu Y, Wen J, et al. Combination of functional magnetic resonance imaging and histopathologic analysis to evaluate interstitial fibrosis in kidney allografts. Clin J Am Soc Nephrol 2019;14(9): 1372–80.

52. Mao W, Zhou J, Zeng M, et al. Chronic kidney disease: pathological and functional evaluation with intravoxel incoherent motion diffusion-weighted imaging. J Magn Reson Imag 2018;47(5):1251–9.

53. Mao W, Zhou J, Zeng M, et al. Intravoxel incoherent motion diffusion-weighted imaging for the assessment of renal fibrosis of chronic kidney disease: a preliminary study. Magn Reson Imaging 2018;47: 118–24.

54. Mao W, Ding Y, Ding X, et al. Capability of arterial spin labeling and intravoxel incoherent motion diffusion-weighted imaging to detect early kidney injury in chronic kidney disease. Eur Radiol 2022. https://doi.org/10.1007/s00330-022-09331-z.

55. Liang P, Chen Y, Li S, et al. Noninvasive assessment of kidney dysfunction in children by using blood oxygenation level-dependent MRI and intravoxel incoherent motion diffusion-weighted imaging. Insights Imaging 2021;12(1):146.

56. Sulkowska K, Palczewski P, Furmanczyk-Zawiska A, et al. Diffusion weighted magnetic resonance imaging in the assessment of renal function and parenchymal changes in chronic kidney disease: a preliminary study. Ann Transplant 2020;25:e920232.

57. Liang P, Yuan G, Li S, et al. Non-invasive evaluation of the pathological and functional characteristics of chronic kidney disease by diffusion kurtosis imaging and intravoxel incoherent motion imaging: comparison with conventional DWI. Br J Radiol 2023; 96(1141):20220644.

58. Zhu Q, Ye J, Zhu W, et al. Value of intravoxel incoherent motion in assessment of pathological grade of clear cell renal cell carcinoma. Acta Radiol 2018; 59(1):121–7.

59. Zhu Q, Zhu W, Ye J, et al. Value of intravoxel incoherent motion for differential diagnosis of renal tumors. Acta Radiol. Mar 2019;60(3):382–7.

60. Ding Y, Tan Q, Mao W, et al. Differentiating between malignant and benign renal tumors: do IVIM and diffusion kurtosis imaging perform better than DWI? Eur Radiol 2019;29(12):6930–9.

61. Jian L, Liu Y, Xie Y, et al. MRI-based radiomics and urine creatinine for the differentiation of renal angiomyolipoma with minimal fat from renal cell carcinoma: a preliminary study. Front Oncol 2022;12:876664.

62. Hashim E, Yuen DA, Kirpalani A. Reduced flow in delayed graft function as assessed by IVIM is associated with time to recovery following kidney transplantation. J Magn Reson Imag 2021;53(1):108–17.

63. Ni X, Wang W, Li X, et al. Utility of diffusion-weighted imaging for guiding clinical management of patients with kidney transplant: a prospective study. J Magn Reson Imag 2020;52(2):565–74.

64. Chang YC, Tsai YH, Chung MC, et al. Intravoxel incoherent motion-diffusion-weighted MRI for investigation of delayed graft function immediately after kidney transplantation. BioMed Res Int 2022;2022: 2832996.

65. Udayakumar D, Zhang Z, Xi Y, et al. Deciphering intratumoral molecular heterogeneity in clear cell renal cell carcinoma with a radiogenomics platform. Clin Cancer Res 2021;27(17):4794–806.

66. Dwivedi DK, Xi Y, Kapur P, et al. Magnetic resonance imaging radiomics analyses for prediction of high-grade histology and necrosis in clear cell renal cell carcinoma: preliminary experience. Clin Genitourin Cancer 2021;19(1):12–21 e1.

67. Zhong J, Palkhi E, Buckley DL, et al. Feasibility study on using dynamic contrast enhanced MRI to assess the effect of tyrosine kinase inhibitor therapy within the STAR trial of metastatic renal cell cancer. Diagnostics 2021; 11(7). https://doi.org/10.3390/diagnostics11071302.

68. Humphreys BD. Mechanisms of renal fibrosis. Annu Rev Physiol 2018;80:309–26.

69. Bokacheva L, Rusinek H, Zhang JL, et al. Estimates of glomerular filtration rate from MR renography and tracer kinetic models. J Magn Reson Imaging 2009; 29(2):371–82.

70. Weinreb JC, Rodby RA, Yee J, et al. Use of intravenous gadolinium-based contrast media in patients with kidney disease: consensus statements from

the American College of Radiology and the National Kidney Foundation. Kidney Med 2021;3(1):142–50.

71. de Boer A, Harteveld AA, Stemkens B, et al. Multiparametric renal MRI: an intrasubject test-retest repeatability study. J Magn Reson Imaging 2021; 53(3):859–73.

72. Chandarana H, Amarosa A, Huang WC, et al. High temporal resolution 3D gadolinium-enhanced dynamic MR imaging of renal tumors with pharmacokinetic modeling: preliminary observations. J Magn Reson Imag 2013;38(4):802–8.

73. Pedrosa I, Alsop DC, Rofsky NM. Magnetic resonance imaging as a biomarker in renal cell carcinoma. Cancer 2009;115(10 Suppl):2334–45.

74. Schutter R, Lantinga VA, Borra RJH, et al. MRI for diagnosis of post-renal transplant complications: current state-of-the-art and future perspectives. MAGMA 2020;33(1):49–61.

75. Giral-Classe M, Hourmant M, Cantarovich D, et al. Delayed graft function of more than six days strongly decreases long-term survival of transplanted kidneys. Kidney Int 1998;54(3):972–8.

Magnetic Resonance Perfusion Imaging of Prostate

Qing Yuan, PhD[a],*, Debora Z. Recchimuzzi, MD[a], Daniel N. Costa, MD[a,b]

KEYWORDS

- Prostate cancer • Dynamic contrast-enhanced (DCE) MRI • Multiparametric MRI
- Arterial spin labeled MRI • Intravoxel incoherent motion

KEY POINTS

- Dynamic contrast-enhanced mahnetic resonance (MR) imaging (DCE-MRI) is an important element of the multiparametric MRI in clinical non-invasive assessment of men with suspected prostate cancer.
- While DCE-MRI plays a secondary role in the scoring of focal abnormalities by prostate imaging reporting and data system, it can be used to differentiate between benign and malignant lesions, to stage tumors, and to monitor response to therapy.
- The arterial spin labeled and intravoxel incoherent motion diffusion-weighted MRI are promising non-contrast techniques for tissue perfusion quantification. Their clinical utility and potential as imaging biomarkers is an active area of ongoing research.

INTRODUCTION

Prostate cancer (PCa) is the most common non-cutaneous malignancy and the second most frequent cause of cancer-related death in men. Most men with PCa, however, die with the disease rather than as a result of the disease.[1] With the broad spectrum of aggressiveness and the potential morbidity related to the standard of care management options, accurate pre-treatment prostate cancer risk stratification is crucial for preventing under and overtreatment.[2]

Following the commonly used screening strategy combining results from serum prostate-specific antigen (PSA) and digital rectal examination (DRE), ultrasound (US)-guided biopsy is used to establish a definitive diagnosis of PCa.[3] Pretreatment determination of prostate cancer aggressiveness is inferred from predictive models such as those derived from tables and nomograms combining demographic factors, serum PSA values, DRE, and biopsy findings (Gleason grade group and volume of disease).[4,5] However, these screening strategies have known shortcomings. For example, a normal PSA value does not exclude PCa and several benign conditions such as prostatitis may cause PSA elevation.[6] Moreover, prostate random biopsies use an ultrasound (US)-guided, anatomy-based approach[7] that commonly leads to suboptimal assessment of the disease volume, extent, and aggressiveness, resulting in increased uncertainty and potential undertreatment of men with significant cancers.[8] For these reasons, alternative image-guided biopsy approaches have emerged in recent years.

Multiparametric MRI (mpMRI) integrates anatomic information from T2-weighted imaging (T2WI) and functional information from diffusion-weighted imaging (DWI) and dynamic contrast-enhanced (DCE) imaging. The adoption of mpMRI

a Department of Radiology, University of Texas Southwestern Medical Center, 5323 Harry Hines Boulevard, Dallas, TX 75390, USA; b Department of Urology, University of Texas Southwestern Medical Center, 2201 Inwood Road, TX 75390, USA
* Corresponding author.
E-mail address: Qing.Yuan@UTsouthwestern.edu

Magn Reson Imaging Clin N Am 32 (2024) 171–179
https://doi.org/10.1016/j.mric.2023.09.007
1064-9689/24/Published by Elsevier Inc.

as a prostate biopsy triage and planning tool has transformed the landscape of PCa diagnosis. Interpreted through the increasingly universal language proposed by prostate imaging reporting and data system (PI-RADS),[9] mpMRI has enabled targeted biopsies to improve the detection and characterization of prostate cancers.[10,11] In the PROstate MR Imaging Study (PROMIS) trial, for example, use of an MRI-based triage approach allowed 27% of men to avoid a biopsy while detecting 18% more cases of clinically significant cancers and 5% fewer clinically insignificant cancers.[8,10,11]

In this article, we provide a detailed description of the different techniques available for assessing perfusion of the prostate with MR imaging, including strategies adopted in clinical practice and research areas.

PROSTATE PERFUSION MR IMAGING
Dynamic Contrast-Enhanced MRI

Description
The DCE MRI technique preconized by PI-RADS and widely adopted in clinical practice consists of a series of fast T1-weighted sequences covering the entire prostate before and after rapid injection (3–4 mL/s) of a bolus of a gadolinium-based contrast agent.[12,13] The term "dynamic" is derived from the multiple serial images that are collected after injection of contrast media. Intravenous contrast agents pass from the arteries to the tissue microvasculature and extravasate within seconds to the extravascular extracellular space. Extracellular space is also called the "leakage space." Contrast agents in vessels and in the extracellular space shorten local relaxation times of blood and tissue, leading to a rapid brightening of signal on T1-weighted images. It assesses signal intensity changes to detect areas with pharmacokinetics features seen in angiogenesis. This occurs in PCa and is shown as an area which enhances faster, and to a greater extent compared with normal prostate tissue, also showing earlier contrast washout.[12,13]

Image acquisition and analysis
Dynamic contrast-enhancement techniques typically use 3-dimensional (3D) T1-weighted fast spoiled gradient-echo MRI sequences to repeatedly image a volume of interest after the administration of a bolus of intravenous (i.v.) contrast agent. T1-weighted spoiled gradient-echo sequences provide high sensitivity to T1 changes, high signal-to-noise ratios, adequate anatomic coverage, and rapid data acquisition. PI-RADS version 2.1[9] recommends a minimum temporal resolution of 15 seconds or less because of lack of diagnostic benefit of images obtained at higher temporal resolution and owing to the qualitative nature of enhancement evaluation. This minimizes the potential trade-offs in spatial resolution that may be required with higher temporal resolution. Although a temporal resolution of 7 seconds or less (as recommended in PI-RADS version 2[14]) does not offer advantages, there may be subjective perceptual penalty for some readers when increasing the temporal resolution to approximately 15 seconds.

To be accessible to a broader radiological community, PI-RADS utilizes a simplified, semi-objective analysis. An abnormality is considered to be DCE imaging positive if it has focal enhancement that occurs earlier than or contemporaneously with enhancement of adjacent normal prostatic tissues and corresponds to a suspicious finding on T2WI T2WI or DWI[9] (Fig. 1). The lack of specificity of DCE imaging requires that the interpretation of imaging findings assumes a different approach seen with the other components of the multiparametric MRI examination—DWI and T2WI. Whereas DWI and T2WI represent the 2 main sequences in the definition of a PI-RADS score in lesions located in the peripheral zone (PZ) and transition zone, respectively, DCE imaging has a secondary role in the assessment of the PI-RADS category. If a focal early enhancement is present, its value can only be assessed after consideration of the presence and characteristics of a corresponding abnormality on DWI and T2WI (Fig. 2).

The visual, subjective comparison of pre-contrast and post-contrast images can be challenging because the prostate is a highly vascularized organ.[15] Moreover, hundreds of images are generated per examination and review of such amount of data can prove inefficient and cumbersome (Fig. 3). To overcome this limitation and provide detailed contrast pharmacokinetics information, dedicated post-processing software can be used. These signal intensity changes—generally represented by gadolinium concentration versus time curves[16] (Fig. 4), allow for semi-quantitative assessment of contrast agent concentration or calculation of different quantitative physiologic parameters by using pharmacokinetic compartmental modeling. Washout slope is a semi-quantitative parameter that captures the curve pattern after the first peak enhancement. Other parameters such as peak enhancement, time to peak, wash-in slope, and area under the curve can be calculated. Semi-quantitative parameters have the advantages of being fast, relatively simple to calculate, and more broadly available. However, these parameters depend on imaging acquisition so are less reliable

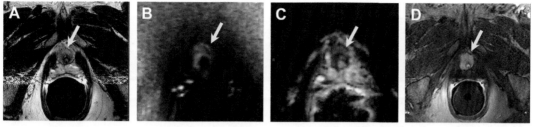

Fig. 1. Dynamic contrast-enhanced (DCE) imaging positivity per prostate imaging reporting and data system (PI-RADS) criteria. MRI reveals a large lesion (*arrows*) located at the apex encasing the urethra, heterogeneous on the axial T2-weighted imaging (T2WI) (*A*), markedly hyperintense on high B-value diffusion-weighted imaging (DWI) (*B*) and markedly hypointense on apparent diffusion coefficient (ADC) (*C*). There is focal enhancement on DCE imaging (*D*) corresponding to the abnormalities seen in the other sequences, constituting a DCE imaging positive finding. Surgery revealed Gleason Grade 2 prostate cancer.

when used to compare the results obtained at different times, different MRI scanners, and different sites. More sophisticated pharmacokinetic modeling, such as the extended Tofts model, can be used to characterize tissue microvasculature[17,18] by formulating the contrast agent exchange between the intravascular space and the extravascular extracellular space. To obtain quantitative DCE imaging–derived vascularity measures, baseline T1 relaxation time mapping is often performed using the variable flip angle technique[19] prior to the contrast injection to convert the DCE imaging signal intensities to the contrast agent concentrations.

A central limitation of DCE imaging in the identification of PCa is the overlapping features with inflammation. Increased vessel leakiness in prostatitis often causes increased enhancement of the involved tissue on imaging (**Fig. 5**). Highly perfused benign prostatic hyperplasia nodules in the transition zone also frequently demonstrate hyperenhancement on DCE imaging.[20] Additionally, the absence of early enhancement can also be a less common presentation of cancer, and therefore cannot be used to exclude the possibility of disease. Thus, DCE imaging must always be viewed in the context of other MRI parameters and cannot stand alone as a diagnostic modality regardless of curve shape or intensity of enhancement. Limitations also result from the lack of consensus in acquisition protocols, standardized approaches for calibration and analysis, and

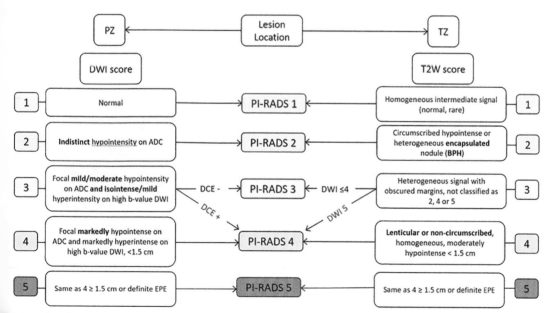

Fig. 2. Flowchart illustrating the PI-RADS version 2.1 scoring algorithm. Note that the impact of DCE imaging status is limited to upgrading lesions in the peripheral zone (PZ) with a DWI score of 3 to an overall PI-RADS category 4. This simplified approach and limited scope may hinder the perceived utility of DCE imaging.

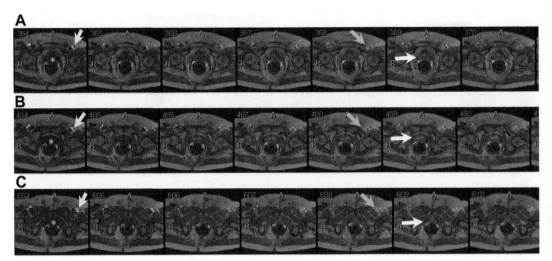

Fig. 3. Example of DCE images acquired as part of a multiparametric MRI. For this particular multiparametric protocol, 30 images are acquired at different time points in each slice location throughout the prostate (*asterisk*), including the base (*A*), mid (*B*), and apex (*C*), during and after the administration of intravenous contrast. In this sample of 21 from a total of 900 images, it is possible to see early images with enhancement of femoral arteries (*yellow arrows*) but no contrast yet reached the prostate gland (*asterisk*). Later images show contrast in veins (*blue arrows*) and in the prostate (*white arrows*).

commercially available tools for pharmacokinetic analysis from different vendors.[15] A potential shortcoming for assessing DCE imaging–derived pharmacokinetic features is its vulnerability to motion, which can result from rectal peristalsis and bladder filling as well as bulk patient movement. Because image acquisition extends over 5 or more minutes, misregistration between consecutive slices can occur, leading to noise in the wash-in and washout curves, difficulty in fitting the curve with pharmacokinetic models.

As previously detailed, the specific scenario in which a DCE imaging finding determines an overall PI-RADS category is a PZ lesion presenting with a DWI score of 3 and a corresponding positive focal early enhancement on DCE imaging—the final assessment must then be upgraded to a PI-RADS category 4. While this approach is supported by evidence that mpMRI and biparametric MRI (ie, T2WI and DWI without DCE imaging) have comparable performances in the diagnosis of PCa,[21] this may be a result of the scoring algorithm and the simplified approach chosen by the expert panel. Another situation in which DCE imaging assumes a more relevant role on PI-RADS assessment is in mpMRI with a nondiagnostic

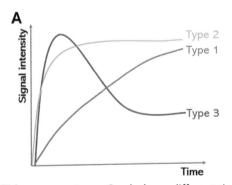

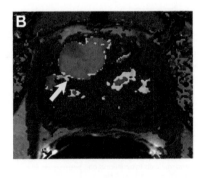

Fig. 4. DCE image curve types. Graph shows different signal intensity versus time curves representing enhancement patterns on DCE imaging (*A*). Type 1 (*blue*, benign) shows progressive enhancement; type 2 (*green*, indeterminate) characterized by rapid enhancement with plateauing, and type 3 (*red*, suspicious for malignancy) revealing rapid enhancement followed by rapid wash-out. Post-processing software may facilitate this analysis by overlaying these color-coded patterns on anatomic T2-weighted images (*B*), in this case revealing an area with suspicious post-contrast features in the right anterior mid gland (*arrow*). This was shown to represent high-grade (Gleason grade group 4) prostate cancer on targeted biopsy informed by the MRI findings.

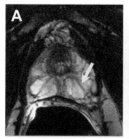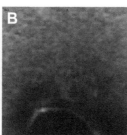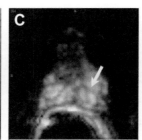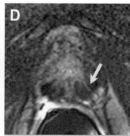

Fig. 5. Abnormal areas of contrast-enhancement in the prostate secondary to prostatitis decrease the specificity of this technique for identification of prostate cancer. In a 67-year-old man with a prostate-specific antigen (PSA) of 4.6 ng/mL, multiparametric MRI for prostate cancer detection revealed a diffusely striated appearance of the PZ with linear hyperintensities on T2WI(*arrow* in A), no corresponding abnormality on high B-value DWI (*B*), and corresponding liner mild hypointensities on ADC (*arrow* in C). DCE (*D*) revealed enhancement of the same abnormalities seen in the other sequences. The distribution and morphology of the abnormalities and lack of restricted diffusion suggest a benign process related to prostatitis and expose the lack of specificity of the DCE imaging findings when analyzed alone.

DWI sequence, most commonly a result of artifacts provoked by the presence of hip prosthesis (**Fig. 6**). Moreover, some argue one of the main benefits of DCE imaging is to help point the radiologist to a potentially abnormal area that was not promptly identified during the review of the T2WI and DWI data sets (**Fig. 7**). Finally, beyond the scope of the clinical applications covered by PI-RADS, DCE imaging sequence has been shown to be a cornerstone sequence in the detection of recurrent PCa lesions.[22]

Arterial Spin Labeled MRI

Arterial spin labeled (ASL) MRI measures tissue perfusion using water protons in the arterial blood as an endogenous diffusible tracer without administration of a contrast agent. In an ASL image acquisition, the magnetization of inflowing blood is selectively inverted using radiofrequency (RF) pulses proximal to the tissue of interest. After the post labeling delay, the labeled blood flows into the tissue, label images of this region measure the blood accumulation in the tissue. Either 2D or 3D image readout using various pulse sequences, such as 2D echo-planar imaging (EPI) and 3D fast/turbo spin echo (FSE/TSE) sequences, can be performed. Control images of the same tissue region are acquired using the same imaging sequence without the spin labeling RF pulses. Subtraction of the label image from the control image generates the perfusion-weighted image (PWI). To quantify absolute perfusion of tissue, proton-density images need to be obtained. Perfusion maps in physiologic value of mL/100 g/min can be calculated pixel-by-pixel from PWI, proton-density image, imaging parameters, and constants.

Different approaches of ASL labeling have been developed. The continuous labeling (CASL) uses 1 single constant RF pulse and a constant gradient to invert the blood as it flows through a single labeling plane.[16] This method was not widely implemented due to hardware limitations. The pseudo-continuous ASL (PCASL) applies a train of slice-selective RF pulses and gradients at the labeling plane,[23] which improves the labeling efficiency compared to CASL and is compatible with modern RF transmission hardware on clinical MRI scanners. PCASL is the recommended implementation for clinical brain perfusion applications by the International Society for Magnetic Resonance in Medicine perfusion study group.[24]

The flow alternating inversion recovery (FAIR) is a pulsed labeling technique (PASL), in which 2 inversion recovery images are acquired: 1 with a non-selective inversion pulse and the other with a slice-selective inversion pulse across the imaging slice.[25] PASL techniques are readily implemented on clinical scanner, however, the inherent signal-to-noise ratio (SNR) of PASL is lower than that of CASL.[26] The FAIR true fast imaging with steady precession (FISP) perfusion sequence has been applied to measure perfusion in abdominal organs.[27]

The velocity-selective ASL (VSASL) also includes a spin labeling phase and image acquisition following a post-label delay.[28] However, the labeling of the blood is based on its velocity instead of the spatial location, in which blood flowing above a cutoff velocity (Vc) is labeled using RF and flow-sensitive gradient pulses. For the control, the flow-sensitive gradient pulses are either turned off or designed for flow-compensation. Similar to spatial-selective labeling methods, the tissue perfusion can be quantified by the signal difference

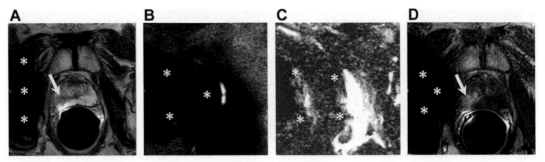

Fig. 6. Role of DCE imaging as a back-up sequence in less common scenarios on clinical practice. In a 76-year-old man with known prostate cancer undergoing multiparametric MRI for monitoring a known cancer (active surveillance), a right-sided metallic hip prosthesis resulted in severe susceptibility artifacts (*asterisks*) on all sequences, particularly DWI (*B*) and ADC (*C*), which were nondiagnostic. The questionable focal abnormality (*arrow*) in the right PZ on the T2-weighted images (*A*), validated by DCE imaging (*D*) as an area of early and focal hyperenhancement (*arrow*), increasing the level of confidence that this did correspond to an area suspicious for cancer and triggered a repeat biopsy of this region. Targeted biopsy of that area revealed high grade (Gleason grade group 3 cancer) and patient was then, appropriately, referred for surgery that validated the biopsy findings. In the absence of the DCE imaging data, reporting this finding may have been less assertive and delayed the diagnosis of this high-risk cancer.

between the label and control images, proton density images, imaging parameters, and constants.

Prostate ASL imaging is still in its early stages of development, and not used in clinical practice. The feasibility study of measuring prostate perfusion using the pulsed labeling approach FAIR by Li and Metzger[29] showed the relatively low total prostate blood flow in 5 healthy subjects (range of 16.4–33.9 mL/100 cm³/min; mean and standard deviation of 25.8 ± 7.1 mL/100 cm³/min). Cai and colleagues[30] compared PASL FAIR perfusion and DCE MRI in 43 patients with histologically proven PCa by transrectal ultrasound -guided systemic biopsy (Gleason score range of 6–9). Significantly higher blood flow was found in cancer than in benign tissues. The ASL-derived blood flow showed significantly strong to moderate correlations with the DCE-MRI quantitative parameters. Another study of 30 patients with biopsy-confirmed PI-RADS 4

and 5 PCa demonstrated both ASL and DCE imaging signals of the index lesion differed significantly from normal prostate tissue. ASL had significantly higher contrast ratio in differentiating cancer from benign tissue in the peripheral and transition zone compared to DCE imaging.[31] To develop the VSASL in prostate, the cutoff velocity for prostate was investigated in healthy volunteers since it determines the sensitivity to perfusion signal.[32]

ASL is a promising noncontrast MRI technique for perfusion quantification. It can be performed repeatedly in patients under active surveillance or treatment without concerns of gadolinium-based contrast agent safety and retention issues. However, it is limited by technical challenges and more research is needed to advance and evaluate its utilization and benefits in patients being evaluated for PCa.

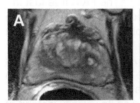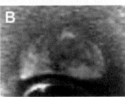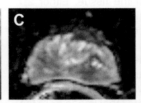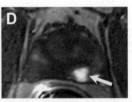

Fig. 7. Role of DCE images in raising awareness of a focal abnormality not as conspicuous on the other MR pulse sequences. In a 58-year-old biopsy-naive man with PSA of 5.1 ng/mL, MRI for biopsy planning revealed 11 mm lesion in the left base PZ, slightly hypointense on T2WI (*A*), not delineated as a focal abnormality on high b-value DWI (*B*), indistinct, and mildly hypointense on ADC (*C*), however, with avid, early enhancement (*arrow* in D). This lesion was initially missed based on T2WI and DWI alone; however, the markedly abnormal DCE image resulted in further review of those images being assigned a score 3 for DWI/ADC, upgraded to overall score 4 given + DCE image. This illustrates the use of DCE image as a "safety net" or "backup" sequence. Targeted biopsy of this finding revealed high-grade cancer (Gleason grade group 3).

Intra-voxel Incoherent Motion

DWI measures random movement of water molecules in biological tissue by acquiring images in the presence of paired diffusion-sensitizing gradients. MR signal attenuation with the increased b-value, which defines the strength and duration of the gradients, allows the calculation of the apparent diffusion coefficient (ADC) of tissue. In clinical practice, a spin echo–echo planar imaging sequence is often used to acquire diffusion-weighted images with fat suppression. Diffusion-sensitizing gradients are applied in 3 orthogonal directions to acquire at least 2 b-values.

On modern commercial MRI scanners, ADC maps can be generated immediately after the DWI acquisition, commonly using a mono-exponential model assuming water diffusion in tissue has a Gaussian distribution. When low b-values are used (less than 200 s/mm^2), the microcirculation of blood in the capillary network mimics a diffusion process called "pseudo-diffusion" and contributes to the signal decay measured by the diffusion-weighted imaging sequence. The intravoxel incoherent motion theory[33] describes this perfusion-related effect by the pseudo-diffusion coefficient, D*, and the perfusion fraction, f, in addition to the tissue diffusion coefficient, D, using a biexponential model in a multiple b-value DWI acquisition. As the b-value increases beyond 1000 s/mm^2, the water diffusion deviates from the Gaussian distribution. This non-Gaussian diffusion effect and the low signal at the "noise floor" due to the high b-value used may lead to errors in estimates of intra-voxel incoherent motion (IVIM) pseudo-diffusion parameters, f and D*.[34]

The IVIM method is appealing since it can potentially extract microvascular perfusion information from a standard diffusion-weighted sequence without the use of exogenous contrast agent. Le Bihan and Turner suggested that the IVIM parameters, f and D*, may provide useful physiologic data for microcirculation. The quantity f represents the fractional volume of the incoherent capillary blood flow at the image voxel level, D* depends on capillary blood flow, so that relative perfusion or blood flow can be estimated from fD*.[35] The interpretation of the IVIM parameters was cautioned by Henkelman[36] who suggested IVIM cannot measure classical tissue perfusion. Nevertheless, the perfusion-driven IVIM imaging has gained interest in oncological applications. Its clinical utility and potential as an imaging biomarker is an active area of ongoing research in phantoms, animal models, and human cancers.[37,38]

Currently, IVIM-DWI is not used in clinical evaluations of PCa. The IVIM method requires multiple b-value image acquisitions which are associated with increased scan time, possible motion artifact, and image registration issues. Reliable estimation of IVIM parameters is challenging due to low SNR in DWI signal, nonlinear model fitting quality and robustness, and a lack of consensus on optimal data acquisition and modeling. Several IVIM-DWI studies have demonstrated the feasibility of IVIM imaging for PCa, and the biexponential model better described the diffusion signal decay in PCa when low b-values are used. However, the perfusion-related IVIM measurements from the in vivo studies showed inconsistent findings.[39–46]

There has been no standardization of IVIM-DWI data acquisition and fitting algorithms for PCa applications. Pang and colleagues[42] demonstrated the choice of b-values had an impact on the estimated f and D* for PCa. Both parameters correlated best with the DCE imaging results when the highest b-value (750 s/mm^2) was not used in the model fitting. Another study involving 50 PCa patients undergoing 2 repeated DWI scans with 12 b-values (0, 10, 25, 50, 80, 100, 200, 500, 1000, and 2000 s/mm^2)[47] showed the optimized b-values distributions improved the repeatability of DWI-derived parameters but not the prediction of PCa aggressiveness.

In general, it is difficult to perform biexponential model fitting reliably to obtain robust fitting results. The "pseudo-diffusion" parameters demonstrated large standard deviation and low repeatability in PCa.[41,43,47] The performance of the IVIM fitting depended on the values of f, D/D* ratio, and noise level.[48] Echo time (TE) also affected the IVIM quantification since blood and tissue have different T2 values.[49] In a multi-site DWI quantification study,[50] 14 sites were involved in analyzing the same whole-mount pathologically validated PCa DWI dataset using site-specific fitting algorithms. The IVIM parameters, D, D*, and f had greater between site variation and lower area under the receiver operating characteristic curve for PCa differentiation. Applying constraints on the fitted IVIM parameters, such as upper and lower bounds, non-negativity constraints, or other error reduction techniques, yielded better performance by having less outliers. The new development of deep learning IVIM modeling showed promising results compared to conventional non-linear least squares fitting approach.[51]

The clinical application of IVIM in oncology has shown its potential and challenges. Technical improvements such as optimal b-value distribution, good SNR, and robust methodology for data modeling are needed for high repeatability and reproducibility of IVIM parameters estimation. Clinical utility and performance in large patient populations is essential before its adoption in clinical practice.

SUMMARY

Dynamic contrast-enhanced MR imaging (DCE-MRI) is an important element of the non-invasive assessment of men being evaluated for prostate cancer. It provides information about tumor vascularity and perfusion, which can be used to differentiate benign from malignant lesions, to stage tumors, and to monitor response to therapy. While it currently plays a secondary role in the scoring of focal abnormalities by PI-RADS, there is growing interest in leveraging its quantitative predictive value to assess tumor aggressiveness and to support artificial intelligence–based automated detection tools. Other non-clinical tools—including IVIM and ASL—remain exploratory and their clinical utility remains an area of active research.

DISCLOSURE

The authors have nothing to disclose.

REFERENCES

1. Surveillance, Epidemiology, and End Results (SEER) Program (www.seer.cancer.gov) SEER*Stat Database: Incidence - SEER 9 Regs Research Data, Nov 2018 Sub (1975-2016). 2019.
2. Schaeffer EM, Srinivas S, Adra N, et al. NCCN Guidelines® Insights: Prostate Cancer, Version 1.2023. J Natl Compr Canc Netw 2022;20(12):1288–98.
3. Matlaga BR, Eskew LA, McCullough DL. Prostate biopsy: indications and technique. Review. J Urol 2003;169(1):12–9.
4. Chun FK, Karakiewicz PI, Briganti A, et al. Prostate cancer nomograms: an update. Eur Urol 2006;50(5):914–26 [discussion 926].
5. Ross PL, Scardino PT, Kattan MW. A catalog of prostate cancer nomograms. J Urol 2001;165(5):1562–8.
6. Hoffman RM. Clinical practice. Screening for prostate cancer. N Engl J Med 2011;365(21):2013–9.
7. Shariat SF, Roehrborn CG. Using biopsy to detect prostate cancer. Reviews in urology. Fall 2008;10(4):262–80.
8. Ahmed HU, El-Shater Bosaily A, Brown LC, et al. Diagnostic accuracy of multi-parametric MRI and TRUS biopsy in prostate cancer (PROMIS): a paired validating confirmatory study. Lancet 2017;389(10071):815–22.
9. Prostate imaging and reporting and data system: version 2.1. American College of Radiology; 2019. Available at: https://www.acr.org/-/media/ACR/Files/RADS/PI-RADS/PIRADS-V2-1.pdf. Accessed June 11, 2021.
10. Siddiqui MM, Rais-Bahrami S, Turkbey B, et al. Comparison of MR/ultrasound fusion-guided biopsy with ultrasound-guided biopsy for the diagnosis of prostate cancer. JAMA 2015;313(4):390–7.
11. Kasivisvanathan V, Rannikko AS, Borghi M, et al. MRI-Targeted or Standard Biopsy for Prostate-Cancer Diagnosis. N Engl J Med 2018;378(19):1767–77.
12. Barentsz JO, Engelbrecht M, Jager GJ, et al. Fast dynamic gadolinium-enhanced MR imaging of urinary bladder and prostate cancer. J Magn Reson Imaging 1999;10(3):295–304.
13. Engelbrecht MR, Huisman HJ, Laheij RJ, et al. Discrimination of prostate cancer from normal peripheral zone and central gland tissue by using dynamic contrast-enhanced MR imaging. Radiology 2003;229(1):248–54.
14. Prostate imaging and reporting and data system: version 2. American College of Radiology; 2015. Available at: http://www.acr.org/~/media/ACR/Documents/PDF/QualitySafety/Resources/PIRADS/PIRADS%20V2.pdf. Accessed June 5, 2015.
15. Hoeks CM, Barentsz JO, Hambrock T, et al. Prostate cancer: multiparametric MR imaging for detection, localization, and staging. Radiology 2011;261(1):46–66.
16. Williams DS, Detre JA, Leigh JS, et al. Magnetic resonance imaging of perfusion using spin inversion of arterial water. Proc Natl Acad Sci U S A 1992;89(1):212–6.
17. Tofts PS. Modeling tracer kinetics in dynamic Gd-DTPA MR imaging. Research Support, Non-U.S. Gov't Review. J Magn Reson Imaging 1997;7(1):91–101.
18. Tofts PS, Brix G, Buckley DL, et al. Estimating kinetic parameters from dynamic contrast-enhanced T(1)-weighted MRI of a diffusable tracer: standardized quantities and symbols. J Magn Reson Imaging 1999;10(3):223–32.
19. Wang HZ, Riederer SJ, Lee JN. Optimizing the precision in T1 relaxation estimation using limited flip angles. Magn Reson Med 1987;5(5):399–416.
20. Jager GJ, Ruijter ET, van de Kaa CA, et al. Local staging of prostate cancer with endorectal MR imaging: correlation with histopathology. AJR Am J Roentgenol 1996;166(4):845–52.
21. Kang Z, Min X, Weinreb J, et al. Abbreviated Biparametric Versus Standard Multiparametric MRI for Diagnosis of Prostate Cancer: A Systematic Review and Meta-Analysis. AJR Am J Roentgenol 2019;212(2):357–65.
22. Tanaka T, Yang M, Froemming AT, et al. Current Imaging Techniques for and Imaging Spectrum of Prostate Cancer Recurrence and Metastasis: A Pictorial Review. RadioGraphics 2020;40(3):709–26.
23. Dai W, Garcia D, de Bazelaire C, et al. Continuous flow-driven inversion for arterial spin labeling using

pulsed radio frequency and gradient fields. Magn Reson Med 2008;60(6):1488–97.

24. Alsop DC, Detre JA, Golay X, et al. Recommended implementation of arterial spin-labeled perfusion MRI for clinical applications: A consensus of the ISMRM perfusion study group and the European consortium for ASL in dementia. Magn Reson Med 2015;73(1):102–16.

25. Kim SG. Quantification of relative cerebral blood flow change by flow-sensitive alternating inversion recovery (FAIR) technique: application to functional mapping. Magn Reson Med 1995;34(3):293–301.

26. Wong EC, Buxton RB, Frank LR. A theoretical and experimental comparison of continuous and pulsed arterial spin labeling techniques for quantitative perfusion imaging. Magn Reson Med 1998;40(3):348–55.

27. Fenchel M, Martirosian P, Langanke J, et al. Perfusion MR imaging with FAIR true FISP spin labeling in patients with and without renal artery stenosis: initial experience. Radiology 2006;238(3):1013–21.

28. Wong EC, Cronin M, Wu WC, et al. Velocity-selective arterial spin labeling. Magn Reson Med 2006;55(6):1334–41.

29. Li X, Metzger GJ. Feasibility of measuring prostate perfusion with arterial spin labeling. NMR Biomed 2013;26(1):51–7.

30. Cai W, Li F, Wang J, et al. A comparison of arterial spin labeling perfusion MRI and DCE-MRI in human prostate cancer. NMR Biomed 2014;27(7):817–25.

31. Boschheidgen M, Schimmoller L, Kasprowski L, et al. Arterial spin labelling as a gadolinium-free alternative in the detection of prostate cancer. Magn Reson Imaging 2021;80:33–8.

32. Liu D, Zhu D, Xu F, et al. Prostate perfusion mapping using Fourier-transform based velocity-selective arterial spin labeling: Choice of cutoff velocity and comparison with brain. Magn Reson Med 2023;90(3):1121–9.

33. Le Bihan D, Breton E, Lallemand D, et al. Separation of diffusion and perfusion in intravoxel incoherent motion MR imaging. Radiology 1988;168(2):497–505.

34. Le Bihan D. What can we see with IVIM MRI? Neuroimage 2019;187:56–67.

35. Le Bihan D, Turner R. The capillary network: a link between IVIM and classical perfusion. Magn Reson Med 1992;27(1):171–8.

36. Henkelman RM. Does IVIM measure classical perfusion? Magn Reson Med 1990;16(3):470–5.

37. Federau C. Intravoxel incoherent motion MRI as a means to measure in vivo perfusion: A review of the evidence. NMR Biomed 2017;30(11). https://doi.org/10.1002/nbm.3780.

38. Iima M. Perfusion-driven Intravoxel Incoherent Motion (IVIM) MRI in Oncology: Applications, Challenges, and Future Trends. Magn Reson Med Sci 2021;20(2):125–38.

39. Riches SF, Hawtin K, Charles-Edwards EM, et al. Diffusion-weighted imaging of the prostate and rectal wall: comparison of biexponential and monoexponential modelled diffusion and associated perfusion coefficients. NMR Biomed 2009;22(3):318–25.

40. Döpfert J, Lemke A, Weidner A, et al. Investigation of prostate cancer using diffusion-weighted intravoxel incoherent motion imaging. Magn Reson Imaging 2011;29(8):1053–8.

41. Shinmoto H, Tamura C, Soga S, et al. An intravoxel incoherent motion diffusion-weighted imaging study of prostate cancer. AJR Am J Roentgenol 2012;199(4):W496–500.

42. Pang Y, Turkbey B, Bernardo M, et al. Intravoxel incoherent motion MR imaging for prostate cancer: an evaluation of perfusion fraction and diffusion coefficient derived from different b-value combinations. Magn Reson Med 2013;69(2):553–62.

43. Valerio M, Zini C, Fierro D, et al. 3T multiparametric MRI of the prostate: Does intravoxel incoherent motion diffusion imaging have a role in the detection and stratification of prostate cancer in the peripheral zone? Eur J Radiol. Apr 2016;85(4):790–4.

44. Pesapane F, Patella F, Fumarola EM, et al. Intravoxel Incoherent Motion (IVIM) Diffusion Weighted Imaging (DWI) in the Periferic Prostate Cancer Detection and Stratification. Med Oncol 2017;34(3):35.

45. Beyhan M, Sade R, Koc E, et al. The evaluation of prostate lesions with IVIM DWI and MR perfusion parameters at 3T MRI. Radiol Med 2019;124(2):87–93.

46. Kooreman ES, van Pelt V, Nowee ME, et al. Longitudinal Correlations Between Intravoxel Incoherent Motion (IVIM) and Dynamic Contrast-Enhanced (DCE) MRI During Radiotherapy in Prostate Cancer Patients. Front Oncol 2022;12:897130.

47. Merisaari H, Toivonen J, Pesola M, et al. Diffusion-weighted imaging of prostate cancer: effect of b-value distribution on repeatability and cancer characterization. Magn Reson Imaging 2015;33(10):1212–8.

48. Merisaari H, Movahedi P, Perez IM, et al. Fitting methods for intravoxel incoherent motion imaging of prostate cancer on region of interest level: Repeatability and gleason score prediction. Magn Reson Med 2017;77(3):1249–64.

49. Feng Z, Min X, Wang L, et al. Effects of Echo Time on IVIM Quantification of the Normal Prostate. Sci Rep 2018;8(1):2572.

50. McGarry SD, Brehler M, Bukowy JD, et al. Multi-Site Concordance of Diffusion-Weighted Imaging Quantification for Assessing Prostate Cancer Aggressiveness. J Magn Reson Imaging 2022;55(6):1745–58.

51. Kaandorp MPT, Barbieri S, Klaassen R, et al. Improved unsupervised physics-informed deep learning for intravoxel incoherent motion modeling and evaluation in pancreatic cancer patients. Magn Reson Med 2021;86(4):2250–65.

Perfusion Imaging of the Musculoskeletal System

James F. Griffith, MD, MRCP (UK), FRCR, FHKCR, FHKAM (Radiology)[a],*,
Stefanie W.Y. Yip, MBBS, FRCR, FHKCR, FHKAM (Radiology)[a],
Rianne A. van der Heijden, MD, PhD[b,c], Raul F. Valenzuela, MD[d], David K.W. Yeung, PhD[a]

KEYWORDS

• MR imaging • Perfusion • Musculoskeletal • Tumors • Inflammation • Avascular necrosis

KEY POINTS

• Perfusion and blood flow represent different physiologic process.
• Perfusion is an excellent readily obtainable measure of metabolic activity.
• Perfusion in the musculoskeletal system is measured by dynamic contrast-enhanced-MR imaging, intravoxel incoherent motion, and arterial spin labeling.
• Perfusion is clinically useful to:
1. quantify tumor treatment response, predict/recognize recurrence, differentiate hematopoietic rests from metastatic infiltration.
2. detect bone ischemia before osteonecrosis occurs and assess response to therapy.
3. quantify degree of synovial inflammation and treatment response.
• Automated consolidated analysis of perfusion data will lead to more widespread clinical usage.

INTRODUCTION

Although high-resolution structural imaging will continue to be the bedrock of musculoskeletal radiology, functional imaging will undoubtedly be more widely used when issues related to standardization of acquisition and automated assessment can be resolved. Functional imaging addresses tissue function rather than structure. Currently, perfusion imaging is the type of functional imaging that is most applicable to musculoskeletal imaging.

First and foremost, the terms "blood flow" and "perfusion" should be clarified. Blood flow refers to flow in vessels where no exchange occurs between the intra- and extravascular spaces (**Fig. 1**). Blood flow is measured experimentally by intravascular microspheres and clinically by spectral or color Doppler imaging on ultrasound (**Fig. 2**) or phase contrast MR imaging. Perfusion is a much more encompassing and physiologically relevant process, which is highly dependent on blood flow. Perfusion refers both to capillary flow, where free exchange with the extravascular space occurs, and interstitial diffusion (see **Fig. 1**). In other words, perfusion encompasses both capillary flow and interstitial diffusion. Perfusion is measured on MR imaging with (1) dynamic contrast-enhanced (DCE)-MR imaging, (2) dynamic susceptibility contrast-enhanced MR imaging, (3) arterial spin labeling (ASL), or (4) intravoxel incoherent motion (IVIM). In musculoskeletal (MSK) imaging, DCE-MR imaging is most used with an increasing use of IVIM, whereas ASL is infrequently used. CT perfusion imaging is also possible. Contrast-enhanced ultrasound measures both intravascular

[a] Department of Imaging and Interventional Radiology, Prince of Wales Hospital, The Chinese University of Hong Kong; [b] Department of Radiology and Nuclear Medicine, Erasmus University Medical Center, Rotterdam, The Netherlands; [c] Department of Radiology, University of Wisconsin-Madison, Madison, WI, USA; [d] Department of Musculoskeletal Imaging, The University of Texas, MD Anderson Cancer Center, USA
* Corresponding author. Department of Imaging and Interventional Radiology, Prince of Wales Hospital, The Chinese University of Hong Kong, 30-32 Ngan Shing Street, Shatin, New Territories, Hong Kong.
E-mail address: griffith@cuhk.edu.hk

mri.theclinics.com

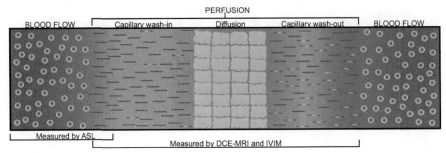

Fig. 1. Illustrating differences between blood flow and perfusion. Blood flow is flow in the intravascular space. Perfusion is a measure of capillary washin, interstitial diffusion, and capillary washout. Perfusion depends on blood flow, though encompasses capillary exchange and interstitial diffusion. The components of blood flow and tissue perfusion measured by ASL, DCE-MR imaging, and IVIM are also shown.

and vascular flow as well as capillary perfusion but not diffusion, whereas infrared spectroscopy, T2* and BOLD, and MR imaging provide indirect measures of, mainly muscle, perfusion through measurement of oxygenated and deoxygenated hemoglobin.[1–3] This review focuses on DCE, IVIM, and ASL.

DYNAMIC CONTRAST-ENHANCED MR IMAGING

DCE-MR imaging captures the passage and concentration of gadolinium contrast agent through the tissues under investigation over time.

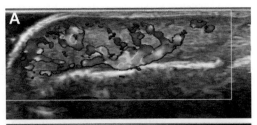

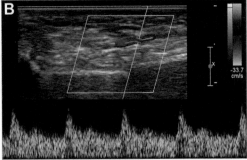

Fig. 2. (A) Longitudinal color Doppler image of normal apical pulp flow. Red indicates flow toward the transducer, blue indicates flow away from the transducer. (B) Spectral Doppler ultrasound analysis showing normal arterial waveform. This is a measure of blood flow rather than perfusion.

DCE-MR imaging interrogates T1-relaxation time. T1-relaxation times shorten relative to tissue gadolinium concentration. Quantitative Imaging Biomarker Alliance (QIBA) guidelines outline acquisition protocols for performing DCE MR imaging. DCE-MR imaging analysis can be qualitative, semiquantitative, or quantitative.[4,5] *Qualitative analysis* is the subjective analysis of the time–signal intensity curve (TIC), which visually depicts changing contrast in-flow and clearance during passage of the gadolinium bolus.[6] For DCE, there are typically three stages of perfusion reflected in the TIC: (1) upslope, which reflects contrast washin; (2) plateau, which represents the steady state of contrast within the interstitial fluid though may not be seen in all lesions; and (3) downslope, which reflects contrast washout as gadolinium passes out of the tissues under interrogation[7] (**Fig. 3**). TIC shape is subjectively assigned to one of five curve types (**Fig. 4**). *Semiquantitative analysis* measures empirical perfusion parameters derived from the TIC morphology and includes maximum enhancement (E_{max}) (ie, curve peak), rate of enhancement (E_{slope}) (ie, upslope gradient), area under the curve (AUC), and time to peak enhancement (TTP) (ie, time between base of upslope and E_{max})[8–11] (see **Fig. 3**). *Quantitative analysis* uses pharmacokinetic modeling, which requires arterial input function to gauge feeding artery changes in gadolinium concentration over time.[12,13] The most widely used pharmacokinetic model in MSK imaging is the extended Tofts model.[14] This generates four perfusion parameters: (1) transfer constant (K_{trans}), that is, the volume delivered into the tissue per unit time, interpreted as the washin rate, reflecting the early upslope to maximum enhancement (ie, the initial area under the time–intensity curve); (2) exchange rate constant (K_{ep}), which is the exchange rate between the plasma and the interstitium, interpreted as the washout rate reflecting the shape from maximum enhancement to the last timepoint

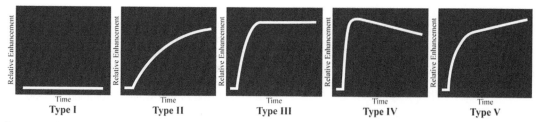

Fig. 3. Qualitative analysis of DCE-MR imaging time–intensity curve (TIC) classified into five types: Type I: no demonstrable enhancement, which may be seen in necrotic tissue. Type II: slow gradually progressive enhancement with no enhancement peak, may be seen in peri-tumoral edema. Type III: rapid steep enhancement followed by sustained plateau. Type IV: rapid steep enhancement followed by washout. Type V: rapid steep enhancement followed by progressive gradual enhancement. Type IV enhancement is caused by a small interstitial compartment due to high cellularity and is most specific curve for malignancy, whereas Types III and V enhancement also indicate hyperperfusion but are less specific for malignancy as they may be seen in both benign (eg, giant cell tumor, Langerhans cell histiocytosis) and malignant (eg, sarcomas, metastases) hypervascular tumors.

measured; (3) extravascular extracellular space fractional volume (V_e), which reflects the interstitial space volume; and (4) plasma fractional volume (V_P)[15] (**Fig. 5**). Tissue perfusion in the selected region of interest (ROI) is often compared with that of adjacent normal bone marrow or muscle.

ARTERIAL SPIN LABELING

For ASL, water protons in arterial blood are selectively magnetically labeled and used as endogenous tracers.[16] Control and labeled image data sets are acquired over the ROI, separated by a time delay based on the expected transit time of the labeled arterial blood into the tissue of interest. Subtraction of the labeled images from the control images provides a signal proportional to blood flow. ASL does not require intravenous gadolinium and provides information on intravascular flow and capillary perfusion but no information on interstitial diffusion because the magnetization of labeled arterial blood is short. Effective uniform marrow

fat suppression is essential for bone marrow ASL imaging.[17] ASL has an inherent low signal-to-noise ratio (SNR) despite efforts to increase labeling efficiency with pseudo-continuous labeling. ASL can recognize neo-angiogenesis, which reflects tumor aggressiveness, metastatic potential, and poor treatment response.[18]

INTRAVOXEL INCOHERENT MOTION

IVIM refers to the random motion of water molecules in the extravascular intercellular space and the capillary microcirculation within each voxel on MR images over time.[19] IVIM requires no contrast administration. IVIM imaging is based on a diffusion-weighted model, using multiple b-values and bi-exponential fitting, which can generate perfusion maps. As blood water in the capillary network is randomly oriented, capillary microcirculation mimics a pseudo-diffusion process.[20] The two main perfusion parameters obtained by IVIM are the pseudo-diffusion

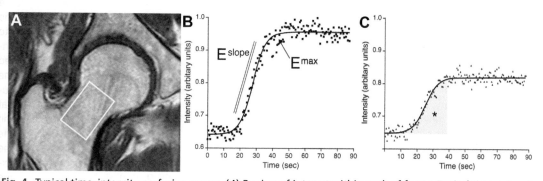

Fig. 4. Typical time–intensity perfusion curves. (A) Region of interest within neck of femur. Typical time–intensity perfusion curves of marrow perfusion from dynamic contrast-enhanced MR imaging examination in subject with (B) normal perfusion, (C) reduced perfusion. E_{slope} and E_{max} are shown as are the initial area. Curve from initial upslope to Emax is known as the initial area under the curve (IAUC) (shaded *).

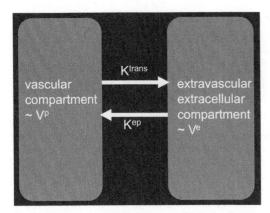

Fig. 5. Bi-compartmental Tofts model and rate constants. Volume transfer constant K_{trans} ("wash-in rate") is influenced mainly by perfusion and permeability. Extravascular extracellular space fractional volume, V_e, reflects interstitial space volume. Exchange rate constant, K_{ep} ("wash-out rate") is not an independent parameter since $K_{ep} = K_{trans}/V_e$. Fractional plasma volume V_p is more consequential in highly vascular tumors.

coefficient (D*), which represents perfusion-related diffusion, and the perfusion fraction (f), which is the flowing capillary blood fraction in each voxel.[20,21] The pseudo-diffusion coefficient (D*) is 10 times higher than the true diffusion coefficient (D), with a corresponding exponential decay. Hence, D* is only a small percentage of overall diffusivity; similarly, the f fraction is usually tiny [19,20] Hence, the SNR of IVIM is low, making it susceptible to motion and pulsation artifacts. Also, it lacks standardization for both image acquisition and measurement.[21] Nonetheless, IVIM does not require intravenous gadolinium administration and is quick to perform. With improved MR technology, the limitations of IVIM are being gradually overcome, resulting in an increased use of IVIM imaging recently.[22]

NORMAL BONE PERFUSION

Bone receives 5% to 10% of cardiac output.[23–25] Two arterial systems supply bone. The periosteal system on the bone surface supplies the periosteum and the outer one-third of the cortex. The nutrient, or medullary, system supplies the medullary canal and the inner two-thirds of the cortex. Normal bone marrow blood flow is about 15 times higher than cortical blood flow.[26] The nutrient and periosteal arterial systems are connected by small arterioles and capillaries passing through the cortex in Volkmann's and Haversian canals.[27] In older patients, periosteal arteries supply a greater proportion of cortical blood flow.[28–30] Nutrient arteries

usually enter the diaphysis of long tubular bones and course along the center of the medullary cavity, giving off smaller thin-walled arterioles that extend to the cortex.[31] Arterioles further divide into smaller (5 μm) meta-arterioles with precapillary sphincters, which flow into the capillaries and a plexus of thin-walled prominent (15–60 μm) venous sinusoids. Capillaries and venous sinusoids have a discontinuous basement membrane facilitating exchange of molecules and cells. Venous sinuses drain into small emissary veins, which drain into nutrient veins[31] (see **Fig. 1**). Pressure in the bone marrow, enclosed within the rigid cortical shell, is about three times that of extraosseous pressure facilitating transcortical venous blood flow.[29]

SOFT TISSUE PERFUSION

Musculoskeletal soft tissue perfusion has not been quantified to the same degree as bone perfusion. Muscle and synovium are soft tissue's most actively perfused components, with fat and fibrous tissue being relatively poorly perfused[32] (**Fig. 6**). Muscle perfusion depends highly on muscle activity and the relative amount of lean versus fatty muscle tissue present. The normal synovium is extremely thin and only demonstrates hyperaemia and increased perfusion when inflamed and thickened due to synovitis and synovial proliferation.

PHYSIOLOGIC CHANGES IN BONE PERFUSION

The cellular bone marrow is much more metabolically active and more highly vascularized than the relatively inert mineralized cortical and trabecular bone.[33] Normally, hematopoietic (red) red marrow is the primary driver of bone marrow blood perfusion.[34] Red marrow is at least six times more metabolically active and more vascularized than fatty (yellow) marrow.[30,35] As the proportion of hematopoietic marrow declines with increasing age, from 90% at birth, 50% at 30 years, and 30% at 70 years,[36,37] the marrow cavity in young subjects is much better perfused than elderly subjects.[38–40] Women less than 50 years have higher bone marrow perfusion than comparably aged men. However, women suffer a sharp decline in marrow perfusion at the time of menopause paralleling changes in marrow fat content and bone mineral density (BMD).[41] As BMD decreases, marrow fat increases and red cell mass decreases. Hence, osteopenic and osteoporotic bone is less well-perfused than bone of normal density. Anatomic variation also occurs. For example, vertebral body perfusion decreases slightly from the upper to the lower lumbar levels, most likely attributable

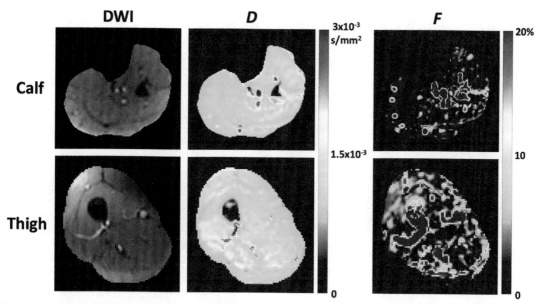

Fig. 6. IVIM perfusion of healthy muscle in the calf and thigh using IVIM maps of diffusion coefficient (D) and perfusion fraction (f). The diffusion coefficient (D) reflects the amount of free water molecules diffusing across a voxel, which reflects tissue cellularity. The perfusion fraction (f) reflects the fraction of flowing capillary blood or microperfusion in each voxel. (*Courtesy of* Gregory Simchick, University of Wisconsin-Madison).

to greater weight-bearing and higher physical stress at the lower lumbar levels.[26]

MARROW PERFUSION IN SYSTEMIC CONDITIONS

Bone marrow perfusion is reduced in systemic conditions such as chronic renal impairment, diabetes mellitus, and hypertension.[42–45] Nonetheless, physiologic or other variations in perfusion related to age, sex, fat fraction, biomechanical stress levels, and underlying chronic systemic disease are relatively small and unlikely to confound the more profound perfusion changes seen in malignancy, infection, inflammation, or ischemia.[46]

CLINICAL APPLICATIONS OF PERFUSION IMAGING

The remainder of this review addresses some current and potential musculoskeletal clinical applications of perfusion imaging looking (a) at soft tissue and bone tumors and then (2) other non-tumoral applications.

Soft Tissue and Bone Tumors

Differentiating benign from malignant soft tissue tumors

It is feasible that perfusion imaging may someday be able to differentiate benign and malignant soft tissue tumors, which can be difficult to distinguish on morphologic grounds alone.[47–53] Malignant soft tissue tumors typically show Type IV enhancement curve starting within 6 seconds of injection and with more pronounced enhancement peripherally rather than centrally[48] (**Fig. 7**). Malignant soft tissue tumors also generally have higher semiquantitative (initial AUC [iAUC], E_{slope}, E_{max}) and quantitative (K_{trans}, K_{ep}) parameters than benign tumors.[47,54–56] Among DCE-MR imaging parameters, $K_{trans} > 110$ min^{-1} × 10^3 had the highest sensitivity of 81% for predicting soft tissue malignancy, followed by a $K_{ep} > 368$ min^{-1} × 10^3, which yielded a sensitivity of 78% and a specificity of 71%.[47] Higher K_{trans} and K_{ep} values in malignant tumors reflect higher perfusion and vascular permeability due to cell proliferation and neoangiogenesis. That said, Leplat and colleagues found no differences between perfusion parameters of benign and malignant bone and soft tissue tumors with the best performance being for Ve (extravascular extracellular space fractional volume), which had a 79% sensitivity and 38% specificity for differentiating benign from malignant tumors. When only soft-tissue tumors were considered, K_{trans} (volume transfer constant) differentiated benign from malignant tumors with a sensitivity of 79% and a specificity of 27%.[57]

DCE-MR imaging iAUC, TTP, K_{trans}, and K_{ep} parameters are also significant predictors of soft tissue sarcoma histologic grade with K_{trans} having the highest diagnostic value for differentiating between high-grade and low-grade sarcomas.[16] In

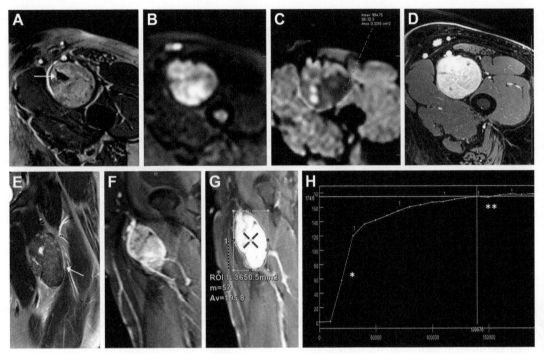

Fig. 7. Treatment-naïve soft tissue sarcoma. A 40-year-old woman with high-grade undifferentiated pleomorphic sarcoma thigh. (*A*) Axial post-contrast T2* contrast-enhanced susceptibility-weighted imaging (CE-SWI) shows solid enhancing mass with areas of T2* hypointense hemorrhage (*arrow*). (*B*) Axial DWI b800 and (*C*) ADC map showing restricted diffusion in solid areas with apparent diffusion coefficient (ADC) minimum of 0.9 × 10 to 3 mm²/seg. (*D*) Axial post-contrast Dixon-water sequence shows solid-enhancing tumor. (*E*) Coronal partial Tau T2 short tau inversion recovery (STIR) shows intermediate T2 signal (*arrows*) with (*F*) hypervascular arterial phase enhancement on sagittal DCE-MR imaging. (*G*) DCE-MR imaging with ROI encompassing soft tissue enhancing lesion and (*H*) Type V enhancement curve with a rapid washin phase (*), followed by a continued progressive enhancement (**).

neurofibromatosis, type 1 (NF-1) patients, DCE may help differentiate neurofibroma from malignant peripheral nerve sheath tumor (MPNST) as MPNST tends to have early enhancement, whereas neurofibroma displays a more delayed enhancement pattern.[58] Nevertheless, many benign tumors, such as vascular malformation, leiomyoma, and nerve sheath tumors, can be highly vascularized and some malignant tumors, such as fibrosarcoma or myxofibrosarcoma are usually poorly vascularized, leading to overlapping perfusion dynamics.[18] Also, using average measures on 2D imaging can lead to considerable misrepresentation of tumor perfusion in heterogenous lesions. For example, a poorly perfused homogenous non-necrotic tumor can have the same mean K_{trans} as a highly vascular partially necrotic malignant tumour though the latter is likely to be more aggressive.[59] In general, serial perfusion imaging data are often more helpful than stand-alone data, particularly in determining treatment response. Therefore, although DCE-MR imaging parameters can differentiate between benign and malignant soft tissue tumors and

indicate their histologic grade with reasonable accuracy,[16,21,56] one should currently still only rely on percutaneous tissue biopsy to determine malignant potential.

Differentiating benign from malignant bone lesions

Perfusion imaging is less helpful in distinguishing benign from malignant bone tumors than soft tissue tumors as physiologic marrow changes from red marrow reconversion and other marrow variations confound differentiation from malignant bone infiltration. Although bony metastases, multiple myeloma, hematological malignancy, and lymphoma show more rapid and higher enhancement with faster washout than normal marrow,[60–63] substantial overlap still exists between benign and malignant lesions.[48,64] For example, benign hypervascular tumors such as giant cell tumor, osteoid osteoma, Brodie abscess, and Langerhans cell histiocytosis may exhibit a Type III enhancement curves and can sometimes display elevated perfusion parameters similar to bone sarcomas (**Figs. 8** and **9**). Quantitative DCE-MR imaging parameters

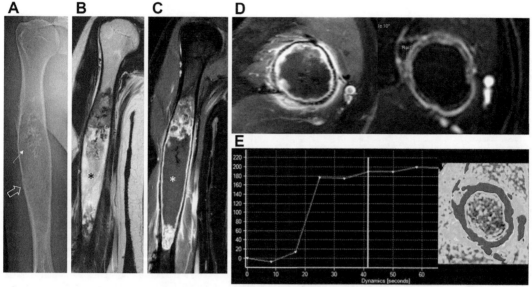

Fig. 8. Treatment-naïve bone sarcoma. A 33-year-old man with biopsy-proven chondrosarcoma humerus. (A) Frontal radiograph showing expansile lytic lesion (open *arrow*) mid-humeral diaphysis with chondroid-type mineralization (*arrow*). (B) T2-weighted coronal, (C) T1-fat-suppressed coronal, and (D) T1-fat-suppressed axial images show severe peripheral tumoral enhancement with a large fluid-rich central area (*asterisk*). (E) DCE-MR imaging with region-of-interest (ROI) placed on enhancing peripheral tumor margin shows rapid steep enhancement followed by plateau (Type III enhancement curve), consistent with aggressive tumor. (*Courtesy of* Dr Rosy Setiawati, Universitas Airlangga).

such as K_{trans}, K_{ep}, and V_p are generally much higher in malignant bone tumors and can act as an adjunct, rather than a definitive measure, to improve sensitivity and specificity in differentiating benign from malignant bone lesions.[60,65–69] The single most practical clinical benefit for perfusion imaging in bone tumors may be distinguishing between hematopoietic cell rests and tumor infiltrate, as percutaneous biopsy of these smaller marrow infiltrates is not straightforward. On IVIM-imaging, nodular hyperplastic marrow had lower diffusion coefficient D values ($0.22 \pm 0.08 \times 10^{-3}$ mm²/s) than malignant marrow infiltration ($0.79 \pm 0.29 \times 10^{-3}$ mm²/s, $P < .001$) with an AUC of 1.[70] Nodular hyperplastic marrow also had a higher f factor (19.8 ± 8.7) than malignant infiltration (10.2 ± 4.6, $P < .001$).[70] On DCE-MR imaging, applying a threshold of greater than 1.888/min, K_{trans} had an 82% sensitivity and 93% specificity (AUC 0.90) at differentiating pelvic bone prostatic metastases from hyperplastic hematopoietic marrow, whereas K_{ep} at a threshold of greater than 2.551/min had a sensitivity of 82% and specificity Of 86% (AUC 0.84)[71]

Prognostication for soft tissue tumors

Percutaneous biopsy is a standard procedure for any suspicious soft tissue or bone tumor. As such, rather than using perfusion imaging to confirm benignity or malignancy, it seems more applicable to study the use of perfusion imaging to help predict prognosis, metastatic potential, delineate margins, and identify tumor recurrence. On conventional MR imaging, high-grade soft tissue sarcomas are typically larger (≥ 5 cm) with more T2W heterogeneity, peritumoral edema, and tumor necrosis (>50%) than low-grade sarcomas[16] (**Fig. 10**). On perfusion imaging, iAUC, K_{trans}, and K_{ep} can help predict histologic grade (see **Fig. 10**). A K_{trans} greater than 0.163 (min⁻¹) had a 73% sensitivity and 88% specificity for differentiating low-grade (grade 1) from high-grade (grade 2 or 3) soft tissue sarcoma.[16]

Prognostication for bone tumors

For bone sarcoma, bone metastasis, acute leukemia, and multiple myeloma, reduced perfusion parameters are associated with a higher chance of remission, better disease-free and overall survival.[72,73] Patients with osteosarcomas who had a washin rate (K_{trans}) of greater than 0.262 min⁻¹ had increased mortality.[74] Also, osteosarcomas with a washout rate (K_{ep}) of ≥ 1.167/min at baseline are more likely to recur postoperativity.[75] Conversely, osteosarcomas with a lower washin rate (K_{trans}) at 10 weeks posttreatment have greater tumor necrosis ($P = .024$) and longer event-free survival ($P = .034$).[76] A decrease in Vp

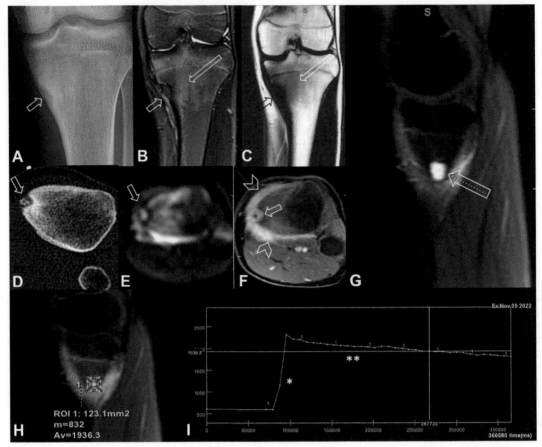

Fig. 9. Osteoid osteoma. A 15-year-old man with biopsy-proven osteoid osteoma. (*A*) Frontal radiograph shows cortical-based lucent lesion with sclerotic rim proximal tibial metaphysis. (*B*) Coronal T2 partial TAU STIR sequence shows intermediate lesion (*arrow*) with moderate perilesional bone marrow and soft tissue edema (long *arrow*). (*C*) Coronal Dixon-fat sequence demonstrates water signal from the cortical-based lesion (*arrow*), with moderate perilesional bone marrow edema (long *arrow*). (*D*) Axial CT image shows a cortical-based lucent lesion with central mineralization (*arrow*). (*E*) Axial DWI b800 demonstrates nidus signal hyperintensity (*arrow*). (*F*) Axial post-contrast Dixon-water sequence demonstrates marked enhancement of the nidus periphery (*arrow*) and thickened periosteum (*G*) DCE-MR imaging shows avid arterial phase enhancement of nidus, (*H*) DCE-MR imaging with ROI encompassing lesion, and (*I*) Type IV enhancement curve with a rapid washin phase (***), followed by a slow washout (****).

of less than 20% for bone metastases predicted posttreatment recurrence with 100% sensitivity and 98% specificity.[66] IVIM-derived fractional perfusion (f) correlated moderately with PET-derived SUV metabolic activity and may also be useful in gauging the treatment response of bone metastases.[70] In acute myelogenous leukemia, high bone marrow vascularity is associated with poor prognoses.[72,77] An IVIM-derived perfusion fraction (f) of greater than 31% or DCE-MR imaging-derived washout rate (K_{ep}) of ≥0.0082/min were both independent predictors of a poor overall survival in leukemic patients with clinical remission.[72,77] Similarly, for multiple myeloma, higher washout rate (K_{ep}) values are associated with shorter overall survival ($P = .02$).[78]

Delineating margins of bone and soft tissue tumors and biopsy planning

The leading edges of malignant bone and soft tissue tumors tend to be the most perfused with necrosis and hemorrhage tending to occur deep in the tumor matrix. Perfusion imaging enables more accurate delineation of tumor margins, as enhancement occurs sooner in tumoral than peritumoral edematous or compressed tissues.[7] Bone marrow and soft tissue edema tends to have Type II enhancement curves, reflecting accumulation of contrast in the edematous extravascular extracellular space.[79] Targeting well-perfused areas on DCE-MR imaging may improve biopsy yield.[80,81] Using DCE-MR imaging to guide soft tissue tumor, biopsies had a 100% diagnostic

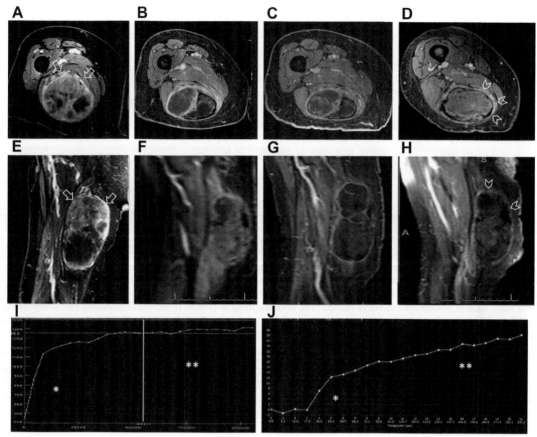

Fig. 10. Treatment-related changes in undifferentiated pleomorphic sarcoma (UPS): A 75-year-old woman with high-grade pleomorphic sarcoma thigh treated with chemotherapy and irradiation followed by resection. (*A*) Axial post-contrast Dixon-water sequence at baseline, (*B*) during and (*C*) after chemoradiotherapy treatment and (*D*) later showing progressive reduction in solid-enhancing components from large heterogeneous contrast-enhancing areas at baseline to peripheral enhancement post-therapy (open *arrowheads*). Sagittal DCE-MR imaging in arterial phase at baseline (*E*), during chemoradiotherapy treatment (*F*), and (*G*) early (*G*) as well as (*H*) later posttreatment phases show substantial reduction in solid-enhancing components from heterogenous arterial phase hypervascular enhancement (*E*, *arrows*) to only residual peripheral ring-like enhancement after the completion of chemoradiation (*G*, *H*, open *arrowheads*). There was a significant change in the TIC curve at (*I*) baseline Type V enhancement with a rapid washin phase (*) followed by continued peak enhancement (**), to (*J*) post-chemotherapy Type II enhancement with a slow gradual washin (*) followed by slow continuous enhancement (**) with a much shallower upslope.

yield when biopsies were performed in the highest "wash-in" rate areas.[82]

Posttreatment response

The single most useful oncological application of perfusion imaging to likely to be determining tumor response to neoadjuvant chemotherapy ± radiotherapy, as sarcomas (particularly bone sarcomas) may not decrease and may even increase in size after effective treatment due to intra-tumoral hemorrhage, edema, or necrosis, rendering tumor size a poor indicator of tumor response[83] (Fig. 11). Functional changes in tumor metabolism proceed changes in tumor size particularly with

newer cytostatic, rather than cytotoxic, chemotherapy agents targeting tumor metabolism rather than tumor necrosis.[83] Ideally, perfusion imaging to gauge neoadjuvant chemotherapy effectiveness should be performed (1) before biopsy, (2) during chemotherapy, and (3) immediately before surgery.[84] Viable tumor continues to show Type III or IV time-intensity curves, whereas nonviable tumour will shift to Types I, II, or V curves[85] (see **Fig. 11**). A good treatment response, indicated by greater than 90% intra-tumoral necrosis, is likely to be present when there is a ≥ 60% reduction in the TIC upslope (E_{slope}).[76,84–86] Conversely, poor responders show minimal reduction or even an increase in

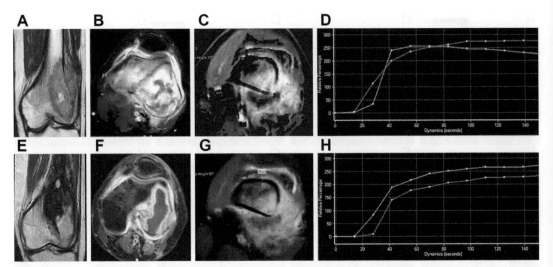

Fig. 11. Bone sarcoma treatment. A 17-year-old man with biopsy-proven giant-cell rich osteosarcoma distal femur. Pre-chemotherapy MR imaging with (*A*) coronal T2-weighted, (*B, C*) axial post-contrast T1-weighted fat-suppressed, (*D*) perfusion sequence showing intraosseous (orange ROI) Type IV enhancement curve and extraosseous (blue ROI) Type III enhancement curve compatible with aggressive tumor. (*E–H*) Corresponding MR imaging sequences post-chemotherapy showing intraosseous and extraosseous Type II enhancement curves with reduced upslope and no washout, consistent with moderate treatment response. (*Courtesy of* Dr Rosy Setiawati, Universitas Airlangga.)

E_{slope}.[84] A good treatment response can be predicted with high specificity if no greater than 5% of the soft-tissue sarcoma volume displays early arterial enhancement.[87] Using textural analysis, specific measurements of perfusion heterogeneity such as coherence may also help discriminate responders from nonresponders, with tumors showing high perfusion coherence at baseline responding best to chemotherapy.[88]

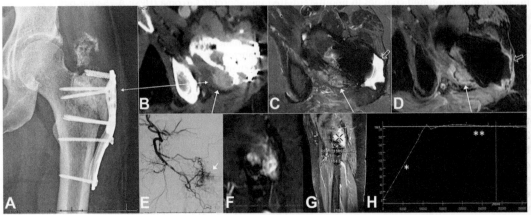

Fig. 12. Recurrent metastatic renal cell carcinoma (RCC): A 53-year-old woman with metastatic RCC to the proximal femur post-curettage and cementation with side plate and interlocking screw stabilization found to have radiographically occult residual/recurrent lesions on follow-up. (*A*) Frontal radiograph proximal femur shows postsurgical changes and mild soft tissue prominence lateral greater trochanter. (*B*) Axial post-contrast CT image shows enhancing soft tissue mass posterior to the cemented area (*arrow*), representing recurrent RCC. (*C*) Axial T2 partial Tau STIR sequence shows solid recurrent RCC tissue with intermediate T2 signal and subtle flow voids (*arrow*). Incidental trochanteric bursitis (block *arrow*). (*D*) Axial post-contrast Dixon-water sequence shows solid-enhancing recurrent metastatic lesion (*arrow*) and capsular-like enhancement of adjacent trochanteric bursitis (block *arrow*). (*E*) Digital subtraction angiogram shows an arterialized vascular lesion with neo-angiogenesis and flow supply from the femur representing hypervascular recurrent RCC. (*F*) DCE-MR imaging post-contrast sagittal sequence demonstrates soft-tissue recurrent RCC with arterial phase hypervascular enhancement. (*G*) DCE-MR imaging with ROI encompassing the recurrent tumor and (*H*) Type III enhancement curve with a rapid washin phase (*), followed by plateau (**).

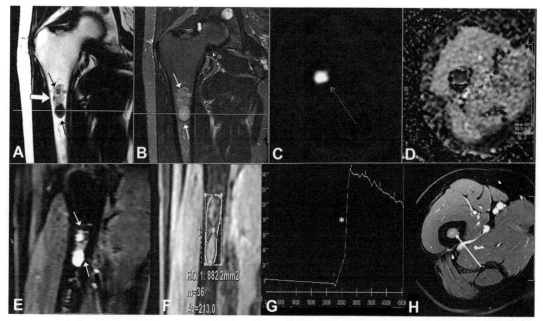

Fig. 13. New active myeloma lesion. A 75-year-old man who had an autologous stem-cell transplant for multiple myeloma 5 years previously and who recently developed a new proximal femoral lesion. (*A*) Coronal T1-Dixon-fat sequence shows two lesions in proximal femoral diaphysis with T1 hypointense water signal suspicious of active disease (*arrows*) and intervening fat-containing lesion (block *arrow*) in favor of a previously treated lesion. Another lesion is present in the acetabulum. (*B*) Coronal partial Tau T2 STIR sequence demonstrates intermediate T2 signal within the diaphyseal lesions compatible with active myeloma. (*C*) Corresponding axial DWI b800 shows nodular hyperintensity indicating active disease. (*D*) ADC map shows restricted diffusion (0.7 × 10–3 mm²/seg). (*E*) Sagittal DCE-MR imaging shows active arterial enhancement of active myeloma lesions. (*F*) DCE-MR imaging with ROIs encompassing intramedullary lesions and (*G*) Type IV enhancement curve with rapid washin phase (*), followed by washout (**). (*H*) axial post-contrast Dixon-water image shows homogenous enhancement of active myeloma lesion.

For bone metastases, mean fractional plasma volume (V_P), a measure of tumor vascularity in the intravascular compartment, decreased by 66% in lesions successfully treated with stereotactic radiotherapy and increased by 145% to 207% in unsuccessfully treated lesions, even before morphologic changes were apparent on conventional MR images.[65,89] For multiple myeloma bone lesions, responders had a lower exchange rate constant K_{ep} values ($P < .001$) as well as a more pronounced decrease in E_{max} ($P < .001$) and f values ($P < .001$) compared with nonresponders.[89] One can potentially use a "combined skeletal score" comprising morphologic features on conventional MR sequences and DCE or IVIM perfusion parameters to enable an earlier, more accurate confirmation of treatment response, earlier detection of relapse, and better disease prognostication for bone and soft tissue tumors.[90]

For treated metastatic disease, traditional analysis based on size criteria cannot judge ultimate disease progression, whereas DCE-MR imaging analysis of spinal metastatic sarcoma 2 months after radiotherapy provided excellent correlation with local control.[91] Similarly, bone marrow peak enhancement ratio is significantly lower in patients with hematological malignancies in remission than in patients with residual active disease following treatment. Similar results are seen for soft tissue sarcomas, where quantitative and semiquantitative MR (DCE or IVIM) perfusion parameters can distinguish good from poor responders with high accuracy, ranging from 85.7% to 100%.[84,92] Such quantitative assessments, while helpful, are currently time-consuming and largely impractical in everyday busy clinical settings, potentially becoming more widely used with the advent of fully automated pre- and posttreatment MR treatment evaluation.

Detection of tumor residual or recurrent tumor

Residual or recurrent tumor posttreatment can be challenging to distinguish from inflammation, fibrosis, and marrow reconversion on conventional MR imaging. Residual or recurrent tumor or

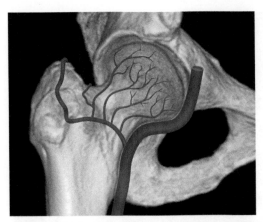

Fig. 14. Arterial supply femoral head. Main arterial supply to the femoral head is via branches from the medial and lateral circumflex femoral arteries, which arise from the profunda femoris artery, a branch of the femoral artery. These ascending branches encircle the femoral neck to supply the femoral head. The other artery providing arterial supply to the femoral head is the ligamentum teres artery (not shown), but its role diminishes with age such that it has only a minor contribution in adults. The femoral head is innately prone to ischemia, particularly after displaced femoral neck fractures which can tear the ascending arterial branches.

myelomatous infiltration typically has Type III or IV enhancement curves as opposed to reactive tissue change, which tends to have a Type II curve, similar to normal muscle[7,79,93] (**Figs. 12** and **13**). In a study of 37 patients, six of whom had recurrence, the presence of a surgical bed mass-like lesion was only 52% specific for tumor recurrence. However, a mass-like lesion and Type III or IV enhancement curve increased specificity to 97% with a sensitivity of 100%.[94] DCE-MR imaging differentiation of recurrent STS from posttreatment change can also be attained by addressing the steepest slope ratio between the artery and the lesion. A ratio of less than 1.05 indicates recurrence, whereas a ratio of greater than 9.28 favors no recurrence. In other words, the more highly perfused the lesion, the greater the likelihood of tumor recurrence.[95]

Other Non-Tumoural Applications

Avascular necrosis

The early detection of avascular necrosis (AVN) before the appearance of structural change was one of the earliest applications of MR perfusion imaging.[96] Varying levels of potentially recoverable bone ischemia can be present before a critical level is reached, which results in osteonecrosis. Perfusion imaging helps predict the likelihood of

developing osteonecrosis after scaphoid and femoral neck fractures,[79,97] which can facilitate surgical decision-making as earlier intervention can prevent or delay the late sequelae of advanced collapse and secondary osteoarthritis (OA).

Femoral head Even in normal subjects, femoral head perfusion is about one-third that of the femoral neck and one-fifth that of the acetabulum.[98] Given this low inherent perfusion, a double or treble gadolinium dose may be necessary to gauge femoral head perfusion.[98] The medial and lateral femoral circumflex arteries, which supply the femoral head, ascend along the surface of the femoral neck (**Fig. 14**). As such, femoral head blood supply can be compromised by displaced femoral neck fractures predisposing to AVN.[99,100] AVN risk is greatest for subcapital or transcervical fractures and least for basal neck fractures. Femoral head AVN occurs in about 15% to 25% of femoral neck fractures following internal fixation.[101] Steroid use, high alcohol intake, systemic vasculitis, and hyperviscosity syndromes are additional risk factors for femoral head AVN. The defining feature of femoral head AVN is articular surface collapse. Once surface collapse occurs, restoration is not possible and secondary OA/total hip replacement usually ensues. Femoral neck E_{max} values were lower (median 2.74%, range 1.7%–4%, $P = .009$) in patients at risk of femoral head osteonecrosis than normal subjects though without visible osteonecrosis on MR imaging [102] (**Fig. 15**). Similarly, femoral head E_{max} values were 55% lower in patients with osteonecrosis than in normal-appearing hips (mean 4.2 vs 1.9 seconds, $P < .0001$)[102] (**Fig. 16**). Bone marrow edema surrounding the osteonecrotic area increases the risk of subchondral bone resorption and articular surface collapse. Osteonecrotic hips with marrow edema exhibit substantially higher perfusion parameters, particularly E_{max}, AUC, and TTP in the femoral head, indicative of hyperperfusion adjacent to osteonecrotic areas, which can serve as a prognostic marker.[102] Perfusion imaging may help detect impaired perfusion before the onset of osteonecrosis in at-risk patients or predict which patients with early-stage osteonecrosis are more likely to proceed to articular surface collapse, though this potential has not yet been fully investigated.[103–105] Perfusion parameters in the femoral head can be compared with those in the acetabulum, the unaffected part of the femoral head, or the femoral neck. One can still obtain good quality DCE-MR images with femoral neck metallic fixation screws in situ. Once moderate to severe femoral head

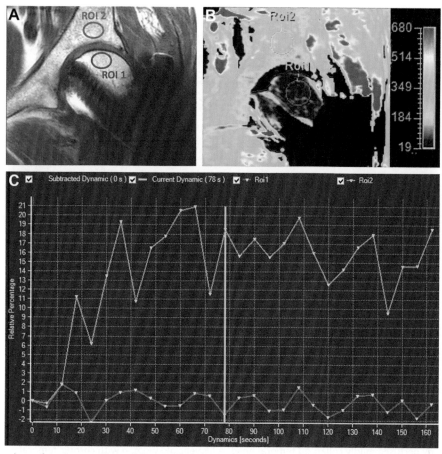

Fig. 15. Poorly perfused non-collapsed femoral head. A 70-year-old woman with traumatic fracture femoral neck and internal screw fixation. (*A*) T1-weighted MR imaging shows normal femoral head with gamma nail in situ. (*B*) DCE-MR imaging and (*C*) with global poor perfusion in the femoral head (blue ROI) compared with the acetabulum (orange ROI), though no morphologic features avascular necrosis were present. Patient developed progressive left hip pain and later required left total hip replacement.

collapse has occurred, perfusion imaging will not likely affect management.

Scaphoid Scaphoid waist fractures predispose to proximal pole ischemia and osteonecrosis as the proximal pole receives its arterial supply retrogradely from the distal pole[104] (**Fig. 17**). Variable ischemia and osteonecrosis of the proximal pole may occur. Increased osteosclerosis seen in the proximal pole on radiographs and CT can be due to either ischemia[106] ± relative hypodensity of the distal pole.[107] Patients with poor or absent bleeding from the fracture margin of the proximal pole at surgery tend to have much lower perfusion factors than those with good bleeding from the proximal pole fracture margin.[104,108] If proximal pole perfusion parameters (E_{slope}, E_{max}) are less than 50% of those in the distal pole, the likelihood

of proximal pole AVN is very high and vice versa[104,108] (**Figs. 18 and 19**). This was not a universal finding, however, with other studies showing no correlation between qualitative assessment perfusion parameters and proximal pole scaphoid viability.[109,110]

Kienbock's disease

Kienbock's disease, often associated with negative ulnar variance, is thought to result from lunate ischemia. The affected lunate will be normal initially on radiographs through with altered signal intensity on MR imaging (Lichtman stage I). This is followed by sclerosis (seen on radiographs and CT) (Lichtman stage II), probably due to lunate ischemia. Later, lunate bone collapse (Lichtman stage IIIA) and fragmentation (usually into dorsal and volar fragments) occurs, accompanied by

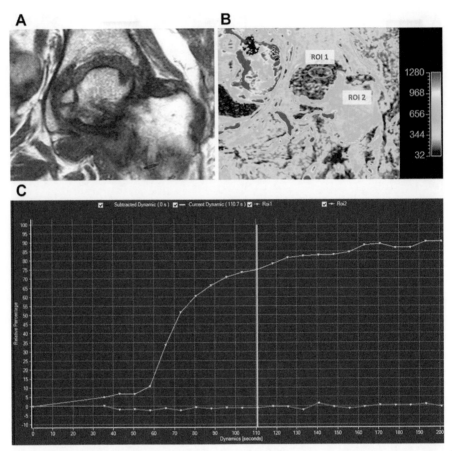

Fig. 16. Poorly perfused mildly collapsed femoral head. A 55-year-old woman with chronic femoral neck fracture following internal fixation and progressive hip pain. (*A*) T1-weighted coronal MR image shows moderate femoral head collapse and fragmentation though no typical demarcation line of osteonecrosis. (*B*) DCE-MR perfusion with (*C*) showing global absence of demonstrable femoral head perfusion, whereas the femoral neck shows normal perfusion. This indicates global avascular necrosis of the femoral head, which was confirmed on subsequent total hip replacement surgery.

carpal collapse (Lichtman stage IIIB) and progressive pan-carpal OA (Lichtman stage IV). Owing to this dorsal–volar lunate fragmentation, it is preferable to perform lunate DCE-MR imaging in the sagittal plane rather than the coronal plane to minimize partial volume averaging.[111]

Histologically, Kienbock's disease demonstrates areas of bone remodeling, fibrous osteoid, viable fatty bone marrow with trabecular necrosis, and normal bone. Reparative and osteonecrotic areas lie at and between the areas of bone fragmentation, whereas normal bone is located on the dorsal and volar aspects of the lunate.[111] In a DCE-MR imaging histology correlative study, reparative and osteonecrotic areas are relatively hyperperfused, whereas normal lunate bone areas have a perfusion profile similar to other carpal bones.[111] Both maximum enhancement (E_{max}

518 vs 28.5) and maximum slope (E_{slope} 10.9 vs 1.1) were substantially higher in areas of fibrous osteoid than in normal bone [111] (**Fig. 20**). Similarly, areas of new bone formation demonstrated increased perfusion compared with normal bone, with E_{max} 170 versus 28.5 and E_{slope} 6.9 versus 1.1, respectively.[111] As such, DCE-MR imaging can provide a more precise assessment of osteonecrotic and reparative bone than standard MR imaging.[111,112] As hyperperfusion also occurs in areas of viable fatty marrow with trabecular necrosis, hyperperfusion is not always a good sign because it does not invariably represent reparative tissue.[111] Early pseudarthrosis with dense fibrous tissue between the lunate fragments shows intense hyperperfusion despite these areas not being well-vascularized.[111] The increased E_{max} and E_{slope} seen in area of pseudarthrosis are

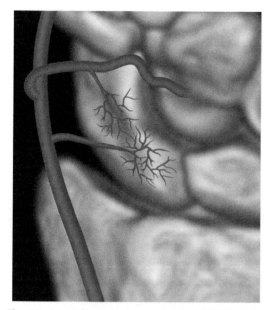

Fig. 17. Arterial supply scaphoid. Most (80%) of the arterial supply to the proximal pole of the scaphoid comes from the dorsal branch of the radial artery, which enters via the distal pole and travels in a retrograde manner toward the proximal pole. The volar branch of the radial artery provides less arterial supply. Owing to this retrograde intraosseous arterial supply, the proximal pole is prone to avascular necrosis after fracture of the scaphoid waist.

more likely due to hyperdiffusion rather than increased blood flow, as neovascularization in this area is scanty.[111] Hand surgeons find lunate DCE-MR imaging helpful in decision-making in patients before lunate collapse (ie, Lichtman stage I and II) but not following lunate collapse (Lichtman stage III and IV).[113] DCE-MR imaging may also be beneficial for patient follow-up after surgical revascularization of Kienbock's disease.

Synovitis: Assessment of disease activity
Perfusion imaging can quantity synovial inflammation ("synovitis") at baseline and follow-up in patients with rheumatological disease more accurately than morphological features. There are two aspects to synovial inflammation on imaging: the degree of synovial thickening (ie, proliferation) present and the degree of synovial inflammation (ie, the severity of inflammation is in the thickened synovium). Although all actively inflamed synovium is thickened, not all thickened synovium is actively inflamed. In general, the greater the degree of inflammation in the synovium, the more perfused the synovium, that is, increased E_{slope} and E_{max} are indicators of increased synovial inflammation.[114–116] Relative

change in perfusion parameters following treatment is a more sensitive indicator of treatment response than absolute values[97,116] (Fig. 21). In early rheumatoid arthritis (RA) patients, after 1 year of treatment, reduced wrist synovial perfusion correlated with a reduction in disease activity ($r = 0.58$) and reduced early morning stiffness ($r = 0.46$).[117] DCE-MR imaging is also helpful in assessing treatment response and disease activity in juvenile idiopathic arthritis (JIA). The rate of early enhancement correlated with clinical disease activity scores and inflammatory serologic markers of disease activity.[118]

Similarly, E_{max} and E_{slope} were significantly higher in JIA patients with active inflammation.[118–120] Applying pharmacokinetic modeling parameters, a reduced washin rate (K_{trans}), washout rate (K_{ep}), and fractional plasma volume (V_P) indicated less severe synovitis in JIA children responding to treatment.[120] For assessing synovial activity, perfusion parameters from DCE-MR imaging seem more valuable and reliable than perfusion parameters derived from IVIM imaging, as IVIM-derived pseudo-diffusion (D^*) and perfusion fraction (f) values were unable to differentiate synovial proliferation from joint effusion. In contrast, IVIM-derived diffusion coefficient (D) and apparent diffusion coefficient (ADC) correlated with synovial proliferation in hand arthritis (Fujimori). Lower diffusion D values (1.81 ± 0.28) in the inflamed synovium of JIA patients were found compared with normal synovium (2.61 ± 0.34, $P < .001$), indicate more restricted diffusion.[121,122]

Osteoarthritis
Synovitis is present in 90% of patients with OA, with a strong correlation between the presence and severity of synovitis and OA symptoms, severity, and progression.[123–125] DCE-MR imaging perfusion parameters, particularly K_{trans}, are more sensitive than synovial volume measurements for detecting OA-related synovial activity changes during treatment and follow-up.[126–128] Improvements in pain score showed a better correlation with reduction in perfusion parameters than changes in synovial volume.[127]

Signal alterations in the infrapatellar fat pad are scored as "Hoffa synovitis" in the MR imaging Osteoarthritis Knee Score, although they do not always represent inflammation.[129,130] DCE-MR imaging-based study has shown that increased blood perfusion in Hoffa's fat pad signal abnormalities is only present in patients with knee OA, but not in patients with patellofemoral pain.[131] DCE-MR imaging also reflected the severity of inflammation in the infrapatellar fat pad[132,133]

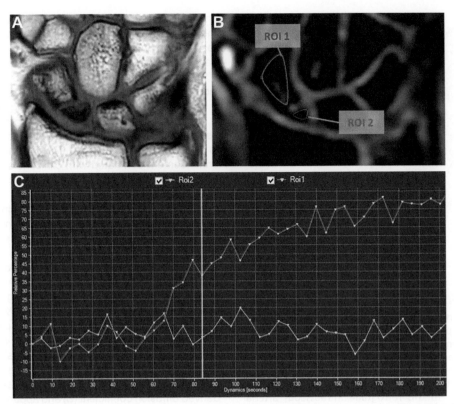

Fig. 18. Poorly perfused proximal pole. A 30-year-old man with traumatic nonunion proximal one-third scaphoid bone. (*A*) MR imaging T1-weighted sequence shows diffusely hypointense of non-collapsed proximal fragment. (*B*) DCE-MR imaging with (*C*) TIC showing no enhancement of proximal fragment (orange ROI) consistent with severe ischemia, with good enhancement of the distal fragment (blue ROI). Subsequent surgery revealed osteonecrosis of the proximal fragment with no bleeding evident and a viable distal fragment with active bleeding. Bone grafting was performed.

Bone marrow lesions (BMLs), typically seen as areas of T2 hyperintensity in the subchondral bone marrow, are another prevalent feature in OA. Increased DCE perfusion parameters are seen in epimetaphyseal bone, subchondral bone, and BMLs in unicompartmental knee OA, with BMLs likely accounting for most of the higher subchondral bone perfusion seen in knee OA.[131] Higher perfusion in BMLs containing subchondral cysts was associated with pain in patients with knee OA though not in BMLs without cysts, indicating the likelihood of separate BML subtypes related to cystic change, perfusion, and pain.[134]

Osteochondritis dissecans
In a small group of normal juveniles and those with osteochondritis dissecans (OCD) of the knee, it was shown how ASL, while technically demanding, could be used to gauge capillary perfusion around the knee and how hyperperfusion was present alongside OCD lesions, potentially due to reparative revascularization.[16] In the

limbs, low inherent normal marrow perfusion can potentially be increased by using physiologic hyperaemia following temporary vascular occlusion by air cuff compression.[1]

Septic arthritis and transient synovitis of hip
Ultrasound-guided joint aspiration is the usual means of distinguishing hip septic arthritis from transient synovitis in children but is invasive and not always feasible.[135] DCE-MR imaging may help to differentiate both conditions. In septic arthritis, the femoral capital epiphysis of the infected hip shows reduced perfusion compared with the contralateral normal side.[136,137] Transient synovitis, conversely, shows similar enhancement on both the affected and normal sides.[136]

Diabetic foot
Distinguishing diabetic foot osteomyelitis from acute Charcot's neuroarthropathy can be difficult, especially in the midfoot. It is helpful to appreciate that diabetic neuroarthropathy tends to undergo

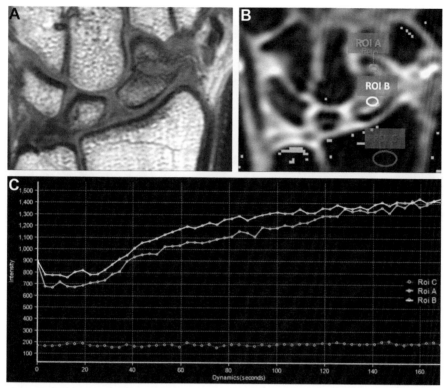

Fig. 19. Well-perfused proximal pole: A 33-year-old man with (A) T1-weighted coronal MR image showing moderately displaced transverse fracture waist of scaphoid (B) DCE-MR imaging with (C) TIC showing good perfusion of both the proximal and distal poles of scaphoid with no evidence of ischemia.

an orderly pattern of destruction ("organised chaos") with deviation from this expected pattern being a helpful imaging sign of midfoot osteomyelitis.[138] As osteomyelitis seems to induce a more intense cellular infiltrate response with more increased vascularity and permeability than neuroarthropathy, perfusion imaging may help in distinguishing between these two entities. A Type II enhancement curve was apparent in 94% of osteomyelitis feet compared with all osteomyelitis-negative feet having a Type I curve.[139] K trans, K_{ep}, and V_e values in osteomyelitic foot regions were significantly higher than those of acute neuropathoarthropathy.[140] K_{trans} (cutoff 0.11 mL/min) and Kep (cutoff 0.19 mL/min) both had sensitivities of 80% and specificities of 93% (AUC 0.94) for differentiating osteomyelitis from acute neuropathic arthropathy.[140] In another study, although K_{trans} and iAUC60 allowed reliable differentiation of diabetic foot osteomyelitis, especially for large ROIs, it did not perform better than diffusion-weighted imaging (DWI) or visual assessment of PET-CT imaging.[141]

ASL imaging is helpful in assessing blood flow around diabetic foot ulcers. When a "near border" is defined as the area of ulceration plus 25%, a "far border" as the area of ulceration plus 50% and a "remote area" as a foot area far removed from the ulceration,[142] ASL showed that blood flow at the wound (96.1 ± 10.7) and near border (92.7 ± 9.4) was about 30% greater than that the far border (73.4 ± 8.2) and remote areas (62.8 ± 2.7 mL/100 g/min).[142] Blood flow in remote areas of the diabetic foot with active foot ulceration was more than twice that of normal healthy subjects.[142] Another ASL-based study showed conflicting results regarding remote diabetic blood flow with muscle perfusion being lower in diabetics with foot ulcers (1.12 ± 0.35) than diabetics without foot ulcers (1.48 ± 0.71) and control subjects (2.58 ± 0.67, $P < .001$).[143] This study, however, showed that peri-ulcer muscle blood flow was greater (41.1 ± 8.5 mL/min/100g) in ulcers that healed in the subsequent 3 months than ulcers that did not heal (27.6 ± 12.0 mL/min/100g).[143]

Osteoporosis

As bone becomes more osteoporotic, marrow fat content increases, red marrow content decreases, and marrow diffusivity increases.[34,144] Perfusion imaging, chemical shift imaging, spectroscopy, and diffusion-weighted imaging can all be used

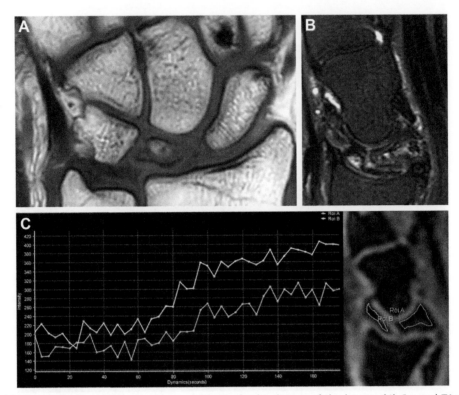

Fig. 20. Kienbock's disease. A 23-year-old man with Kienbock's disease of the lunate. (*A*) Coronal T1-weighted and (*B*) sagittal T2-fat-saturated MR images showing collapse and fragmentation of lunate bone into volar and dorsal fragments with moderate marrow edema, compatible with Kienbock's disease. (*C*) DCE-MR imaging with ROIs on the dorsal and volar fragments shows hyperperfusion of the bone fragments with Type V enhancement curves, a common finding in Kienbock's disease that reflects a mixture of both osteonecrotic and reparative bone.

to quantify osteoporosis severity.[145] Perfusion parameters (E_{max}, E_{slope}) in the proximal femur and vertebral bodies are significantly lower in osteoporosis than in osteopenic subjects, which in turn have lower bone perfusion than normal subjects.[144] Perfusion parameters are higher in acute osteoporotic fractures than in malignant vertebral fractures.[146] A mean interstitial volume of less than 11.72 mL/100 mL, a mean extracellular volume of less than 35.83 mL/100 mL, and a mean extraction flow of less than 6.52 mL/100 mL/min differentiated malignant from benign acute osteoporotic vertebral fractures with a specificity of 96%, 92%, and 92%, respectively.[147] Similarly, a higher washin rate (K_{trans}) and higher plasma volume fraction (V_P) are seen in pathologic vertebral fractures than benign fractures.[148]

Paget's disease

Paget's disease is characterized by dysregulated heightened bone turnover with cortical and trabecular thickening. Bone vascularity in Pagetic bone is inhomogeneous, with hypervascularity tending to be a feature of the advancing peripheral zone.[149]

Bone perfusion on DCE-MR imaging directly correlates with the rate of Pagetic bone turnover,[149] with perfusion parameters reducing significantly on bisphosphonate therapy.[150]

CHALLENGES AND OPPORTUNITIES FOR MSK PERFUSION IMAGING

DCE-MR imaging involves an inevitable trade-off between temporal and spatial resolution. For example, musculoskeletal tumor imaging typically requires high spatial resolution and large field-of-view (FOV) imaging, which compromises the high temporal resolution needed by DCE-MR imaging. For quantitative analysis, a large feeding artery for arterial input function needs to be incorporated and reliably identified in the FOV, which is not always the case. A typical single-plane DCE-MR imaging takes 3 to 7 minutes scan time using a temporal resolution of 5 to 30 seconds to avoid further lengthening of scan time. However, QIBA, in general, recommends a temporal resolution of 5 to 10 seconds and about 6 minutes scan time to capture the wash-out phase. Scan duration is

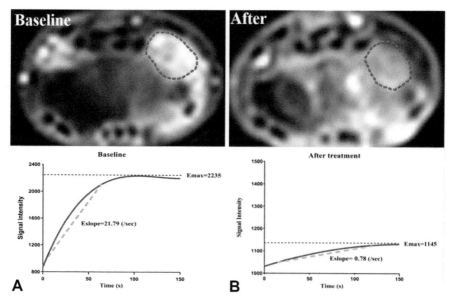

Fig. 21. Synovitis response to treatment. A 54-year-old woman with early rheumatoid arthritis. Axial DCE-MR imaging images at near similar level (*A*) pretreatment and (*B*) posttreatment with anti-biologic agents. Although the amount of synovial enhancement is similar, the degree of synovial enhancement is much less charging from a Type 4 curve pretreatment to a Type 2 curve posttreatment consistent with a good treatment response.

also a limitation of IVIM. As the pseudo-diffusion coefficient (D*) has a much greater exponential decay than the standard true diffusion coefficient (D), a longer scan time is needed to compensate for the low intrinsic SNR to ensure sufficient SNR for reliable IVIM imaging. The reliability of IVIM-derived perfusion parameters has been less extensively studied than those of DCE-MR imaging.

This said, inherent trade-offs between temporal and spatial resolution in DCE-MR imaging can be improved by using parallel imaging techniques to accelerate acquisition. Although parallel imaging lowers SNR and potentially increases artifact, modest acceleration factors are beneficial for DCE-MR imaging with a range of acceleration factors suggested by QIBA. Ultrashort TE (UTE) sequencing uses TEs 100 to 1000 times shorter than conventional gradient-echo sequences, with time-to-echo (TE) as short as 8 μs, enabling low-level perfusion to be assessed.[151–153] The use of an adiabatic inversion recovery pulse can augment cortical bone contrast enhancement by up to 60%.[16,154] Two-dimensional IR-UTE sequencing can feasibly be included in the routine 3T scanning protocol for DCE-MR imaging.[154] Higher field strength MR imaging provides better spatial, temporal, and contrast resolution, which are advantageous for DCE-MR imaging and IVIM.

Although core needle biopsy is used for preoperative diagnosis and evaluation of bone and soft tissue sarcomas, tumor heterogeneity can confound assessment. Quantitative techniques enable the whole tumor to be noninvasively evaluated. Rather than looking at perfusion in isolation, the ideal will be a multiparametric approach encompassing all components of functional imaging (such as diffusion, perfusion, spectroscopy, elastography, and PET imaging) along with clinical characteristics and a radiomic approach incorporated into a prognostication pipeline to optimize prognosis prediction and guide clinical decision making.[155] Standardization is of utmost importance for clinical implementation. QIBA seeks to standardize acquisition, whereas the Open Science Initiative for Perfusion Imaging group aims to standardize the analysis and reporting of perfusion MR imaging studies (osipi.ismrm.org)

SUMMARY

Perfusion is essential to the metabolism all viable tissues and is an extremely useful measure of tissue activity. The most vascularized musculoskeletal tissues are the hematopoietic bone marrow and the synovium. Perfusion can be evaluated with DCE-MR imaging, IVIM, and to a lesser degree ASL. As outlined in this review, it has a lot of potential clinical musculoskeletal applications, though is generally underused currently. The standardization of data acquisition and a more automated approach to data analysis, using artificial intelligence to consolidate the various perfusion factors into a few perfusion indices will, no doubt, lead to more widespread clinical usage.

CLINICS CARE POINTS

- As tissue perfusion is one of the best measures of tissue biological activity on MR imaging, it is currently most appropriately used during to quantify treatment response of tumors and synovitis, differentiate hematopoietic rests from metastatic infiltration, and detect bone ischemia.
- Serial standardized MR examinations of tissue perfusion are much more useful than a stand-alone examination.
- Empirical time–intensity curve measurements (such as Emax, Eslope) are generally adequate for most clinical purposes and are easier to obtain than pharmacokinetic measures.

CONFLICT OF INTEREST

The authors declare that they have no conflicts of interest.

FUNDING STATEMENT

No funding was received for this study.

DISCLOSURE

The University of Wisconsin receives research support from Bracco, unrelated to this work.

REFERENCES

1. Yeung DK, Griffith JF, Li AF, et al. Air pressure-induced susceptibility changes in vascular reactivity studies using BOLD MRI. J Magn Reson Imaging 2013;38(4):976–80.
2. Partovi S, Schulte AC, Jacobi B, et al. Blood oxygenation level-dependent (BOLD) MRI of human skeletal muscle at 1.5 and 3 T. J Magn ResonImaging 2012;35(5):1227–32.
3. Luck JC, Sica CT, Blaha C, et al. Agreement between multiparametric MRI (PIVOT), Doppler ultrasound, and near-infrared spectroscopy-based assessments of skeletal muscle oxygenation and perfusion. Magn Reson Imaging 2023;96:27–37.
4. Khalifa F, Soliman A, El-Baz A, et al. Models and methods for analyzing DCE-MRI: A review. Med Phys 2014;41(12):1–32.
5. Sourbron SP, Buckley DL. On the scope and interpretation of the Tofts models for DCE-MRI. Magn Reson Med 2011;66(3):735–45.
6. Geirnaerdt MJA, Hogendoorn PCW, Bloem JL, et al. Cartilaginous tumors: fast contrast-enhanced MR imaging. Radiology 2000;214(2):539–46.
7. Drapé JL. Advances in magnetic resonance imaging of musculoskeletal tumours. Orthop Traumatol Surg Res 2013;99(1 Suppl):S115–23.
8. Lavini C, de Jonge MC, van de Sande MG, et al. Pixel-by-pixel analysis of DCE MRI curve patterns and an illustration of its application to the imaging of the musculoskeletal system. Magn Reson Imaging 2007;25:604–12.
9. Toms AP, White LM, Kandel R, et al. Limitations of single slice dynamic contrast enhanced MR in pharmacokinetic modeling of bone sarcomas. Acta Radiol 2009;50(5):512–20.
10. van Rijswijk CS, Geirnaerdt MJ, Hogendoorn PC, et al. Dynamic contrast-enhanced MR imaging in monitoring response to isolated limb perfusion in high-grade soft tissue sarcoma: initial results. Eur Radiol 2003;13(8):1849–58.
11. Hawighorst H, Libicher M, Knopp MV, et al. Evaluation of angiogenesis and perfusion of bone marrow lesions: role of semiquantitative and quantitative dynamic MRI. J Magn Reson Imaging 1999;10(3):286–94.
12. Yankeelov TE, Gore JC. Dynamic contrast enhanced magnetic resonance imaging in oncology: theory, data acquisition, analysis, and examples. Curr Med Imaging Rev 2007;3(2):91–107.
13. Calamante F. Arterial input function in perfusion MRI: a comprehensive review. Prog Nucl Magn Reson Spectrosc 2013;74:1–32.
14. perfusionTofts PS. Modeling tracer kinetics in dynamic. J Magn Reson Imaging 1997;7:91–101.
15. Sourbron SP, Buckley DL. Classic models for dynamic contrast-enhanced MRI. NMR Biomed 2013;26(8):1004–27.
16. Li X, Wang Q, Dou Y, et al. Soft tissue sarcoma: can dynamic contrast enhanced (DCE) MRI be used to predict the histological grade? Skeletal Radiol 2020 Nov;49(11):1829–38.
17. Li X, Xie Y, Hu Y, et al. Soft tissue sarcoma: correlation of dynamic contrast-enhanced magnetic resonance imaging features with HIF-1α expression and patient outcomes. Quant Imaging Med Surg 2022;12(10):4823–36.
18. Bajaj G, Callan AK, Weinschenk RC, et al. Multiparametric Evaluation of Soft Tissue Sarcoma: Current Perspectives and Future Directions. Semin Roentgenol 2022;57(3):212–31.
19. Le Bihan D. What can we see with IVIM MRI? Neuroimage 2019;15(187):56–67.

20. Le Bihan D, Breton E, Lallemand D, et al. Separation of diffusion and perfusion in intravoxel incoherent motion MR imaging. Radiology 1988; 168(2):497–505.

21. Li X, Johnson CP, Ellermann J. Measuring Knee Bone Marrow Perfusion Using Arterial Spin Labeling at 3 T. Sci Rep 2020 24;10(1):5260–8.

22. Simchick G, Geng R, Zhang Y, et al. b value and first-order motion moment optimized data acquisition for repeatable quantitative intravoxel incoherent motion DWI. Magn Reson Med 2022;87(6): 2724–40.

23. Cumming JD, Nutt ME. Bone-marrow blood flow and cardiac output in the rabbit. J Physiol 1962; 162:30–4.

24. Ray RD, Kawabata M, Galante J. Experimental study of peripheral circulation and bone growth. An experimental method for the quantitative determination of bone blood flow. 3. Clin Orthop Relat Res 1967;54:175–85.

25. Gross PM, Heistad DD, Marcus ML. Neurohumoral regulation of blood flow to bones and marrow. Am J Physiol 1979;237:H440–8.

26. Hillengass J, Stieltjes B, Bauerle T, et al. Dynamic contrast-enhanced magnetic resonance imaging (DCE-MRI) and diffusion-weighted imaging of bone marrow in healthy individuals. Acta Radiol 2011;52:324–30.

27. Whiteside LA, Ogata K, Lesker P, et al. The acute effects of periosteal stripping and medullary reaming on regional bone blood flow. Clin Orthop Relat Res 1978;131:266–72.

28. Shim SS. Bone and joint circulation. Physiological basis for clinical practice. Yonsei Med J 1986; 27(2):91–9.

29. Brookes M, Revell WJ. Blood vessels in Bone Marrow. In: Brookes M, Revell, editors. Blood supply of bone, scientific aspects. Cambridge, UK: Springer; 1998. p. 75–107.

30. Bridgeman G, Brookes M. Blood supply to the human femoral diaphysis in youth and senescence. J Anat 1996;188:611–21.

31. Marenzana M, Arnett TR. The Key Role of the Blood Supply to Bone. Bone Res 2013 Sep 25;1(3): 203–15.

32. Greif DN, Kouroupis D, Murdock CJ, et al. Infrapatellar Fat Pad/Synovium Complex in Early-Stage Knee Osteoarthritis: Potential New Target and Source of Therapeutic Mesenchymal Stem/Stromal Cells. Front Bioeng Biotechnol 2020;8:860.

33. Clark B. Normal Bone Anatomy and Physiology. Clin J Am Soc Nephrol 2008;3(Supl 3):S131–9.

34. Griffith JF, Wang YX, Zhou H, et al. Reduced bone perfusion in osteoporosis: likely causes in an ovariectomy rat model. Radiology 2010;254(3):739–46.

35. Wilson JW. Blood supply to developing, mature, and healing bone//Sumner. In: -Smith G, editor.

Bone in clinical orthopedics. 2nd edition. Stuttgart New York: Georg Thieme Verlag; 2002. p. 23–116.

36. Hartsock RJ, Smith EB, Petty CS. Normal Variations with Aging of the Amount of Hematopoietic Tissue in Bone Marrow from the Anterior Iliac Crest. A Study Made from 177 Cases of Sudden Death Examined by Necropsy. Am J Clin Pathol 1965; 43:326–31.

37. Ricci C, Cova M, Kang YS, et al. Normal age-related patterns of cellular and fatty bone marrow distribution in the axial skeleton: MR imaging study. Radiology 1990;177(1):83–8.

38. Chen WT, Shih TT, Chen RC, et al. Vertebral bone marrow perfusion evaluated with dynamic contrast-enhanced MR imaging: significance of aging and sex. Radiology 2001;220:213–8.

39. Vande Berg BC, Malghem J, Lecouvet FE, et al. Magnetic resonance imaging of the normal bone marrow. Skeletal Radiol 1998;27:471–83.

40. Vande Berg BC, Malghem J, Lecouvet FE, et al. Magnetic resonance imaging of normal bone marrow. Eur Radiol 1998;8:1327–34.

41. Griffith JF, Yeung DK, Ma HT, et al. Bone marrow fat content in the elderly: a reversal of sex difference seen in younger subjects. J Magn Reson Imaging 2012;36(1):225–30.

42. Zhang YF, Wang YX, Griffith JF, et al. Proximal femur bone marrow blood perfusion indices are reduced in hypertensive rats: a dynamic contrast-enhanced MRI study. J Magn Reson Imaging 2009;30:1139–44.

43. Malyszko J. Mechanism of endothelial dysfunction in chronic kidney disease. Clin Chim Acta 2010; 411(19-20):1412–20.

44. Aref MW, Swallow EA, Chen NX, et al. Skeletal vascular perfusion is altered in chronic kidney disease. Bone Rep 2018 May 4;8:215–20.

45. Oikawa A, Siragusa M, Quaini F, et al. Diabetes mellitus induces bone marrow microangiopathy. Arterioscler Thromb Vasc Biol 2010;30:498–508.

46. Breault SR, Heye T, Bashir MR, et al. Quantitative dynamic contrast-enhanced MRI of pelvic and lumbar bone marrow: effect of age and marrow fat content on pharmacokinetic parameter values. AJR Am J Roentgenol 2013;200:W297–303.

47. Lee JY, Ahn KJ, Lee YS, et al. Differentiation of grade II and III oligodendrogliomas from grade II and III astrocytomas: a histogram analysis of perfusion parameters derived from dynamic contrast-enhanced (DCE) and dynamic susceptibility contrast (DSC) MRI. Acta Radiol 2018;59(6): 723–31.

48. van der Woude HJ, Verstraete KL, Hogendoorn PC, et al. Musculoskeletal tumors: does fast dynamic contrast-enhanced subtraction MR imaging contribute to the characterization? Radiology 1998;208:821–8.

49. Kransdorf MJ, Jelinek JS, Moser RP, et al. Soft-Tissue masses: diagnosis using MR imaging. AJR Am J Roentgenol 1989;153:541–7.

50. Crim JR, Seeger LL, Yao L, et al. Diagnosis of soft-tissue masses with MR imaging: can benign masses be differentiated from malignant ones? Radiology 1992;185:581–6.

51. Benedikt RA, Jelinek JS, Kransdorf MJ, et al. Mr imaging of soft-tissue masses: role of gadopentetate dimeglumine. J Magn Reson Imaging 1994;4:485–90.

52. Moulton JS, Blebea JS, Dunco DM, et al. Mr imaging of soft-tissue masses: diagnostic efficacy and value of distinguishing between benign and malignant lesions. AJR Am J Roentgenol 1995;164: 1191–9.

53. Gielen JLMA, De Schepper AM, Vanhoenacker F, et al. Accuracy of MRI in characterization of soft tissue tumors and tumor-like lesions. A prospective study in 548 patients. Eur Radiol 2004;14:2320–30.

54. Zhang Y, Yue B, Zhao X, et al. Benign or Malignant Characterization of Soft-Tissue Tumors by Using Semiquantitative and Quantitative Parameters of Dynamic Contrast-Enhanced Magnetic Resonance Imaging. Can Assoc Radiol J 2020 Feb;71(1):92–9.

55. Bian Y, Jin P, Wang Y, et al. Clinical Applications of DSC-MRI Parameters Assess Angiogenesis and Differentiate Malignant From Benign Soft Tissue Tumors in Limbs. Acad Radiol 2020 Mar;27(3): 354–60.

56. Choi YJ, Lee IS, Song YS, et al. Diagnostic performance of diffusion-weighted (DWI) and dynamic contrast-enhanced (DCE) MRI for the differentiation of benign from malignant soft-tissue tumors. J Magn Reson Imaging 2019 Sep;50(3):798–809.

57. Leplat C, Hossu G, Chen B, et al. Contrast-Enhanced 3-T Perfusion MRI With Quantitative Analysis for the Characterization of Musculoskeletal Tumors: Is It Worth the Trouble? AJR Am J Roentgenol 2018;211(5):1092–8.

58. Soldatos T, Fisher S, Karri S, et al. Advanced MR imaging of peripheral nerve sheath tumors, including diffusion imaging. Semin Musculoskelet Radiol 2015;19(2):179–90.

59. Spinnato P, Kind M, Le Loarer F, et al. Soft Tissue Sarcomas: The Role of Quantitative MRI in Treatment Response Evaluation. Acad Radiol 2022; 29(7):1065–84.

60. Guan Y, Peck KK, Lyo J, et al. T1-weighted Dynamic Contrast-enhanced MRI to Differentiate Nonneoplastic and Malignant Vertebral Body Lesions in the Spine. Radiology 2020;297(2):382–9.

61. Moulopoulos LA, Maris TG, Papanikolaou N, et al. Detection of malignant bone marrow involvement with dynamic contrast-enhanced magnetic resonance imaging. Ann Oncol 2003;14:152–8.

62. Zhang L, Mandel C, Yang ZY, et al. Tumor infiltration of bone marrow in patients with hematologic malignancies: dynamic contrast-enhanced magnetic resonance imaging. Chin Med J (Engl) 2006;119:1256–62.

63. Zha Y, Li M, Yang J. Dynamic contrast enhanced magnetic resonance imaging of diffuse spinal bone marrow infiltration in patients with hematological malignancies. Korean J Radiol 2010;11: 187–94.

64. Koo JH, Yoon YC, Kim JH. Diffusion-weighted and Dynamic Contrast-enhanced MRI of Metastatic Bone Tumors: Correlation of the Apparent Diffusion Coefficient, Ktrans and ve values. J Korean Soc Magn Reson Med 2014 Mar;18(1):25–33.

65. Chu S, Karimi S, Peck KK, et al. Measurement of blood perfusion in spinal metastases with dynamic contrast-enhanced magnetic resonance imaging: evaluation of tumor response to radiation therapy. Spine (Phila Pa 1976) 2013;38(22):E1418–24.

66. Kumar KA, Peck KK, Karimi S, et al. A pilot study evaluating the use of dynamic contrast-enhanced perfusion MRI to predict local recurrence after radiosurgery on spinal metastases. Technol Cancer Res Treat 2017;16(6):857–65.

67. Lis E, Saha A, Peck KK, et al. Dynamic contrast-enhanced magnetic resonance imaging of osseous spine metastasis before and 1 hour after high-dose image-guided radiation therapy. Neurosurg Focus 2017;42(1):E9.

68. Morales KA, Arevalo-Perez J, Peck KK, et al. Differentiating Atypical Hemangiomas and Metastatic Vertebral Lesions: The Role of T1-Weighted Dynamic Contrast-Enhanced MRI. AJNR Am J Neuroradiol 2018;39(5):968–73.

69. Oh E, Yoon YC, Kim JH, et al. Multiparametric approach with diffusion-weighted imaging and dynamic contrast-enhanced MRI: a comparison study for differentiating between benign and malignant bone lesions in adults. Clin Radiol 2017;72(7): 552–9.

70. Park S, Yoon JK, Chung NS, et al. Correlations between intravoxel incoherent motion diffusion-weighted MR imaging parameters and 18F-FDG PET/CT metabolic parameters in patients with vertebral bone metastases:initial experience. Br J Radiol 2018;91(1086):20170889.

71. Park S, Park JG, Jun S, et al. Differentiation of bone metastases from prostate cancer and benign red marrow depositions of the pelvic bone with multiparametric MRI. Magn Reson Imaging 2020;73: 118–24.

72. Chen BB, Hsu CY, Yu CW, et al. Dynamic contrast-enhanced MR imaging measurement of vertebral bone marrow perfusion may be indicator of outcome of acute myeloid leukaemia patients in remission. Radiology 2011;258(3):821–31.

73. Kayhan A, Yang C, Soylu FN, et al. Dynamic contrast-enhanced MR imaging findings of bone

metastasis in patients with prostate cancer. World J Radiol 2011;3:241–5.

74. Guo J, Reddick WE, Glass JO, et al. Dynamic contrast-enhanced magnetic resonance imaging as a prognostic factor in predicting event-free and overall survival in pediatric patients with osteosarcoma. Cancer 2012;118:3776–85.

75. Reddick WE, Wang S, Xiong X, et al. Dynamic magnetic resonance imaging of regional contrast access as an additional prognostic factor in pediatric osteosarcoma. Cancer 2001;91(12):2230–7.

76. Guo J, Glass JO, McCarville MB, et al. Assessing vascular effects of adding bevacizumab to neoadjuvant chemotherapy in osteosarcoma using DCE-MRI. Br J Cancer 2015;113(9):1282–8.

77. Li J, Zheng R, Niu J, et al. Correlation of intravoxel incoherent motion parameters and histological characteristics from infiltrated marrow in patients with acute leukemia. J Magn Reson Imaging 2020;51(6):1720–6.

78. Merz M, Ritsch J, Kunz C, et al. Dynamic contrast-enhanced magnetic resonance imaging for assessment of antiangiogenic treatment effects in multiple myeloma. Clin Cancer Res 2015;21(1):106–12.

79. Aaron RK, Dyke JP, Ciombor DM, et al. Perfusion abnormalities in subchondral bone associated with marrow edema, osteoarthritis, and avascular necrosis. Ann N Y Acad Sci 2007 Nov;1117:124–37.

80. Kawakami Y, Kunisada T, Sugihara S, et al. New approach for assessing vascular distribution within bone tumors using dynamic contrast-enhanced MRI. J Cancer Res Clin Oncol 2007;133:697–703.

81. Parkkola RK, Mattila KT, Heikkila JT, et al. Dynamic contrast-enhanced MR imaging and MR-guided bone biopsy on a 0.23 T open imager. Skeletal Radiol 2001;30:620–4.

82. Noebauer-Huhmann IM, Amann G, Krssak M, et al. Use of diagnostic dynamic contrast-enhanced (DCE)-MRI for targeting of soft tissue tumour biopsies at 3T: preliminary results. Eur Radiol 2015 Jul;25(7):2041–8. Epub 2015 Jan 11. PMID: 25577522.).

83. Tirkes T, Hollar MA, Tann M, et al. Response criteria in oncologic imaging: review of traditional and new criteria. Radiographics 2013;33:1323–41.

84. Verstraete KL, Lang P. Bone and soft tissue tumors: the role of contrast agents for MR imaging. Eur J Radiol 2000;34(3):229–46.

85. Barile A, Regis G, Masi R, et al. Musculoskeletal tumours: preliminary experience with perfusion MRI. Radiol Med 2007;112:550–61.

86. Amit P, Patro DK, Basu D, et al. Role of dynamic MRI and clinical assessment in predicting histologic response to neoadjuvant chemotherapy in bone sarcomas. Am J Clin Oncol 2014;37:384–90.

87. Soldatos T, Ahlawat S, Montgomery E, et al. Multiparametric MR imaging assessment of high-grade soft-tissue sarcomas. Radiology 2016;278(3).

88. Alic L, van Vliet M, van Dijke CF, et al. Heterogeneity in DCE-MRI parametric maps: a biomarker for treatment response? Phys Med Biol 2011;56:1601–16.

89. Bourillon C, Rahmouni A, Lin C, et al. Intravoxel incoherent motion diffusion-weighted imaging of multiple myeloma lesions: correlation with whole-body dynamic contrast agent-enhanced MR imaging. Radiology 2015;277(3):773–83.

90. Dutoit JC, Claus E, Offner F, et al. Combined evaluation of conventional MRI, dynamic contrast-enhanced MRI and diffusion weighted imaging for response evaluation of patients with multiple myeloma. Eur J Radiol 2016;85(2):373–82.

91. Spratt DE, Arevalo-Perez J, Leeman JE, et al. Early magnetic resonance imaging biomarkers to predict local control after high dose stereotactic body radiotherapy for patients with sarcoma spine metastases. Spine J 2016;16:291–8.

92. Van Rijswijk CS, Geirnaerdt MJ, Hogendoorn PC, et al. Soft-tissue tumors: value of static and dynamic gadopentetate dimeglumine-enhanced MR imaging in prediction of malignancy. Radiology 2004;233(2):493–502.

93. Lehotska V, Tothova L, Valkovic L. The role of dynamic contrast-enhanced MRI in differentiation of local recurrence and residual soft-tissue tumor versus post-treatment changes. Bratisl Lek Listy 2013;114(2):88–92.

94. Del Grande F, Subhawong T, Weber K, et al. Detection of soft-tissue sarcoma recurrence: added value of functional MR imaging techniques at 3.0 T. Radiology 2014;271(2):499–511.

95. Jaovisidha S, Traiporndeeprasert P, Chitrapazt N, et al. Dynamic contrasted MR imaging in differentiation of recurrent malignant soft tissue tumor from post-treatment changes. J Med Assoc Thai 2011;94(9):1127–33.

96. Nadel SN, Debatin JF, Richardson WJ, et al. Detection of acute avascular necrosis of the femoral head in dogs: dynamic contrast-enhanced MR imaging vs spin-echo and STIR sequences. AJR Am J Roentgenol 1992;159:1255–61.

97. Griffith JF. Functional imaging of the musculoskeletal system. Quant Imaging Med Surg 2015;5(3):323–31.

98. Griffith JF, Yeung DK, Tsang PH, et al. Compromised bone marrow perfusion in osteoporosis. J Bone Miner Res 2008;23:1068–75.

99. Bachiller FG, Caballer AP, Portal LF. Avascular necrosis of the femoral head after femoral neck fracture. Clin Orthop Relat Res 2002;399:87–109.

100. Cahill DG, Yam MKH, Griffith JF. Imaging of the Acutely Injured Hip. Radiol Clin North Am 2023 Mar;61(2):203–17.

101. Han S, Oh M, Yoon S, et al. Risk Stratification for Avascular Necrosis of the Femoral Head After Internal Fixation of Femoral Neck Fractures by Post-Operative Bone SPECT/CT. Nucl Med Mol Imaging 2017 Mar;51(1):49–57.

102. Teixeira PA, Dubois L, Hossu G, et al. Quantitative dynamic contrast-enhanced MRI of bone marrow perfusion at the proximal femur: influence of femoral head osteonecrosis risk factor and overt osteonecrosis. Eur Radiol 2023;33(4):2340–9.

103. Lang P, Mauz M, Schorner W, et al. Acute fracture of the femoral neck: assessment of femoral head perfusion with gadopentetate diglumineenhanced MR imaging. AJR Am J Roentgenol 1993; 160:335–41.

104. Ng AW, Griffith JF, Taljanovic MS, et al. Is dynamic contrast-enhanced MRI useful for assessing proximal fragment vascularity in scaphoid fracture delayed and non-union? Skeletal Radiol 2013;42: 983–92.

105. Tripathy SK, Goyal T, Sen RK. Management of femoral head osteonecrosis: Current concepts. Indian J Orthop 2015 Jan-Feb;49(1):28–45. PMID: 25593355; PMCID: PMC4292325.

106. Downing ND, Oni JA, Davis TR, et al. The relationship between proximal pole blood flow and the subjective assessment of increased density of the proximal pole in acute scaphoid fractures. J Hand Surg Am 2002;27(3):402–8.

107. Madeley NJ, Stephen AB, Downing ND, et al. Changes in scaphoid bone density after acute fracture. J Hand Surg Br 2006 Aug;31(4):368–70.

108. Koc BB, Schotanus M, Jong B, et al. The Role of Dynamic Contrast-Enhanced MRI in a Child with Sport-Induced Avascular Necrosis of the Scaphoid: A Case Report and Literature Review. Case Rep Orthop 2016;2016:7898090. https://doi.org/10.1155/2016/7898090.

109. Larribe M, Gay A, Freire V, et al. Usefulness of dynamic contrast-enhanced MRI in the evaluation of the viability of acute scaphoid fracture. Skeletal Radiol 2014;43:1697–703.

110. Donati OF, Zanetti M, Nagy L, et al. Is dynamic gadolinium enhancement needed in MR imaging for the preoperative assessment of scaphoidal viability in patients with scaphoid nonunion? Radiology 2011;260(3):80816.

111. Müller G, Månsson S, Müller MF, et al. Increased perfusion in dynamic gadolinium-enhanced MRI correlates with areas of bone repair and of bone necrosis in patients with Kienböck's disease. J Magn Reson Imaging 2019 Aug;50(2):481–9.

112. Schmitt R, Heinze A, Fellner F, et al. Imaging and staging of avascular osteonecroses at the wrist and hand. Eur J Radiol 1997;25:92–103.

113. Güvenç K, Asfuroğlu ZM, Yılmaz C, et al. Effect of gadolinium perfusion magnetic resonance imaging on surgeons' management preferences in kienböck's disease. A survey study. Hand Surg Rehabil 2021;40(3):283–7.

114. Tamai K, Yamato M, Yamaguchi T, et al. Dynamic magnetic resonance imaging for the evaluation of synovitis in patients with rheumatoid arthritis. Arthritis Rheum 1994;37:1151–7.

115. Axelsen MB, Poggenborg RP, Stoltenberg M, et al. Reliability and responsiveness of dynamic contrast-enhanced magnetic resonance imaging in rheumatoid arthritis. Scand J Rheumatol 2013; 42:115–22.

116. Tam LS, Griffith JF, Yu AB, et al. Rapid improvement in rheumatoid arthritis patients on combination of methotrexate and infliximab: clinical and magnetic resonance imaging evaluation. Clin Rheumatol 2007;26:941–6.

117. Xiao F, Griffith JF, Ko JKL, et al. MRI wrist in early rheumatoid arthritis: reduction in inflammation assessed quantitatively during treatment period correlates best with clinical improvement. Skeletal Radiol 2021;50(7):1337–45.

118. Malattia C, Damasio Mb, Basso C, et al. Dynamic contrast-enhanced magnetic resonance imaging in the assessment of disease activity in patients with juvenile idiopathic arthritis. Rheumatology 2010;49(1):178–85.

119. Workie Dw, Dardzinski Bj, Graham Tb, et al. Quantification of dynamic contrast-enhanced MR imaging of the knee in children with juvenile rheumatoid arthritis based on pharmacokinetic modeling. Magn. ResonImaging 2004;22(9): 1201–10.

120. Workie Dw, Graham Tb, Laor T, et al. Quantitative MR characterization of disease activity in the knee in children with juvenile idiopathic arthritis: a longitudinal pilot study. Pediatr. Radiol 2007;37(6): 535–43.

121. Fujimori M, Murakami K, Sugimori H, et al. Intravoxel incoherent motion MRI for discrimination of synovial proliferation in the hand arthritis: A prospective proof-of-concept study. J Magn Reson Imaging 2019;50(4):1199–206.

122. Huch B, Stumpf K, Bracher AK, et al. Intravoxel incoherent motion (IVIM) MRI in pediatric patients with synovitis of the knee joint: a prospective pilot study. Pediatr Rheumatol Online J 2022;20(1):99.

123. Baker K, Grainger A, Niu J, et al. Relation of synovitis to knee pain using contrast-enhanced MRIs. Ann Rheum Dis 2010;69:1779–83.

124. Hill CL, Hunter DJ, Niu J, et al. Synovitis detected on magnetic resonance imaging and its relation to pain and cartilage loss in knee osteoarthritis. Ann Rheum Dis 2007;66:1599–603.

125. Atukorala I, Kwoh CK, Guermazi A, et al. Synovitis in knee osteoarthritis: a precursor of disease? Ann Rheum Dis 2016;75:390–5.

126. MacKay JW, Nezhad FS, Rifai T, et al. Dynamic contrast-enhanced MRI of synovitis in knee osteoarthritis: repeatability, discrimination and sensitivity to change in a prospective experimental study. Eur Radiol 2021;31(8):5746–58.

127. Gait AD, Hodgson R, Parkes MJ, et al. Synovial volume vs synovial measurements from dynamic contrast enhanced MRI as measures of response in osteoarthritis. Osteoarthritis Cartilage 2016;24: 1392–8.

128. Riis RGC, Gudbergsen H, Henriksen M, et al. Synovitis assessed on static and dynamic contrast-enhanced magnetic resonance imaging and its association with pain in knee osteoarthritis: a cross-sectional study. Eur J Radiol 2016;85:1099–108.

129. Hunter DJ, Guermazi A, Lo GH, et al. Evolution of semi- quantitative whole joint assessment of knee OA: MOAKS (MRI Osteoarthritis Knee Score). Osteoarthritis Cartilage 2011;19:990–1002.

130. Roemer FW, Guermazi A, Zhang Y, et al. Hoffa's Fat Pad: Evaluation on Unenhanced MR Images as a Measure of Patellofemoral Synovitis in Osteoarthritis. AJR Am J Roentgenol 2009;192: 1696–700.

131. de Vries BA, van der Heijden RA, Verschueren J, et al. Quantitative subchondral bone perfusion imaging in knee osteoarthritis using dynamic contrast enhanced MRI. Semin Arthritis Rheum 2020;50(2): 177–82.

132. Ballegaard C, Riis RG, Bliddal H, et al. Knee pain and inflammation in the infrapatellar fat pad estimated by conventional and dynamic contrast-enhanced magnetic resonance imaging in obese patients with osteoarthritis: a cross-sectional study. Osteoarthritis Cartilage 2014;22(7):933–40.

133. de Vries BA, van der Heijden RA, Poot DHJ, et al. Quantitative DCE-MRI demonstrates increased blood perfusion in Hoffa's fat pad signal abnormalities in knee osteoarthritis, but not in patellofemoral pain. Eur Radiol 2020;30(6):3401–8.

134. Daugaard CL, Riis RG, Bandak E, et al. Perfusion in bone marrow lesions assessed on DCE-MRI and its association with pain in knee osteoarthritis: a cross-sectional study. Skeletal Radiol 2020;49(5):757–64.

135. Lee SK, Suh KJ, Kim YW, et al. Septic arthritis versus transient synovitis at MR imaging: preliminary assessment with signal intensity alterations in bone marrow.

136. Kim EY, Kwack KS, Cho JH, et al. Usefulness of dynamic contrast-enhanced MRI in differentiating between septic arthritis and transient synovitis in the hip joint. AJR Am J Roentgenol 2012;198(2): 428–33.

137. Kwack K, Cho J, Lee J, et al. Septic arthritis versus transient synovitis of the hip: gadolinium-enhanced MRI finding of decreased perfusion at the femoral epiphysis. Am J Roentgenol 2007;189:437–45.

138. Griffith J, Davies AM, Close CF, et al. Organized chaos? Computed tomographic evaluation of the neuropathic diabetic foot. Br J Radiol 1995; 68(805):27–33.

139. Raj S, Prakash M, Rastogi A, et al. The role of diffusion-weighted imaging and dynamic contrast-enhanced magnetic resonance imaging for the diagnosis of diabetic foot osteomyelitis: a preliminary report. Pol J Radiol 2022;87:e274–80.

140. Liao D, Xie L, Han Y, et al. Dynamic contrast-enhanced magnetic resonance imaging for differentiating osteomyelitis from acute neuropathic arthropathy in the complicated diabetic foot. Skeletal Radiol 2018;47(10):1337–47.

141. Diez AIG, Fuster D, Morata L, et al. Comparison of the diagnostic accuracy of diffusion-weighted and dynamic contrast-enhanced MRI with ^{18}F-FDG PET/CT to differentiate osteomyelitis from Charcot neuro-osteoarthropathy in diabetic foot. Eur J Radiol 2020;132:109299.

142. Pantoja JL, Ali F, Baril DT, et al. Arterial spin labeling magnetic resonance imaging quantifies tissue perfusion around foot ulcers. J Vasc Surg Cases Innov Tech 2022;8(4):817–24.

143. Zheng J, Li R, Dickey EE, et al. Regional skeletal muscle perfusion distribution in diabetic feet may differentiate short-term healed foot ulcers from non-healed ulcers. Eur Radiol 2023;33(5): 3303–11.

144. Griffith JF, Yeung DK, Antonio GE, et al. Vertebral bone mineral density, marrow perfusion, and fat content in healthy men and men with osteoporosis: dynamic contrast-enhanced MR imaging and MR spectroscopy. Radiology 2005;236:945–51.

145. Oei L, Koromani F, Rivadeneira F, et al. Quantitative imaging methods in osteoporosis. Quant Imaging Med Surg 2016;6(6):680–98.

146. Biffar A, Schmidt GP, Sourbron S, et al. Quantitative analysis of vertebral bone marrow perfusion using dynamic contrast-enhanced MRI: initial results in osteoporotic patients with acute vertebral fracture. J Magn Reson Imaging 2011;33:676–83.

147. Geith T, Niethammer T, Milz S, et al. Transient bone marrow edema syndrome versus osteonecrosis: perfusion patterns at dynamic contrast-enhanced MR imaging with high temporal resolution can allow differentiation. Radiology 2016;283:478–85.

148. Arevalo-Perez J, Peck KK, Lyo JK, et al. Differentiating benign from malignant vertebral fractures using T1 -weighted dynamic contrast-enhanced MRI. J Magn Reson Imaging 2015;42(4):1039–47.

149. Libicher M, Kasperk C, Daniels M, et al. Dynamic contrast-enhanced MRI in Paget's disease of bone—correlation of regional microcirculation and bone turnover. Eur Radiol 2008;18:1005–11.

150. Libicher M, Kasperk C, Daniels-Wredenhagen M, et al. Dynamic contrast-enhanced MRI for

monitoring bisphosphonate therapy in Paget's disease of bone. Skeletal Radiol 2013;42:225–30.

151. Robson MD, Gatehouse PD, Bydder M, et al. Magnetic resonance: an introduction to ultrashort TE (UTE) imaging. J Comput Assist Tomogr 2003;27: 825–46.

152. Reichert IL, Robson MD, Gatehouse PD, et al. Magnetic resonance imaging of cortical bone with ultrashort TE (UTE) pulse sequences. Magn Reson Imaging 2005;23:611–8.

153. Du J, Bydder GM. Qualitative and quantitative ultrashort-TE MRI of cortical bone. NMR Biomed 2013;26:489–506.

154. Wan L, Wu M, Sheth V, et al. Evaluation of cortical bone perfusion using dynamic contrast enhanced ultrashort echo time imaging: a feasibility study. Quant Imaging Med Surg 2019 Aug;9(8):1383–93.

155. Crombé A, Matcuk GR, Fadli D, et al. Role of Imaging in Initial Prognostication of Locally Advanced Soft Tissue Sarcomas. Acad Radiol 2023;30(2):322–40.

Moving?

Make sure your subscription moves with you!

To notify us of your new address, find your **Clinics Account Number** (located on your mailing label above your name), and contact customer service at:

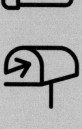

Email: journalscustomerservice-usa@elsevier.com

800-654-2452 (subscribers in the U.S. & Canada)
314-447-8871 (subscribers outside of the U.S. & Canada)

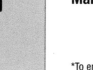

Fax number: 314-447-8029

Elsevier Health Sciences Division
Subscription Customer Service
3251 Riverport Lane
Maryland Heights, MO 63043

ELSEVIER

Printed and bound by CPI Group (UK) Ltd, Croydon, CR0 4YY

08/05/2025

01864750-0011